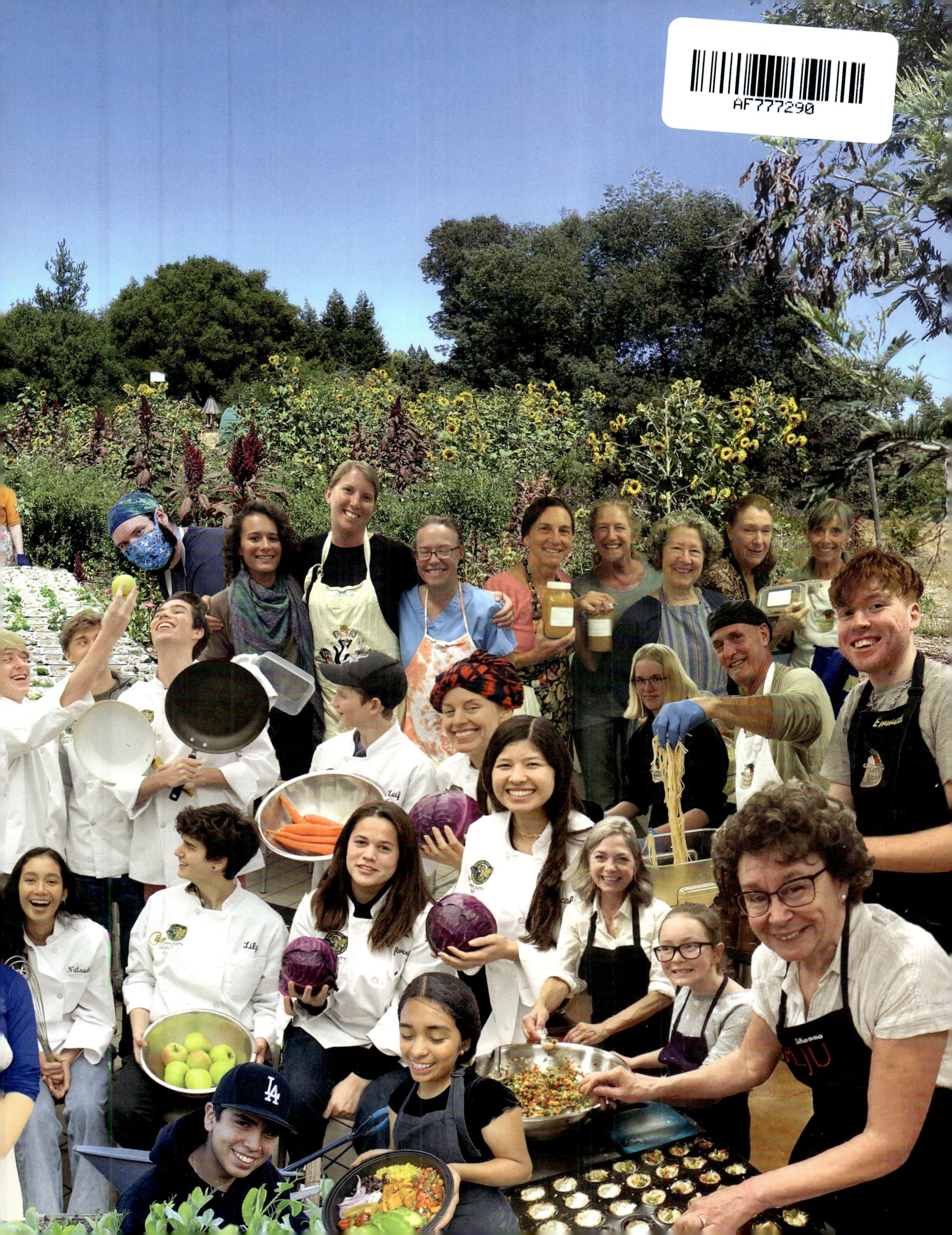

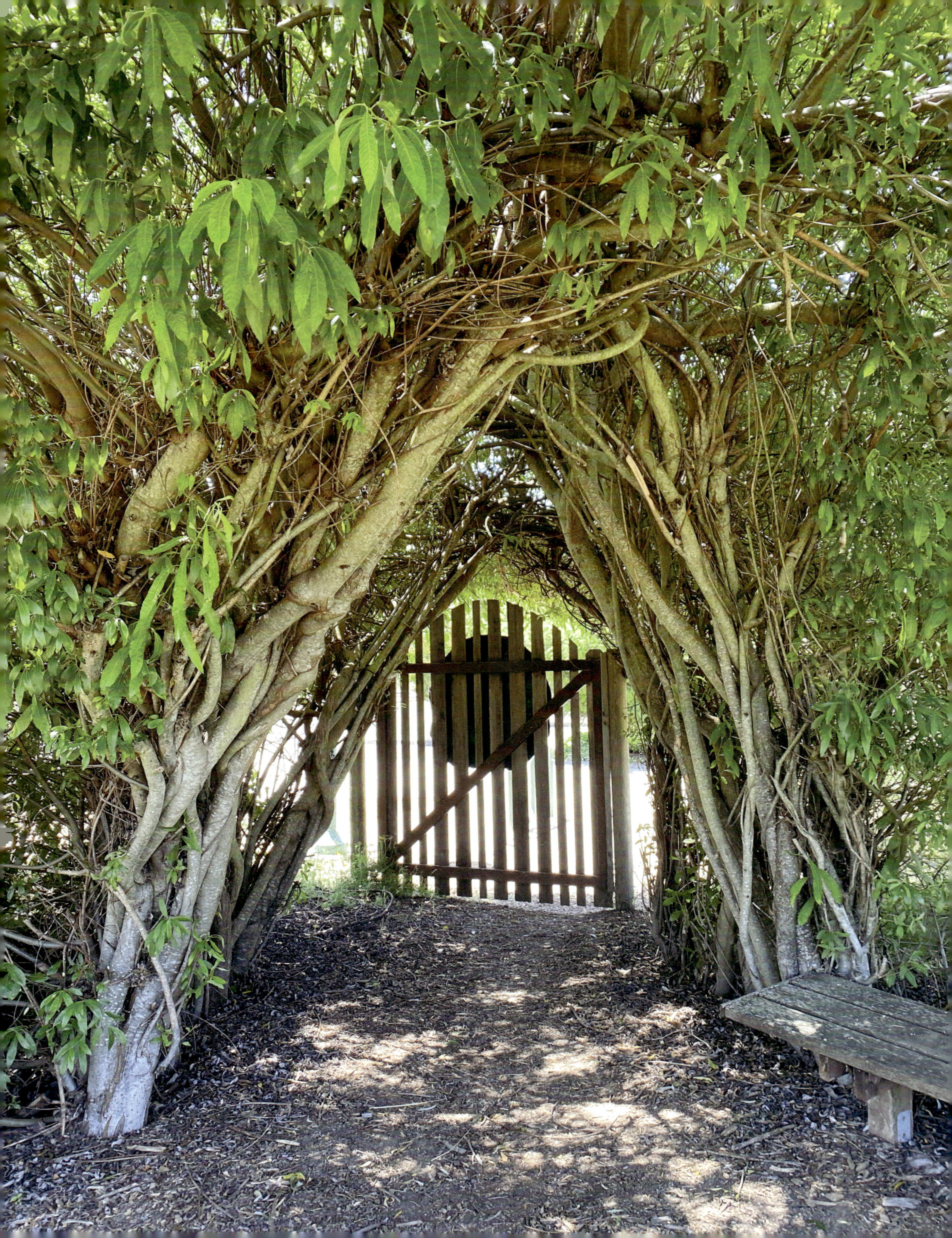

NOURISHING COMMUNITY

Healing Recipes Made with Love

from
The Ceres Affililate Partner Family

Published in the United States by Ceres Community Project, Sebastopol, California
ISBN 978-0-578-96773-8

Edited by Cathryn Couch and Deborah Ramelli
Designed by Felicity Crush

Printed in the United States
www.CeresProject.org

FSC
www.fsc.org
MIX
Paper from responsible sources
FSC® C001755

Previous page: The willow entrance to Ceres Community Garden, Sebastopol, CA.

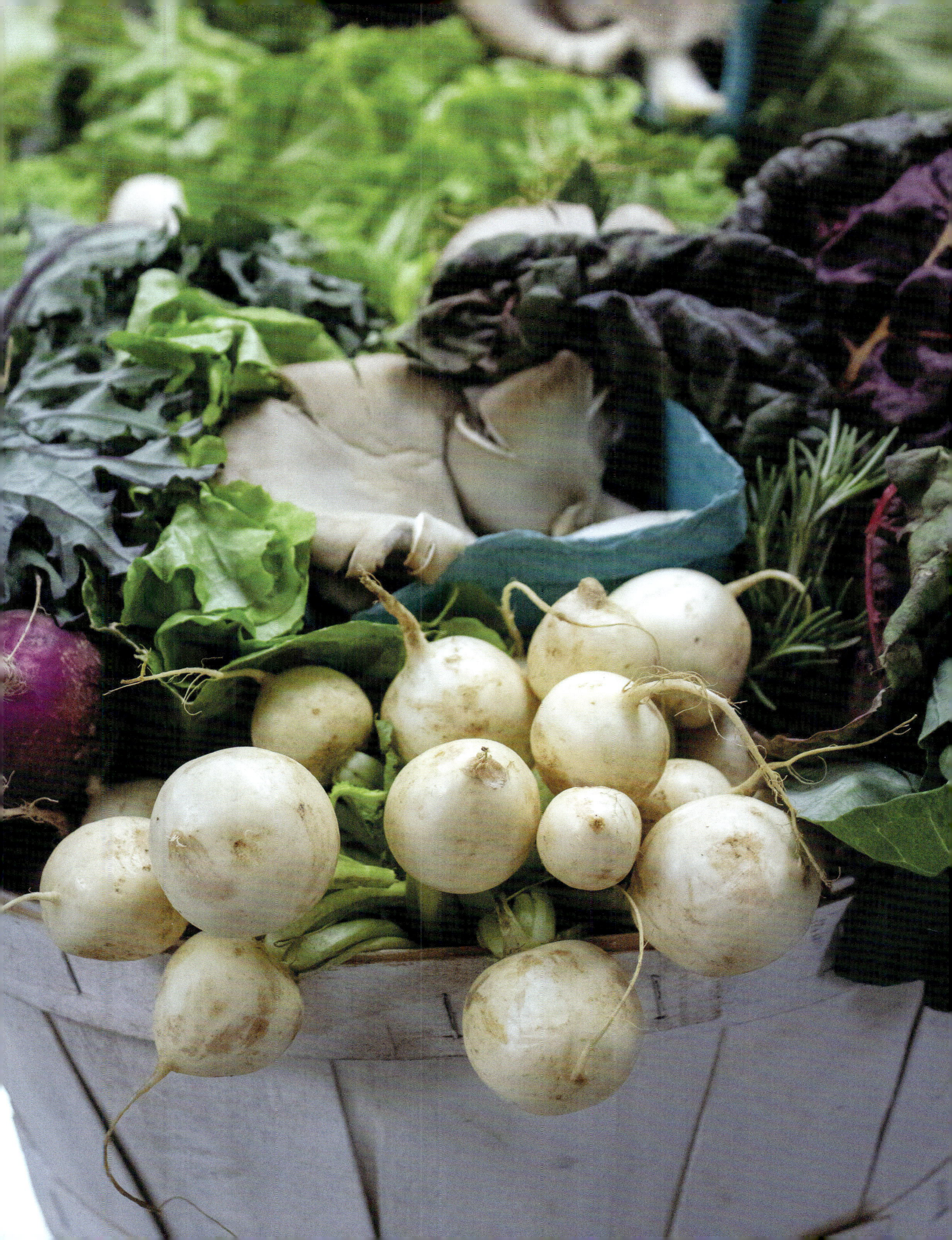

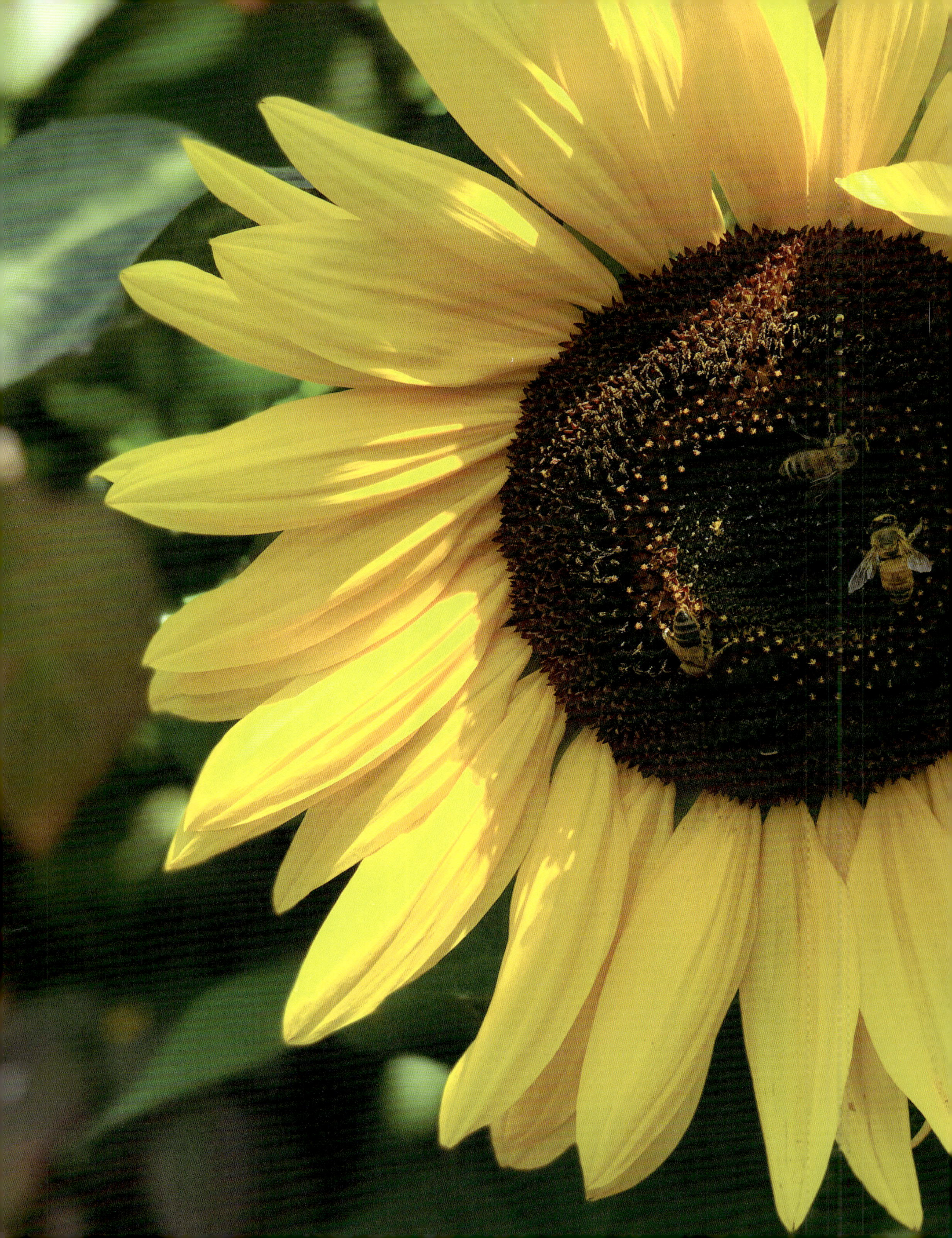

Dedication

To our adult and youth volunteers,
clients, staff, donors and community partners,
who collaborate with us
to model and create
a healthy, caring, just and sustainable world.

CONTENTS

SALADS 79

SOUPS & STEWS 105

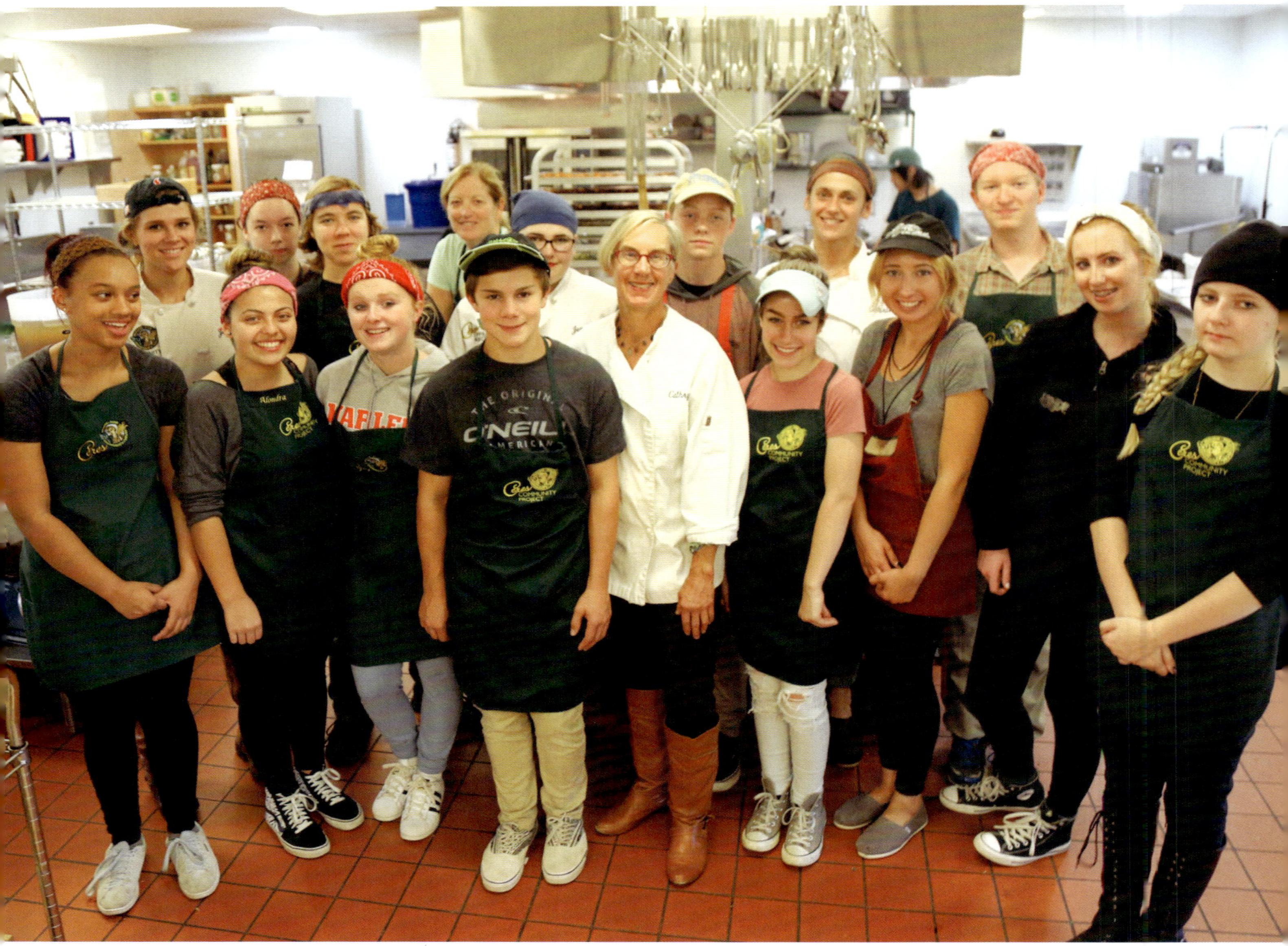

Ceres' Founder Cathryn Couch with a group of teens. Cathryn was the primary chef for the first three years of Ceres' operations.

Introduction

Welcome to the Ceres Affiliate Partner family, a group of non-profit organizations that are bringing nourishment, healing and connection to communities from Nashville to Grand Rapids and Sonoma County, California to Aarhus, Denmark. The recipes in the book are the same tasty, nutritious ones used for the meals we deliver to our clients. We hope you enjoy them!

Our Model Is Simple

Teens volunteer in our gardens and kitchens to grow organic food and prepare healthy meals. We deliver those meals to community members and their families who are living with a serious illness like cancer, heart disease, or diabetes. Adult volunteers mentor teens and deliver meals. Local organizations donate kitchen space, food and more. Other community members support the work financially. There is a place for everyone and together we create a circle of love, connection and healing.

The Impact Is Profound

Our teen volunteers learn to grow, cook and eat healthy foods. They gain job and leadership skills and form empowering bonds with peers and adult mentors. And most importantly, they discover their power to make a difference – in their own life and the lives of others. The fundamental questions for teens are "Who am I outside of my family?" and "Where is my place in the larger community?" In our programs, they experience a sense of belonging, discover their ability to create positive change in their community, and become the future leaders our world needs.

Our meals provide vital nourishment to clients at a time when it's most needed. That nourishment comes in the form of meals *and* in the form of love. Most of the illnesses our clients face – cancer, diabetes, heart disease – are related in part to poor nutrition. Clients who are ill often don't eat much, and as a result many become malnourished. That's why we focus on organic, nutrient-rich whole foods and meals that are, in many cases, medically tailored to meet the nutritional needs of our clients. When every bite counts, our meals need to be both delicious and nourishing.

And while our clients rave about the meals, what we hear even more often is "I can feel the love in the food," or "Knowing that all these people I don't even know are making and delivering meals to me makes me feel like the whole community cares." The research on the power of feeling cared for is profound: When you feel connected to and cared for by others, you are 50% more likely to live an average of eight years longer.

We live in a world that has become increasingly disconnected. Many of us don't live near our families, and we often don't stay at the same jobs for long periods. We gather less often for things like bowling leagues and other organized activities. And yet one of our deepest human needs is to feel connected and to know that we can make a difference for others. At each of our organizations, we build webs of connection and caring across the community. Each volunteer, teen, client, donor and community partner is part of that web. Each of them is contributing, but each of them is also receiving something profound —knowing that they are making a life-saving difference in someone's life. This is the reason we so often hear from our volunteers that they feel they get more from the experience of volunteering than they give. Whether you are 15 or 55, when one of our clients tells you that you saved their life, it changes how you think about yourself and the difference you can and do make in the world.

Food Is Medicine

Our work is part of a growing movement to recognize that food is medicine. Food and nutrition insecurity is directly related to $77 billion annually in health care costs. Poor diets are now the number one risk factor for mortality in the United States. And nearly 85% of health care spending goes to address nutrition-related chronic disease. We are literally eating ourselves into poor health.

Food can be the poison that contributes to diabetes, hypertension, heart disease and cancer. And it can also be the medicine that helps prevent and treat those same illnesses. Highly processed foods laden with sugar, salt and preservatives are making us sick. Whole fresh foods, including lots of vegetables and whole grains, can help us stay healthy and get well.

The good news is that this connection is increasingly being recognized by health care providers and health care plans. Changes at both the federal and state level are creating opportunities for health plans to pay for meals as a health care intervention. Beginning in 2020, Medicare Advantage plans are able to offer and pay for meals for some members. States such as California, New York and North Carolina are using innovation opportunities in Medicaid to address food and nutrition insecurity that contributes to poor health. Organizations like ours are conducting pilots and research studies to demonstrate the impact that medically appropriate meals can have on patients' lives, health outcomes, and health care costs.

The data is promising. Published studies about medically tailored meals consistently demonstrate 16% to 20% net savings in health care costs. A two-year pilot by a health plan in California saved $3.60 for every $1.00 that was spent when Medicaid members were provided twelve weeks of meals after discharge from the hospital. In early 2021, Ceres Community Project completed one of four large-scale randomized control trials on medically tailored meals with our partners at Kaiser Permanente. We look forward to seeing that data soon. These examples demonstrate the tremendous opportunity we have to improve the lives of our friends and neighbors through the work that we do.

Finally, we believe that food is medicine only if it's produced in ways that support the health of those who grow it and of the land itself. For this reason, we use organic ingredients in our meals. Organic food has been shown to have more of the vitamins, minerals, phytochemicals and antioxidants that our bodies need for health. And organic foods are also better for our communities and for the planet. The way we currently produce food in the United States and much of the world is a leading contributor to climate change and loss of topsoil that's crucial for food production. Organic and other sustainable food production methods reduce topsoil erosion, help sequester carbon, and help keep our water, air and farmworkers healthy. If you are interested in learning more, you can visit **Ceresproject.org/Policy.**

Join Us

Thank you for purchasing this book. The proceeds from sales support the clients and teens we serve. There are many other ways to get involved. If you live in one of the communities we serve, please volunteer your time, support our work financially, and spread the word to help us support more clients who need meals and to engage teens who could benefit from being part of our programs.

If you live somewhere else, consider bringing the Ceres Affiliate Partner program to your community. Share what we are doing and see if there are others who want to help. You'll find information about our Affiliate Partner program and training, plus information about all eight of our programs on page 234, including how to donate to support us.

Finally, we encourage you to support your local farmers and food producers and to cook for yourself and those you love. Shop at a nearby farmer's market and get to know the people who are growing food in your community. Buy organic whole foods that are locally grown, and notice how fresh and vibrant they are.

Make time to prepare food from scratch. Eat mindfully, with appreciation for those who grew it and for the nourishment it gives you. Share food with friends and family members. Make and deliver a meal to someone you know who is having a tough time – perhaps because of illness or for some other reason. Notice how good it makes you feel.

Making and sharing food has been central to our human story for hundreds of thousands of years. It's in our DNA. It's how we connect and how we express and feel love. Making and sharing a meal is simple. The impact is profound. This is what Ceres Affiliate Partners do every day, with hundreds of teen and adult helping hands putting thousands of meals on our clients' tables. We invite you to join our circle of nourishment and love. You can support our organizations, bring the Ceres Affiliate Partner program to your community, or simply prepare a nourishing meal with love for yourself or others.

Together we can create the world we want to live in. A world where everyone has access to the food they need to thrive. Where all people are valued. Where food is grown and produced in ways that are sustainable. And where the circle of love, generosity and compassion is ever-widening.

Welcome!

Cathryn Couch

Founder & CEO
Ceres Community Project

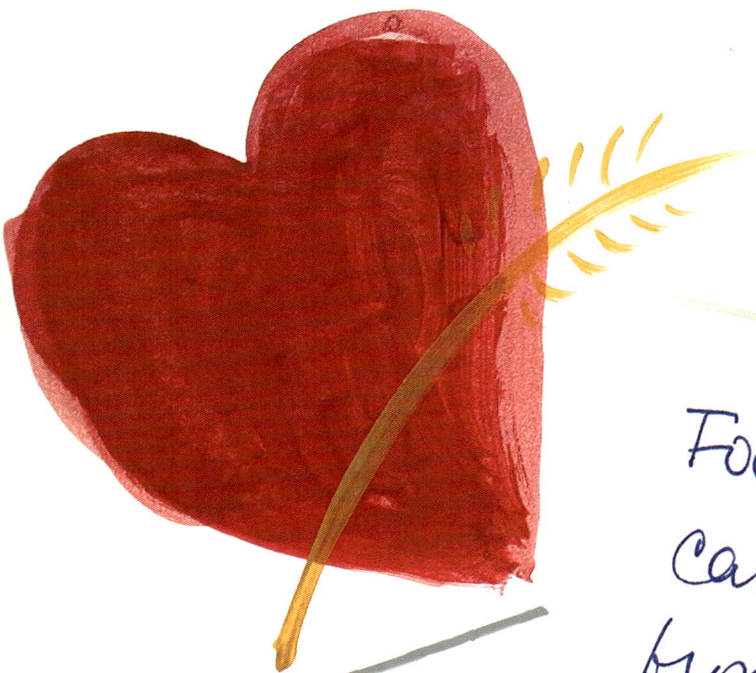

Food is love! Hoping you can feel love and support from all of us here.

Diane,
Delivery Angel

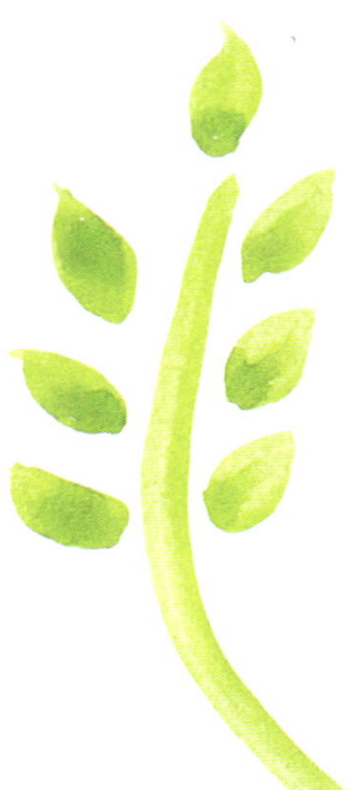

I'm grateful. part of the community that is supporting you during this difficult time.

Love from
Diane, Delivery Angel

CERES AFFILIATE FAMILY

Ceres Community Project

Mission: We create health for people, communities and the planet through love, healing food and empowering the next generation.

In 2006, a friend of Cathryn Couch's implored her to teach her daughter cooking skills, so she rolled up her sleeves and found a few families that needed meals. The first day that the teen met one of the families she was helping, a lightbulb went off for Cathryn. She realized her young friend wasn't just learning to cook, she was learning to take care of her community - and the pride was palpable. At the same time, those families who were struggling with a serious health challenge could take a deep breath, knowing that a healthy and delicious dinner was taken care of. The vision for Ceres Community Project was born.

Eight months later, Ceres began as a small volunteer project operating out of a local church's kitchen. We prepared organic meals for folks with cancer and other health challenges while creating a safe and fun place for teens to learn leadership, cooking, job skills, and the value of community. From that simple beginning, Ceres grew to include two youth-run organic sustainable gardens and three commercial kitchens serving two counties just north of San Francisco. By 2010, we had begun to share our program with others and the Ceres Affiliate Partner Program was launched in 2012.

Food can't be healthy unless it's healthy across the food system - for food and farm workers, our communities, and our environment. That's why we're committed to providing meals that are 100% organic and sustainable, with ingredients sourced locally as much as possible. Our gardens provide a special opportunity for youth volunteers to learn about food systems, from soil to community.

Medically tailored meals—meals specifically designed to meet the nutritional needs of a health condition—make a huge difference in the health and wellbeing of our clients. That's why we're hard at work to have meals like ours covered by insurance. Over the years, we've participated in research studies and pilot projects to "prove the case" for medically tailored meals, and we're a founding member of the California Food is Medicine Coalition.

Now a trusted and valued organization in our community, Ceres Community Project provides more than 180,000 meals per year to over 1,500 clients, engages hundreds of youth volunteers, and provides nutrition education programming at libraries and health centers. Our community leans on us in times of crisis, such as wildfires and COVID-19, because they know we can get delicious, nourishing food to those who need it when it matters most. Thanks to the dedication of our staff, volunteers, and donors, we're helping to create a just and sustainable future where everyone has access to the healthy food they need to thrive.

"Tending our soil organically comes with an understanding that growing food is an act of interdependence with all living things. The health of our bodies depends upon the health of our ecosystems. The two cannot be separated."

—Lee, Garden Coordinator

Teen volunteers learn the importance of tending the earth with organic gardening at the two Ceres gardens.

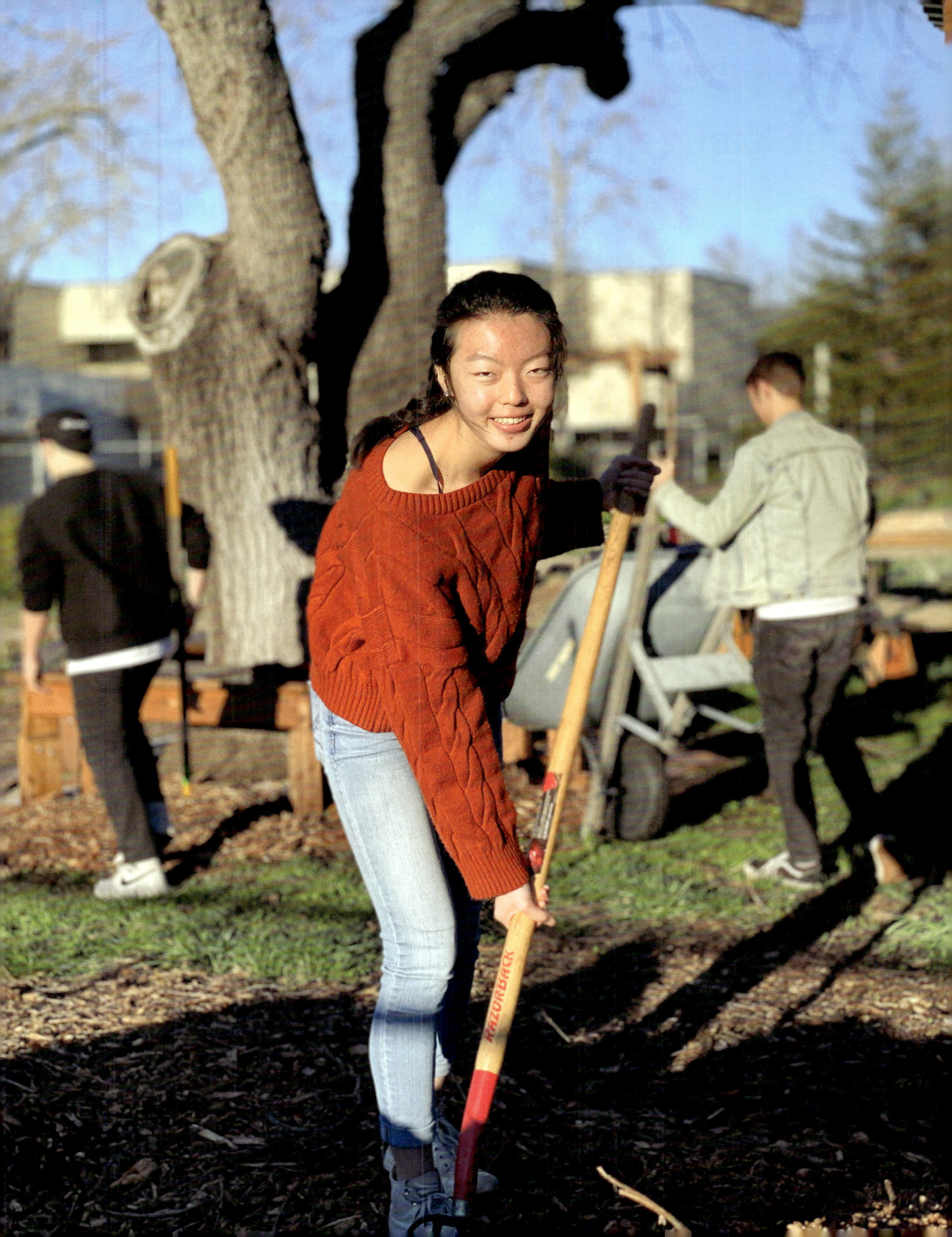
RAZORBACK

Det Kælige Måltid (The Loving Meal)

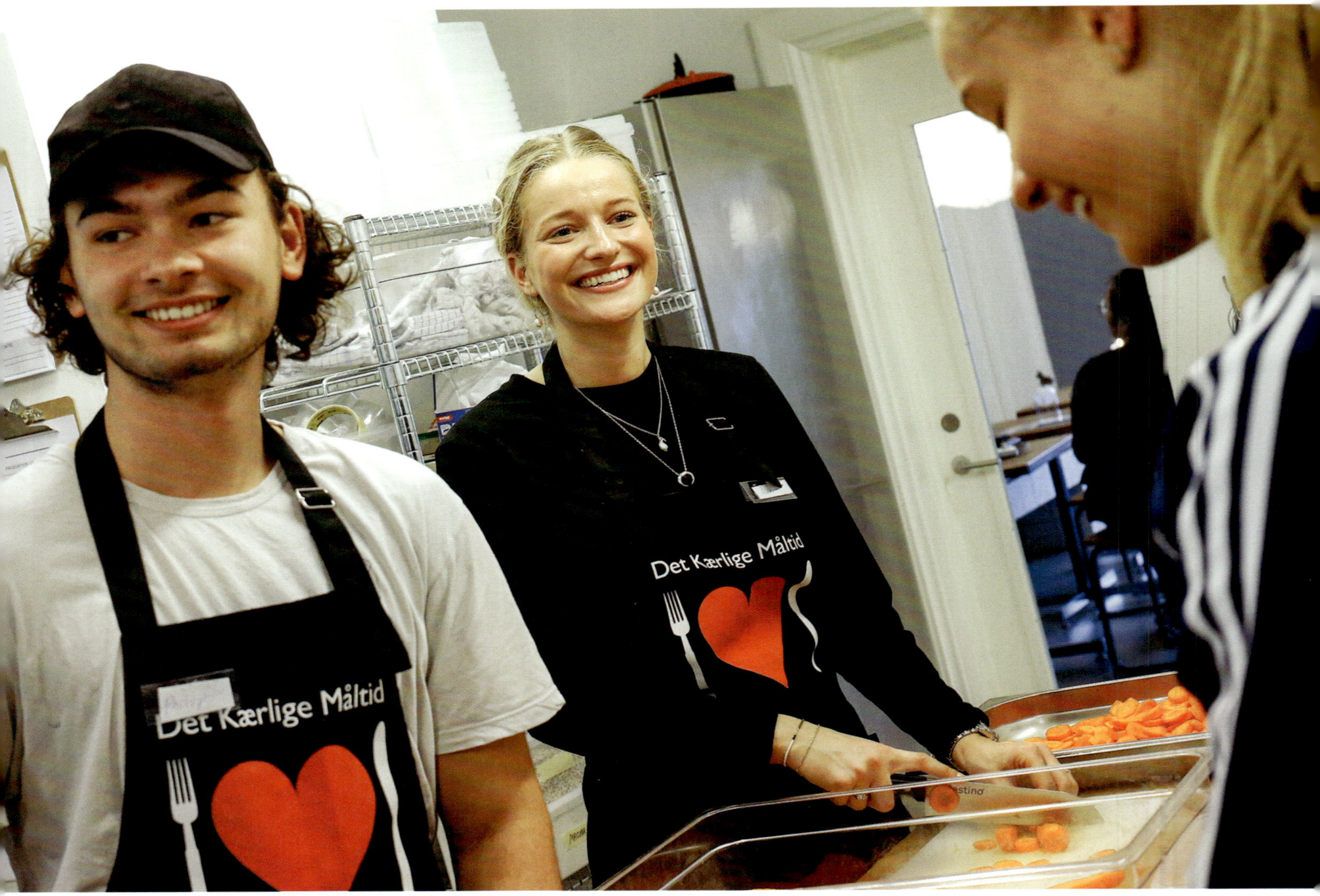

Teen volunteers learn about nourishment and health while gaining culinary skills and contributing to their community.

January 23, 2019 will forever be a memorable day as Det Kærlige Måltid (The Loving Meal) delivered the first meals to clients and their families in Aarhus, Denmark. Five months prior the founder of The Loving Meal, Charlotte Thyberg, left a good and safe job to work fulltime to launch this organization and live out her life-long dream of making a profound impact. She had known about the Ceres Community Project for a long time and seen how it has grown to touch so many people. The time now felt right to do the same in her local community. As Charlotte watched all the wonderful volunteers on a late, cold winter evening drive away to deliver the nourishing and colorful meals, she could not help but shed a few tears.

Since then, all of us at The Loving Meal have spent many busy hours in the kitchen to offer a helping hand to our clients. We have built a

"It is a heartfelt pleasure to help other people and to do something that makes an impact. I love to witness what a difference it makes for the clients and the youth volunteers. It makes it all worth it"

-Trine, Volunteer Mentor

truly unique community of volunteers who all share the same dream of making an impact for other people while gaining new culinary skills. Twice a week, we meet up in the kitchen to prepare meals for our clients. We feel a great responsibility for having the opportunity to pass over our passion for exploring the world of food and equipping our volunteers with tools and skills that demystify the approach to raw ingredients and new techniques. We hope to encourage the youth volunteers to skip quick, easy and often unhealthy options and instead make nourishing and healthy meals that will provide a healthier and happier life in the long run.

At The Loving Meal, we genuinely believe and witness that our meals are not only helping families affected by a medical crisis but also have a profound influence on our youth volunteers' cooking skills and desire to contribute to their community—something that is still very rare in Denmark.

Founder Charlotte Thyberg, living out her dream of making a profound impact with Det Kærlige Måltid.

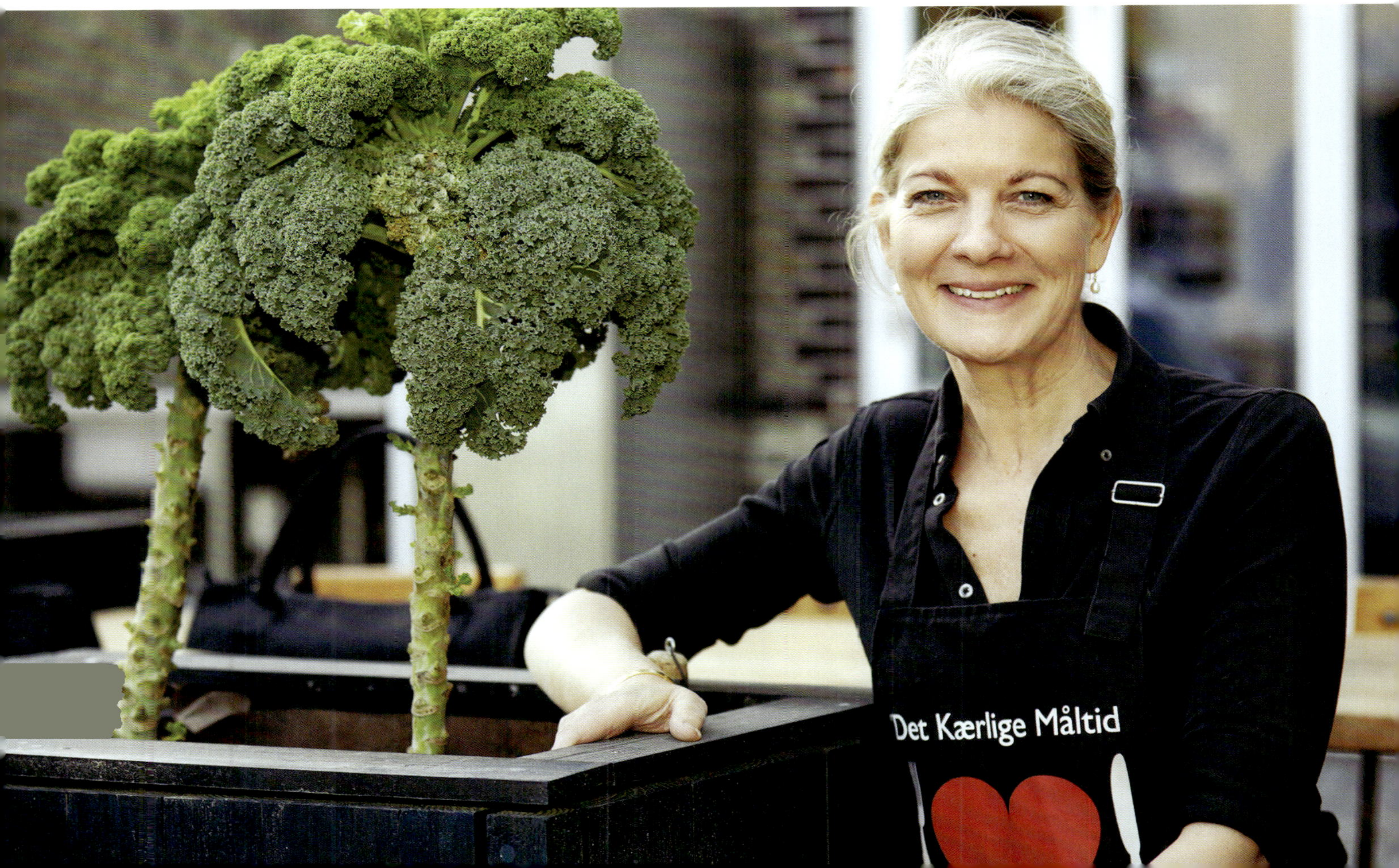

Fox Valley Food for Health

Mission: Fox Valley Food for Health promotes a nutrition-focused community by educating teens and serving those struggling with a health crisis.

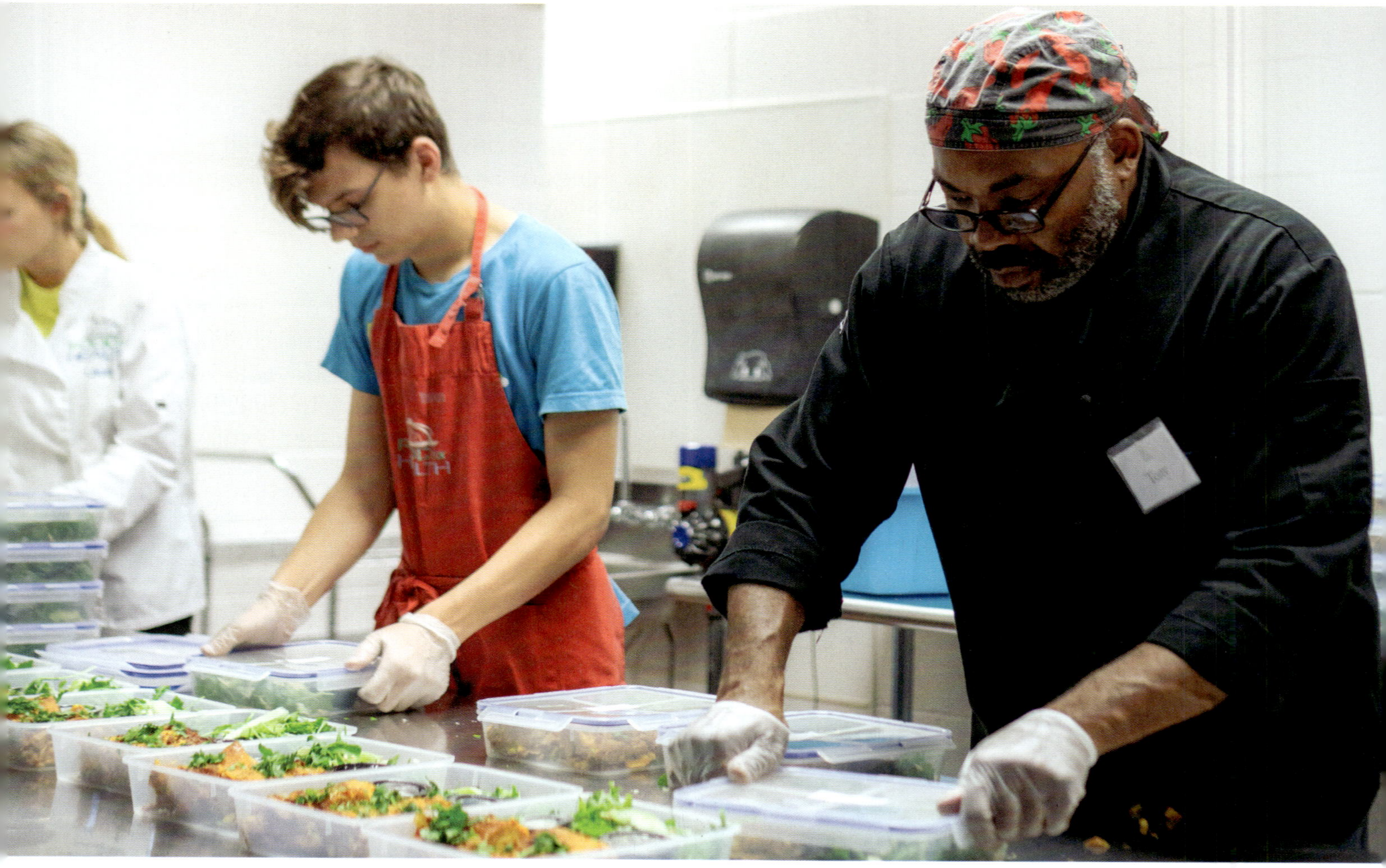

Above and right: Fox Valley brings together teen and adult volunteer chefs to create nourishing, delicious food.

After spending a summer volunteering together at the Living Well Cancer Resource Center's Culinary Comforts Program, Mary Fremgen and Susan Leigh decided to participate in the Ceres Community Project affiliate training. They shared a love for good food, an understanding of the positive impact of nutrition on health, and a passion for seeing families sharing healthy meals together. The need for a program that provided nourishing meals and education to help families experience positive health changes was clear. After their training, Mary and Susan established Fox Valley Food for Health in January 2013.

At the heart of Fox Valley Food for Health is the Healthy Meals Program. Each week, we provide 6 mostly organic, nutrient-rich, and plant-based meals to each of our clients and their families, prepared by our teen and adult chefs. The program is completely free for 12 weeks. Many of our clients receive our meals while they are going through treatment for cancer or navigating other health crises. Every year, we have expanded our program—from serving 41 clients and their families and 2,544 meals in the first year, to serving 292 clients and their families and 17,179 meals in 2020.

Our Teen Chefs stay with us for at least 12 weeks, and during this time they learn valuable cooking skills and go through a nutrition education program to learn about the importance of clean, healthy eating and serving their community. The Teen Program focuses on promoting the overall wellbeing of our Teen Chefs and providing a safe, welcoming atmosphere where they can learn and interact with their peers and adult chef mentors. We even have a special leadership track within the Teen Program where teens can serve on a Teen Board of Directors to help us guide the program to ensure we have a teen-focused kitchen. Community outreach is important, so we offer community education courses like our Caring Cooks Education Series to promote healthful, clean eating to our community. We often partner with like-minded organizations locally to provide support and education throughout the Fox Valley area.

We believe there is nothing more beautiful than bringing people together around healthy food, and we strive to do this in all areas of our program. Whether it's delivering a meal to a family in need, teaching a Teen Chef so they can cook for their family, or developing a cookbook like this so you can experience love and care through our meals, everything we do at Fox Valley Food for Health is about bringing people together in the name of nourishing, delicious food.

"I am excited for the clients to receive our perfectly prepared meals and beyond grateful for the opportunity to give back to the people of my community struggling with a health crisis"

—Ashleigh, teen volunteer

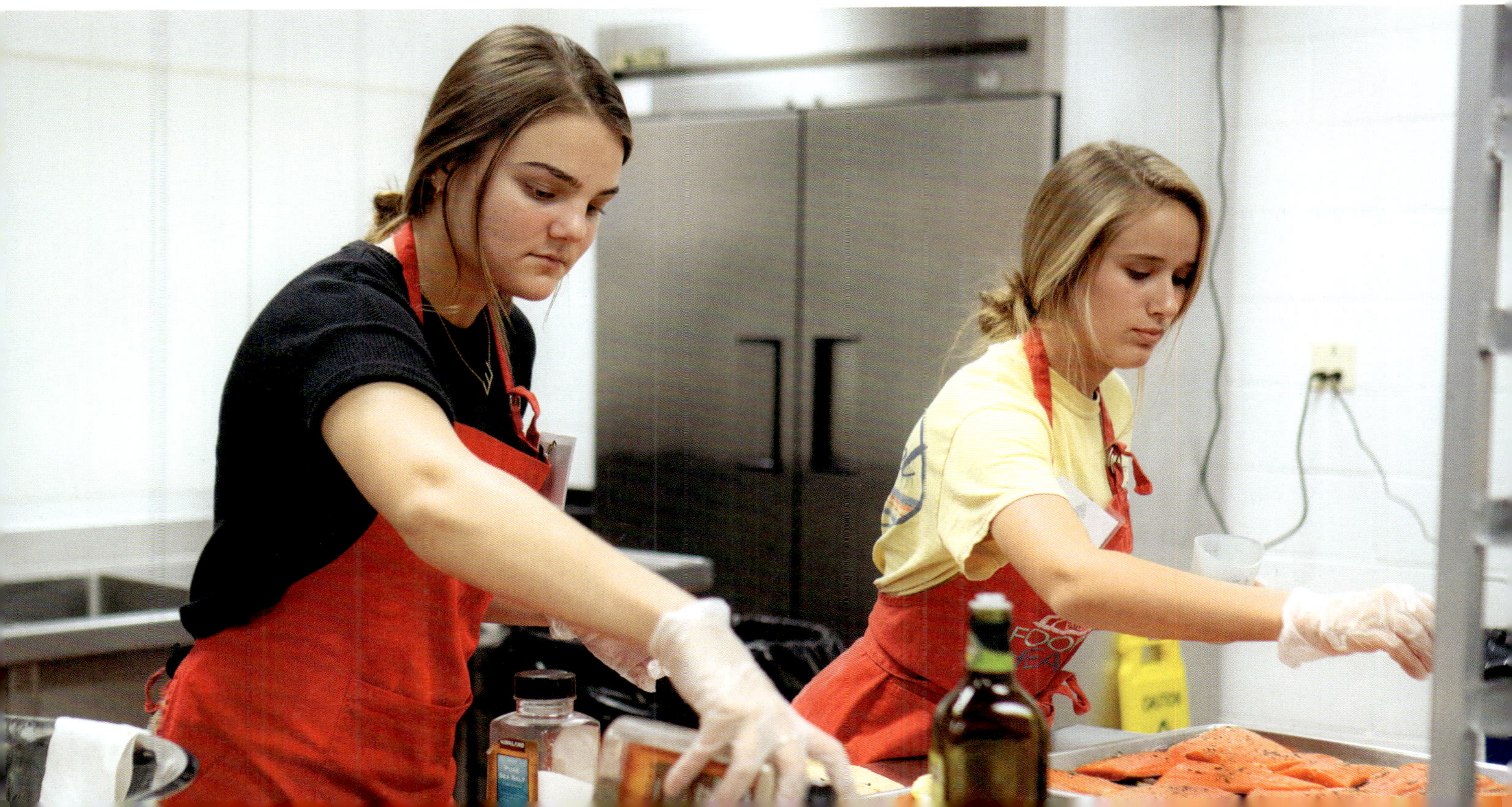

Healing Meals Community Project

Mission: To provide healthy, organic meals to people in a health crisis, while fostering compassion and empowering youth and adult volunteers in our communities.

For many years, founder Sarah Leathers watched her sister Cathryn develop and grow the Ceres Community Project. After their father passed away and having a major health crisis of her own, Sarah knew she wanted to start a similar organization at home in Connecticut. Understanding how food and community support can have a positive impact in someone's life, she decided this dream needed to become a reality. She recruited three other women to join her on this journey—Ellen Palmer, Ellen Deutsch, and Emily Safino. And in November of 2015, they spent a week participating in the Ceres affiliate training in California, launching Healing Meals Community Project (HMCP) in the spring of 2016.

HMCP was built on three certainties: nutrient-rich food is necessary to a person's overall wellbeing, young people must be central participants in shaping our collective future, and when individuals are linked to their community, they have an overall sense of connection. Healing Meals Community Project is focused on creating ripples of kindness in the community.

We nourish with love and understand the power of treating food as medicine. The cornerstone of HMCP is the Organic Meals Program which provides meals and Immune Broth for 12 weeks, enabling clients and their families to enjoy health-boosting meals without the work or stress of buying and preparing food. In addition to their healthy meals, our clients also receive nutrition education and wellness information each week to promote the fact that food is medicine and to encourage healthy eating habits.

The HMCP mission also calls for fostering compassion and empowering youth. Our kitchen brings together youth and adult volunteer chefs in a welcoming place where cross-generational creativity and respect

Healing Meals volunteers package and deliver nutrient dense meals to people dealing with a health crisis.

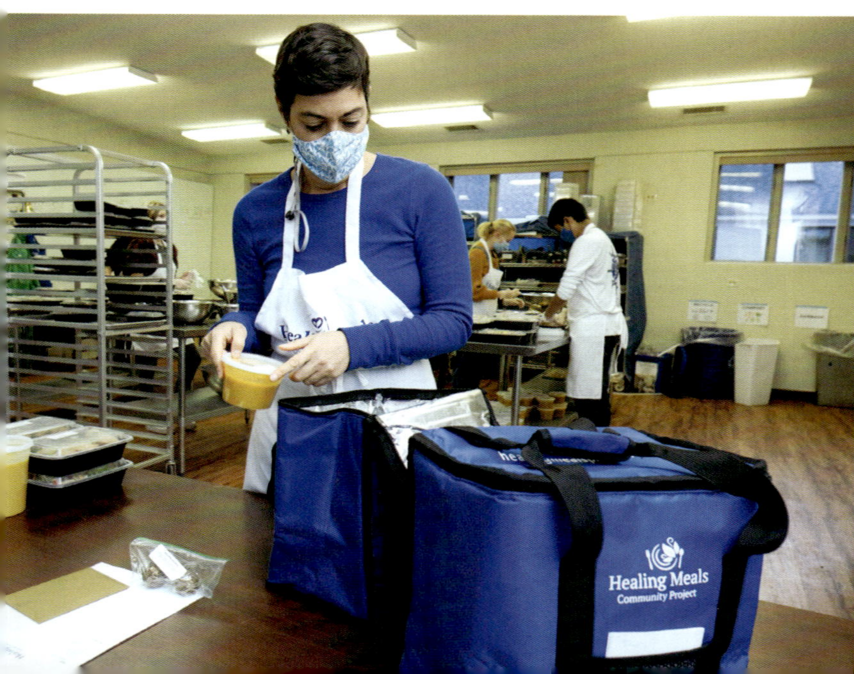

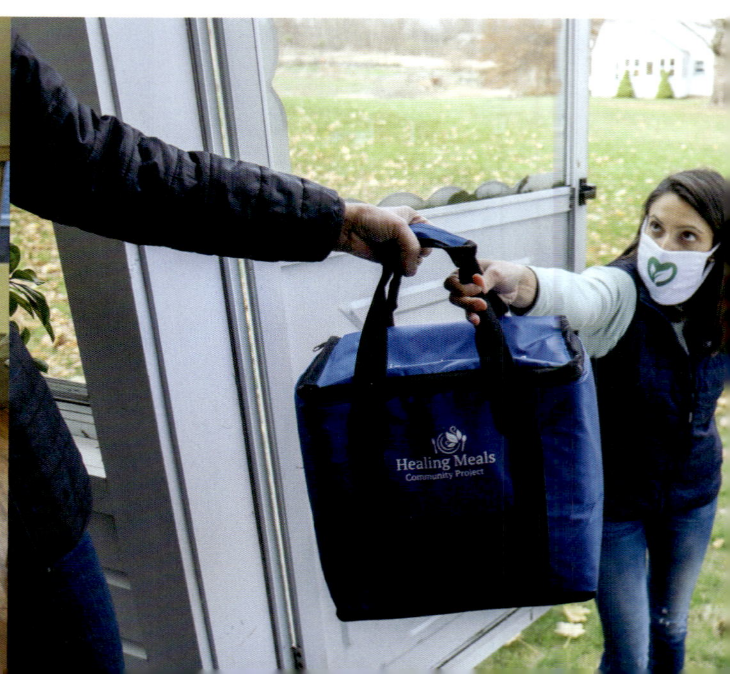

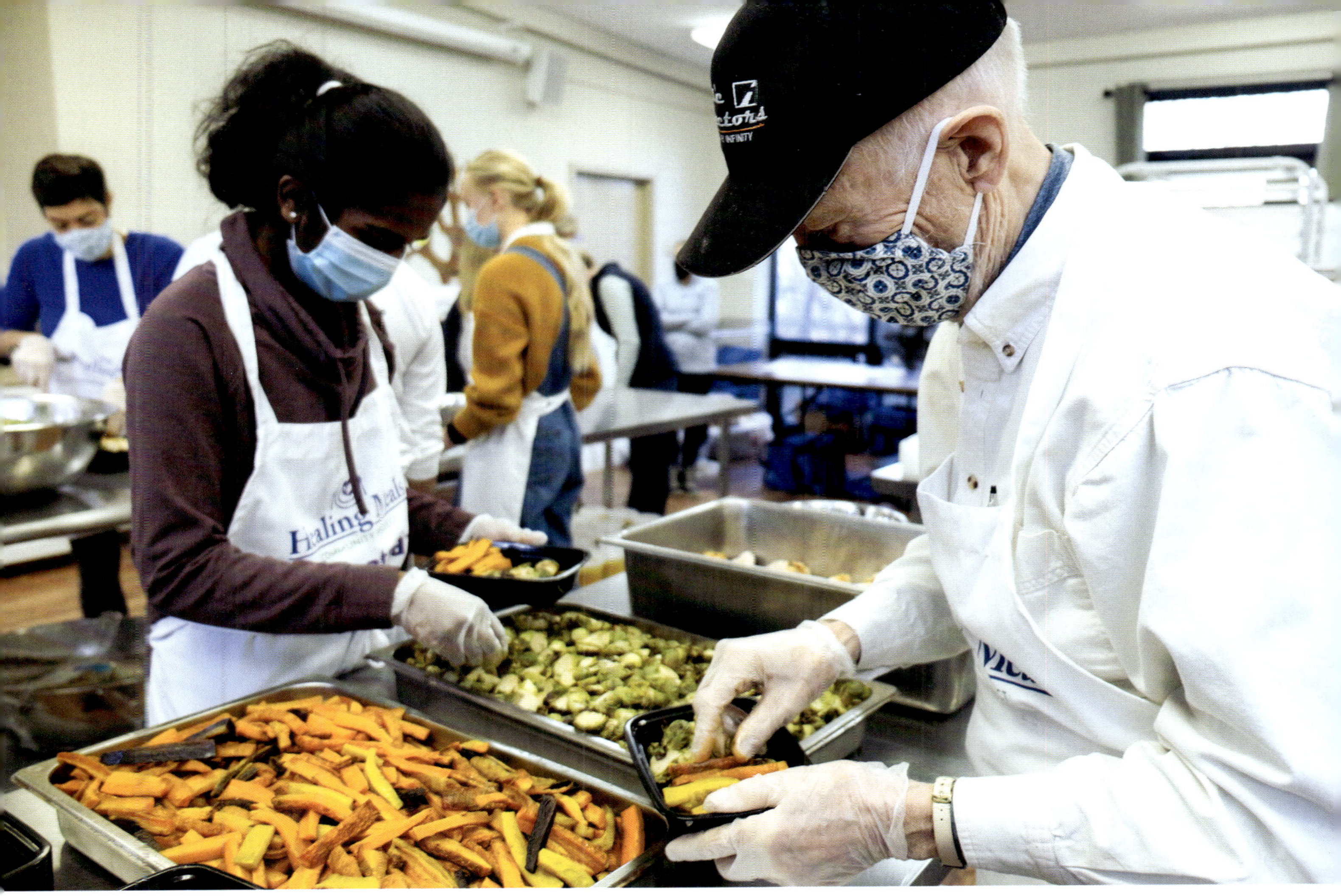

The kitchen brings together youth and adult volunteer chefs for cross-generational creativity and connection.

form the foundation of our culture. With a balance of these "old-fashioned" community values and a recognition of the relationship between nutrition and healing, we support families facing a health crisis. Our youth learn how to prepare healthy food in the kitchen and experience the farm-to-table journey in the garden. They create connections with others as they write notes of encouragement for our clients. They learn important life and leadership skills that demonstrate the values of compassion and service to others while helping to decrease the isolation that many of our clients feel.

We are a small but growing organization that nourishes with love. Focused on addressing a critical need in our community, about 70% of our meals are provided for free to low-income clients. In our first four years, we've served more than 56,000 meals to 940 clients with the support of 12,000 adult volunteer hours and 9,500 youth volunteer hours, and we work every day toward fulfilling the potential to serve all of Connecticut.

"I love the way my heart feels when I finish volunteering at Healing Meals."

—Ana, teen volunteer

Meals 4 Health and Healing

Mission: We are dedicated to raising awareness in our community about healthy lifestyles and nourishing meal preparation. We strive to be a resource for those undergoing cancer treatments by providing guidance, support, and delicious organic meals.

After the passing of her husband, Mike, in 2011 from a rare form of cancer, Kathie Heimerdinger and her family transformed their grief into love and support for others. Many of us know the devastation of a cancer diagnosis, and through her husband's cancer journey and her own journey as his caretaker, Kathie learned first-hand just what a burden it can be on families. She understood that when you need to manage appointments, the stress of the disease, and the raw emotions, that shopping for and preparing nutritious meals falls to the bottom of the list just when you need it most. Through her enormous loss, Kathie and her family founded the Heimerdinger Foundation and started Meals 4 Health and Healing in Nashville, Tennessee in 2013. Her inspiration came from the discovery of the Ceres Community Project, which, after completing the affiliate training, became the template for our program.

In our first six years, we served more than 100,000 meals to clients and families facing cancer treatment. Our clients are in medical and personal crisis. They often have little or no caregiving support or lack the financial means and resources to prepare often-expensive nutritious food. We serve our clients 8 meals per week for up to 6 months. We are able to provide meals to our clients as a result of referral partnerships with local cancer clinics and deep commitment from many partners.

Meals 4 Health and Healing is a caring community of hope and support that helps counter the side effects caused by cancer treatment and promote healing. Our teen and adult volunteers are the weekly pulse of the organization. They spend time in our organic garden, cooking in our kitchen, and delivering meals directly to our clients' homes. In addition to providing healthful, nourishing meals, we also provide education to our clients, volunteers, and community members about healthier food options and how those foods promote health and support healing throughout illness.

Rich community partnerships make our work possible. We are grateful to Calvary United Methodist Church for generously providing our kitchen, work, and organic garden space since we started our program. Our relationships with numerous local farms and gardens not only keep our costs down, but also provide the best fresh, seasonal, organic, and sustainably grown produce and lean meats year-round for our meals. Local universities deepen our Meals 4 Health and Healing program by involving their dietetic interns in our program for hands-on learning in the kitchen as well as completing special projects, such as nutritional content analysis for our meals and creating educational materials to distribute in the community. Within the cancer care community, we partner to conduct informational sessions and cooking demos.

At the heart of Meals 4 Health and Healing is deep partnership with our clients, our volunteers, and our community, because we know that leaning on one another is the best way to get through a challenging period in life.

"Our mission has not only brought joy to many lives, but also changed my life for the better. Being a Teen Chef has left a permanent impact on my life now and for the future, as I carry the philosophy of "food is medicine" to serve and nourish others wherever I go"

—AJ, teen volunteer

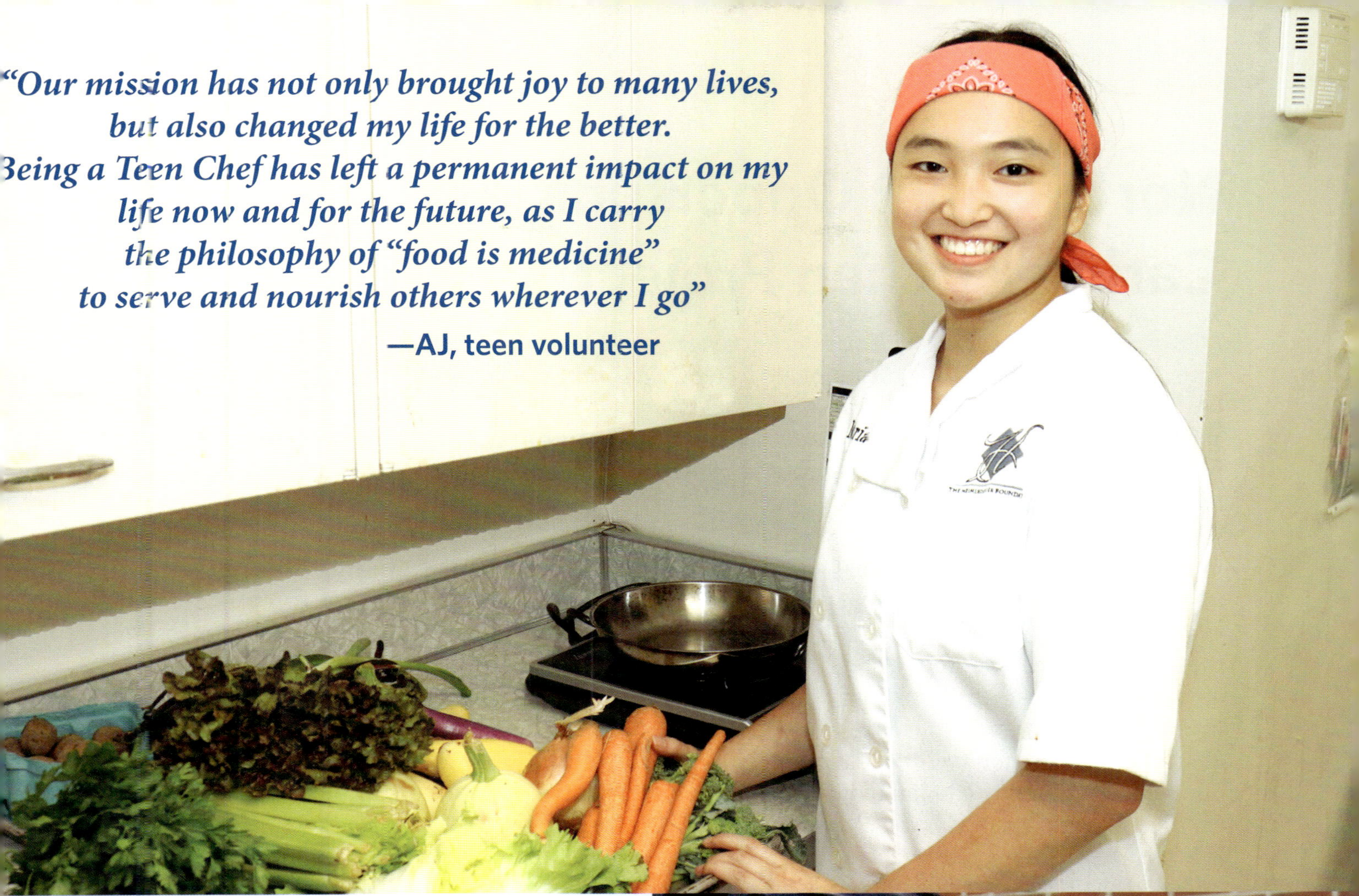

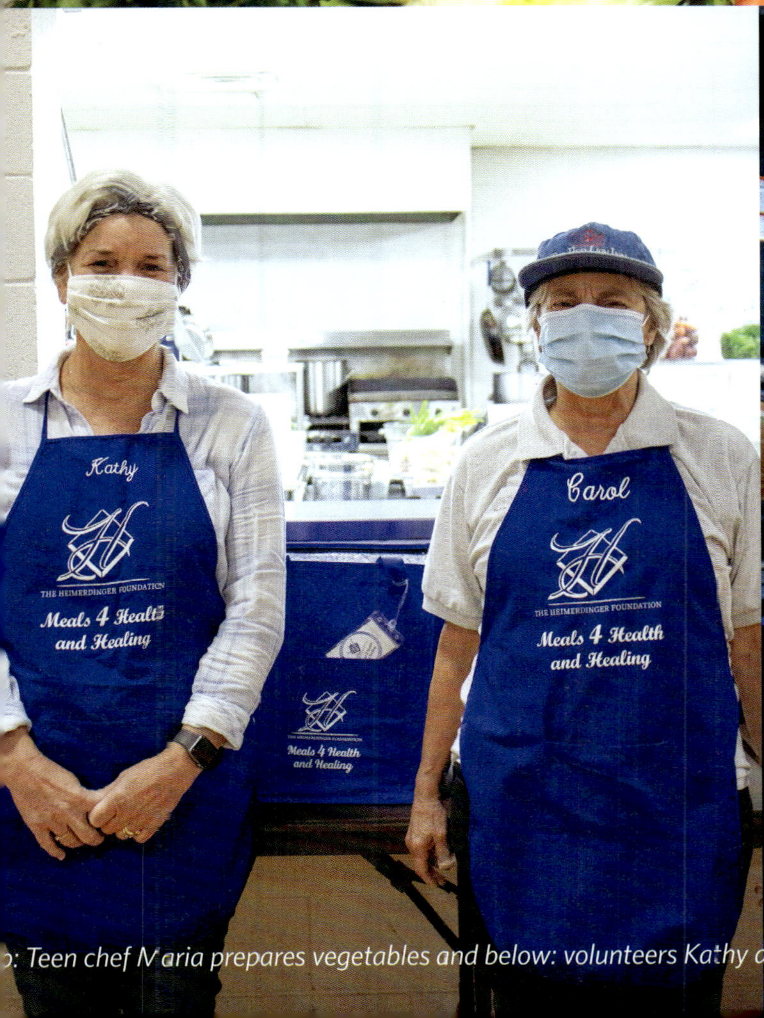

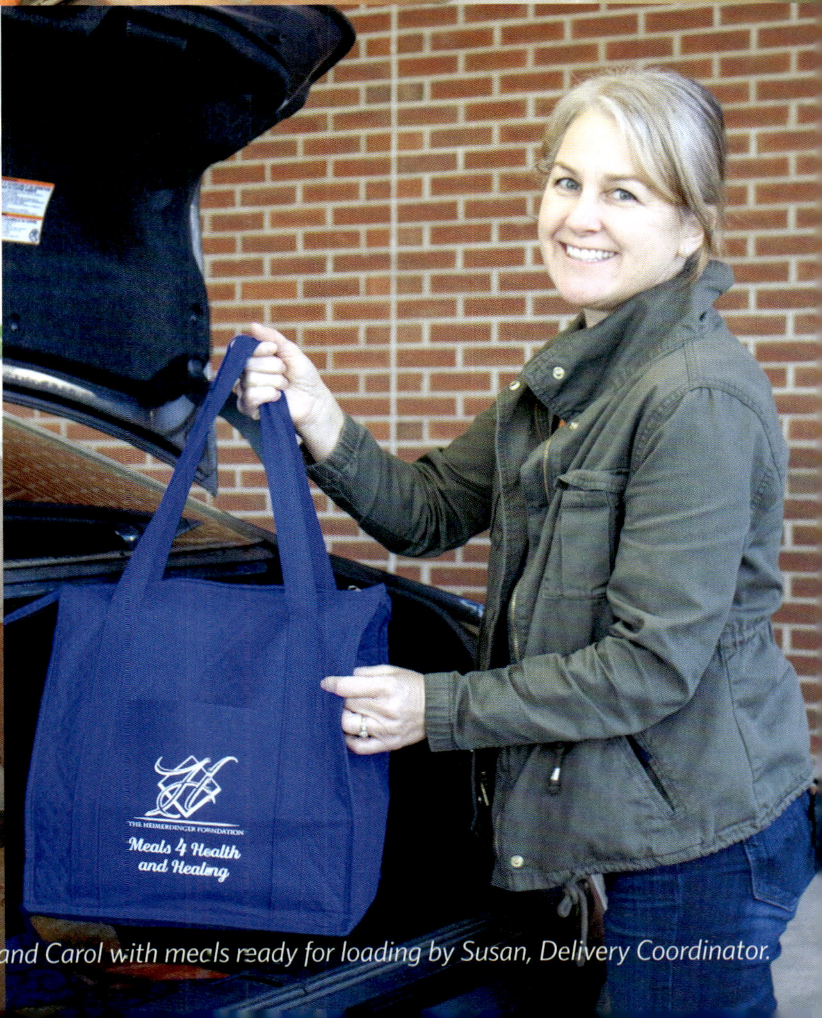

: Teen chef Maria prepares vegetables and below: volunteers Kathy and Carol with meals ready for loading by Susan, Delivery Coordinator.

North Coast Opportunities Caring Kitchen Project

Mission: North Coast Opportunities Caring Kitchen Project supports the health and recovery of individuals with critical health needs and their families by providing organic, vegetable-rich meals designed for healing; trains teen volunteers in nutrition, cooking, and job skills; develops a sense of empathy in the community's youth; fosters meaningful connections and a sense of community for all partners and participants; sources ingredients from local, organic food producers; and promotes "Food as Medicine" in the broader community.

In 2011, Tarney Sheldon was mentoring teens in a peer-nutrition education program in local elementary schools. In addition to their work in the schools, Tarney wanted to show the teens local programs that were making a deep impact in the community, and this is when she learned about Ceres Community Project in our neighboring county. Tarney and the teens were all inspired and dreamed of starting a similar project at home. Five years later, after completing the Ceres affiliate training, she partnered with North Coast Opportunities and a group of community partners to make that dream a reality. In 2016, chef April Cunningham joined the team to help bring the Caring Kitchen Project to life.

The Caring Kitchen Project became a passion project for April when she began to witness the power of healing meals when friends and neighbors were in a health crisis, and she dedicated the founding of the project to a dear friend who had passed away from cancer. She knew that many others facing cancer needed a support network and access to nourishing organic meals, and the Caring Kitchen Project was brought to life to fill this need.

Each week we deliver 5 organic, plant-based meals to cancer patients and others with critical

A vibrant community collaboration of volunteers and staff fosters empathy and connection.

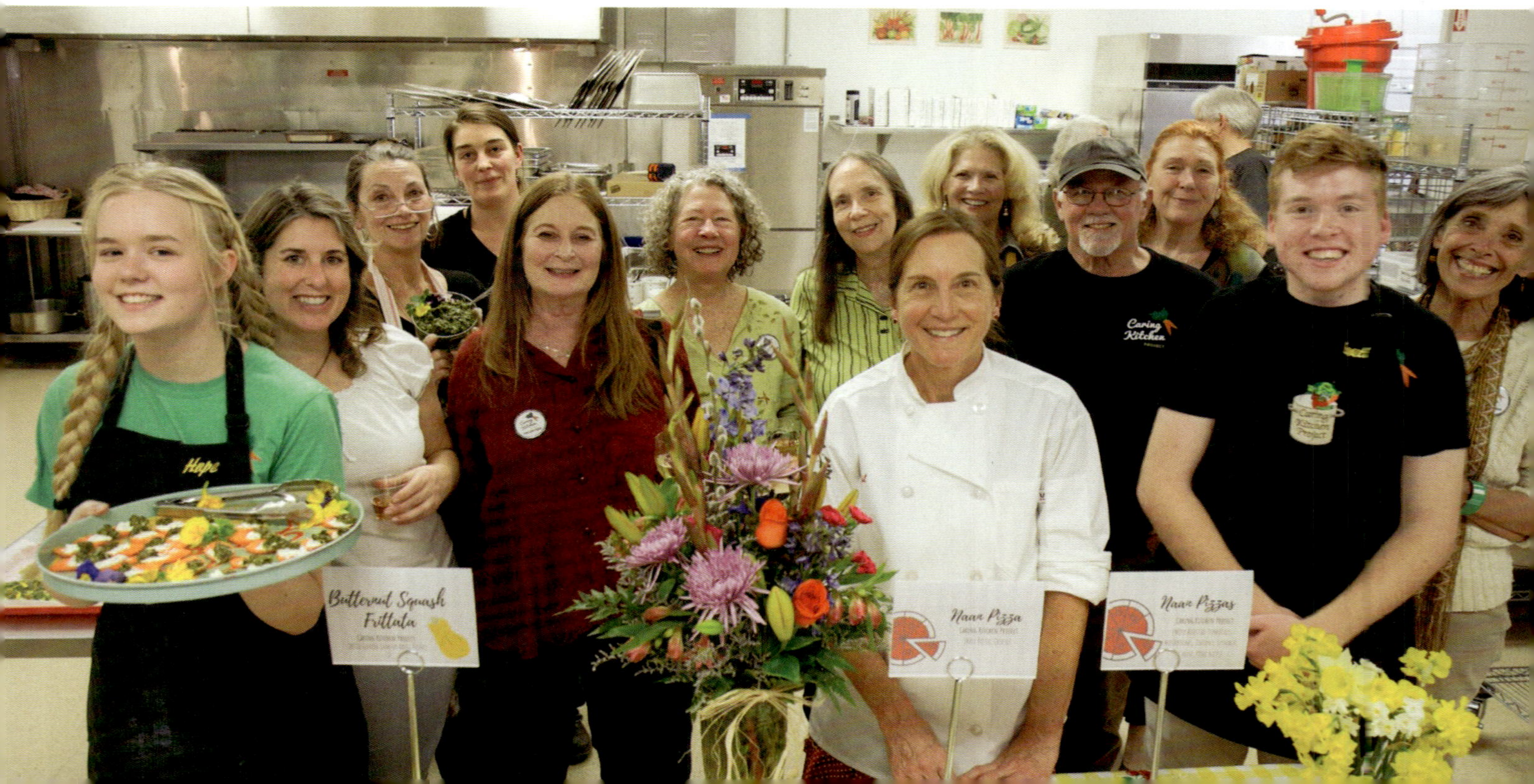

"I wasn't the greatest cook when I came to Caring Kitchen but now I definitely have some skills. I have learned the value of healthy food and eat way better than I did before coming here."

—Hope, teen volunteer

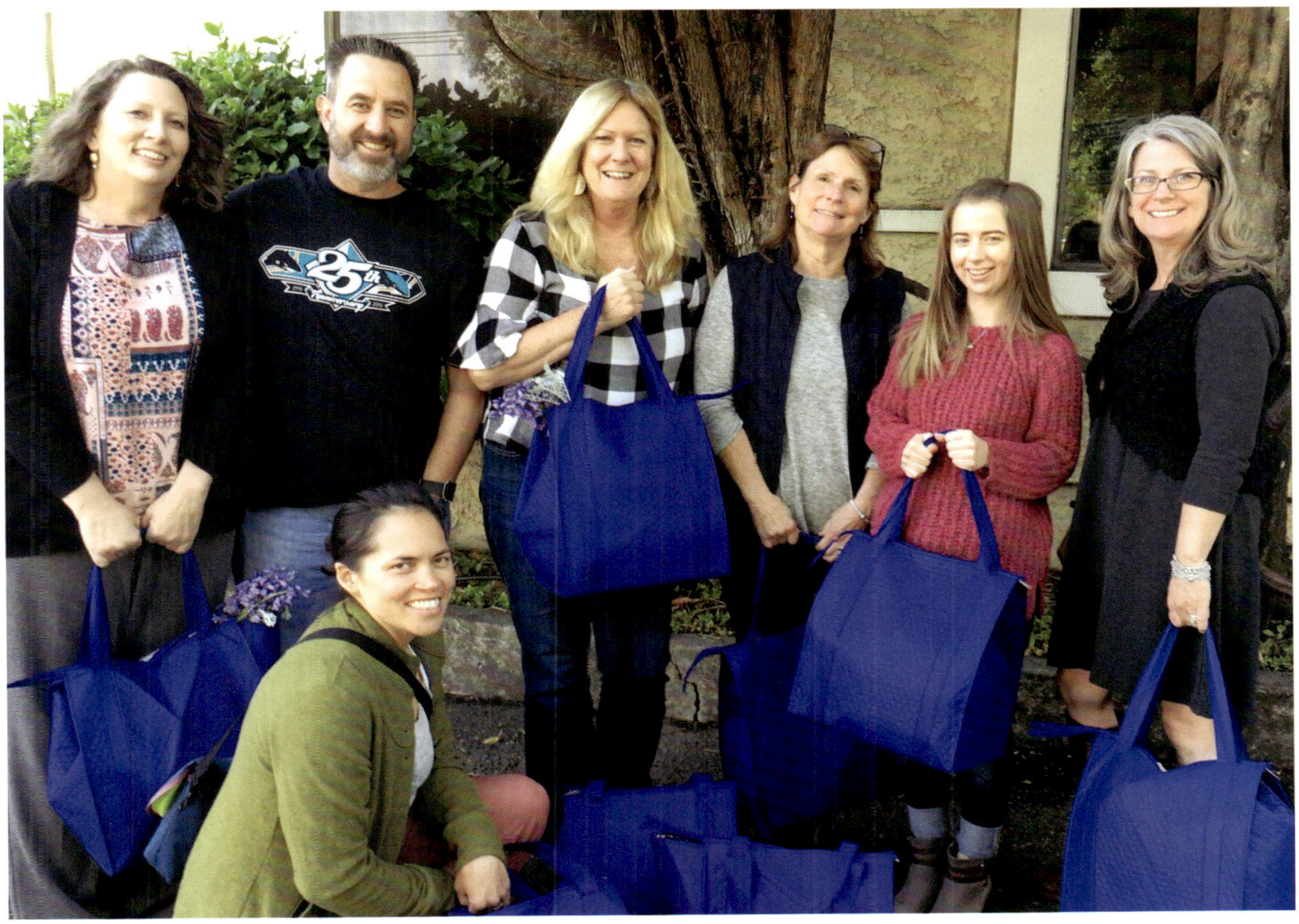

Volunteer Delivery Angels - the majority of the ingredients for the meals are sourced from local farmers.

health needs in our community via volunteer Delivery Angels. We pride ourselves on preparing nutritious meals with the majority of ingredients sourced from local organic farmers, the community college Agriculture Department garden, and community gardeners. We never lost sight of our youth-focused inspiration. We offer training for Teen Chef volunteers to develop life, job, and leadership skills.

Since we started, the Caring Kitchen Project has grown and become recognized and trusted in our community for the high-quality meals we provide, our strong volunteer base, and the vibrant community collaboration. At the heart of our work is fostering genuine empathy and connection through nourishing meals and the opportunity to serve others.

Positive Community Kitchen

Mission: To inspire community wellness through food.

In the winter of 2011, our local community was devastated when two teens tragically drowned while visiting the Oregon coast on a leadership retreat. As a tribute to these teenagers and to facilitate the processing of the collective grief, many parents came together to create a healing garden space at the high school, which served as a transformational space for many years. In the summer of 2013, Wendy Strgar, one of the parents who started the garden, learned about Ceres Community Project and was attracted to the program because of its focus on youth, community, and positivity. Wendy was inspired to nurture our youth community and decided to attend the Ceres affiliate training to channel the energy that this period of transformation and grief had produced. Positive Community Cures, the initial garden at the high school, changed into our current model and the Positive Community Kitchen was established.

Year-round, we deliver free, fresh, organic meals to clients who are experiencing life-threatening illnesses. Our program is unique because we do not require a medical referral, specific diagnosis, demographic, or geographical boundary to qualify for our meals. We believe that simply alleviating stress by providing healthy meals during an overwhelming time can move mountains, and we know that in this same move, we are nourishing our community with love and nutrition, giving all a healing foundation upon which to thrive. Every twelve weeks, we welcome in a new group of teen volunteers to prepare meals for a new cohort of clients. Positive Community Kitchen provides a welcoming space for volunteers of all ages and abilities to gather weekly as a team to explore nourishment, to foster professional and leadership development, and to spread love in our community. We also partner with local schools to provide nutrition education, including time in our kitchen, peer-to-peer lessons, job training, and internships. Third grade classes in our community are the official weekly pen-pals of our meal recipients. Our kitchen doors are open to all youth after school, and we encourage our teen volunteers to bring a friend with them.

We have a partnership with the local cancer foundation, public television, farmers' markets, and grocers called Nourish Food for Life to produce free cooking videos. Our chefs feature local, seasonal ingredients and show how simple it is to prepare healing, nourishing meals at home.

Born from tragedy as a healing space, Positive Community Kitchen strives to nourish our community the best we can. Our teen program, our community outreach, and our healthy, delicious meals allow us to do just that.

"I think my role as a teen chef is very fun and important and I see a lot of meaning in my volunteering and how it contributes to my community. I've also loved making new friends."

—Marco, teen volunteer

Teen volunteers enjoying the welcoming space of the kitchen while preparing meals and learning about leadership.

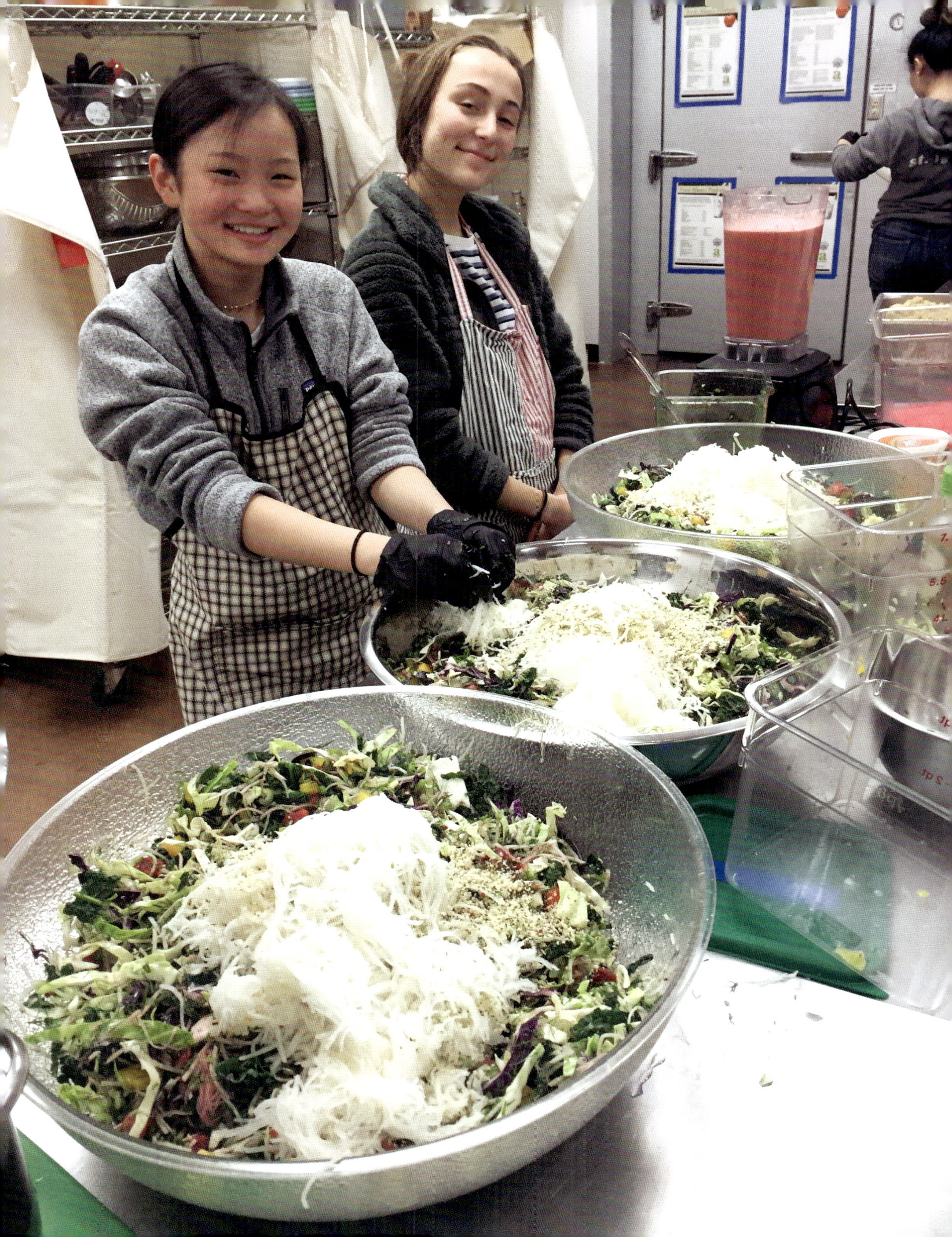

Revive & Thrive Project

Mission: We combine the power of nourishing foods with the heart of community service to provide meals to those facing a health crisis, empower teens, and support a vibrant local food system.

Founder Wendy Borden first learned about Ceres Community Project in 2011 while working on her master's degree in holistic nutrition. She was immediately inspired by the framework and collaborated with Ceres on her final thesis, focusing on nutrition and well-being in teenagers. The more Wendy learned about Ceres, the more she dreamed about starting a similar project in her hometown of Grand Rapids, Michigan—and events in her own life soon confirmed her vision. Two months after finishing her thesis, Wendy was diagnosed with breast cancer. She learned firsthand of the devastation that a serious illness can bring. Her nutrition background equipped her with knowledge of the tremendous benefits that nourishing foods can provide during the healing process, but she lacked the energy and strength to prepare healthy meals. She recognized that many others in West Michigan lack not only the energy, but also knowledge and access to healthy foods during cancer treatment. Her experience affirmed the need to create a Ceres affiliate and in May of 2015, she launched Revive & Thrive Project.

Revive & Thrive Project prepares delicious and nourishing food while empowering high school students with healthy eating and cooking skills. The teens volunteer as Teen Chefs and together with adult mentors, they prepare nutritious meals for individuals with serious illness and their families. We strive to be an intergenerational program, connecting people from diverse walks of life. Participating in the kitchen for an average of 18 months, youth grow in their nutrition knowledge, self-esteem, and leadership abilities. They experience the transformative power of serving those in need and learn valuable life and career skills. Teen Chefs prepare hundreds of meals each week for individuals experiencing the debilitating effects of serious illness. For these individuals, suppressed appetites and side effects of treatment mean they may only be able to eat a few bites at each meal. We seek to provide the most healthy, nourishing, and delicious meals that our clients can find, so that every bite counts. Each client receives twelve weeks of healthy and nourishing meals prepared with ingredients that are whole, fresh, and seasonal. Our local-first philosophy inspires us to source locally whenever possible —from local farm fresh foods to packaging containers and kitchen supplies. We even grow organic produce in our kitchen garden!

Our Delivery Angels bring meals to the homes of clients throughout Grand Rapids and surrounding suburbs, offering a caring connection in addition to healthy food. We often hear that our meals help our clients feel better and give them hope.

Revive & Thrive Project also inspires hope by providing nutrition education programs. These resources promote the understanding that healthy food can reduce the risk of diet-related disease and improve treatment outcomes. We partner with local food growers and healthcare providers to promote the connection between food and wellness.

We're proud to cultivate a community where healthy eating is unifying, simple, and enjoyable. Our goal is to create a culture where wholesome foods are valued, supported, and accessible to all. At Revive & Thrive Project, we embrace community connections through nourishing meals, a robust volunteering program, and a local-sourcing mindset to serve our clients the best way we know—delicious meals made with love.

"I delivered meals one night and handed healthy food to someone in need. That gives you an awesome feeling. I also learned how great-tasting healthy food can be. People think eating healthy is disgusting: it's not."

—Nicole, teen volunteer

Teen chefs at Lubbers Farm, learning in a culture where healthy eating is valued, supported and accessible.

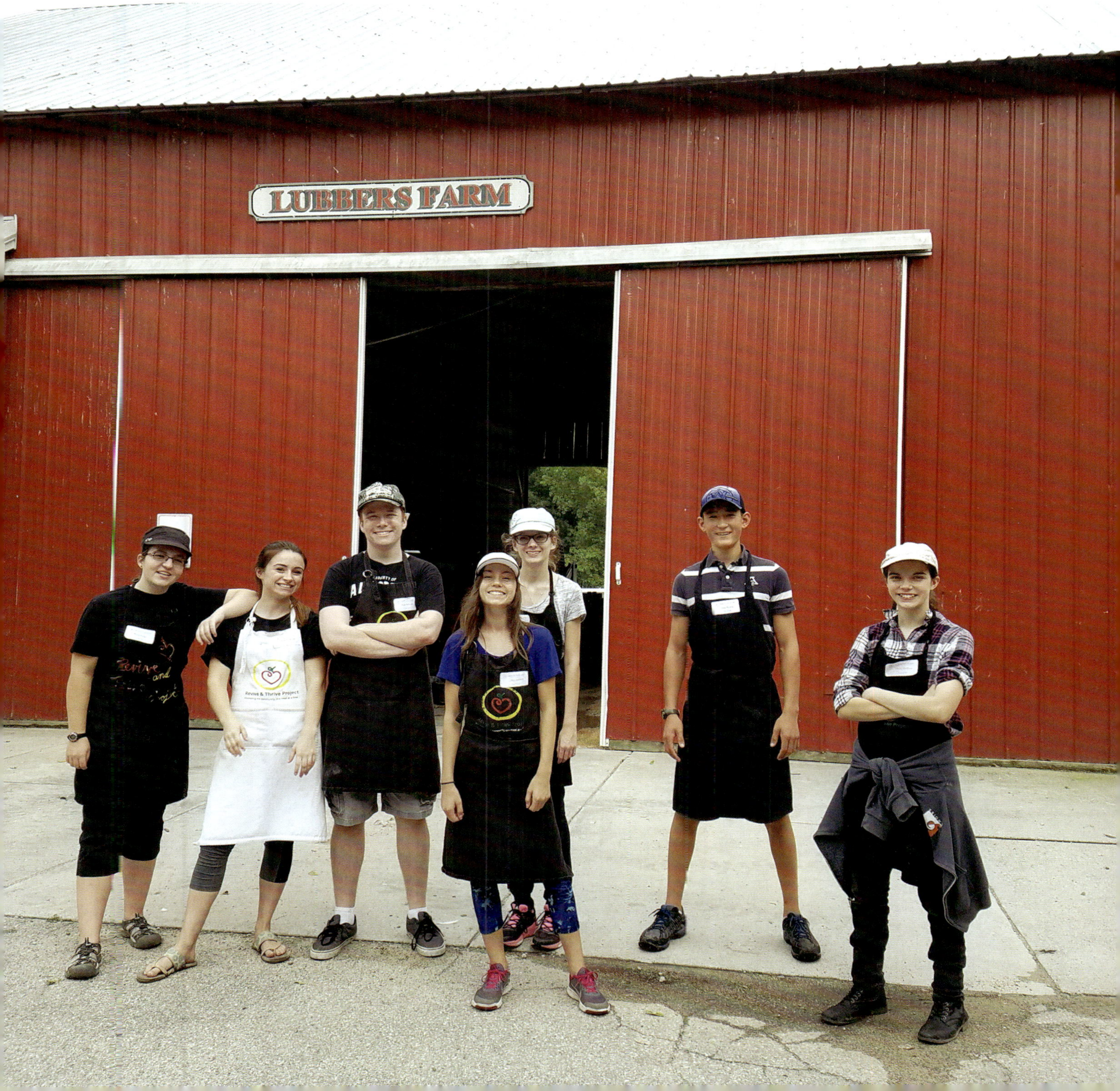

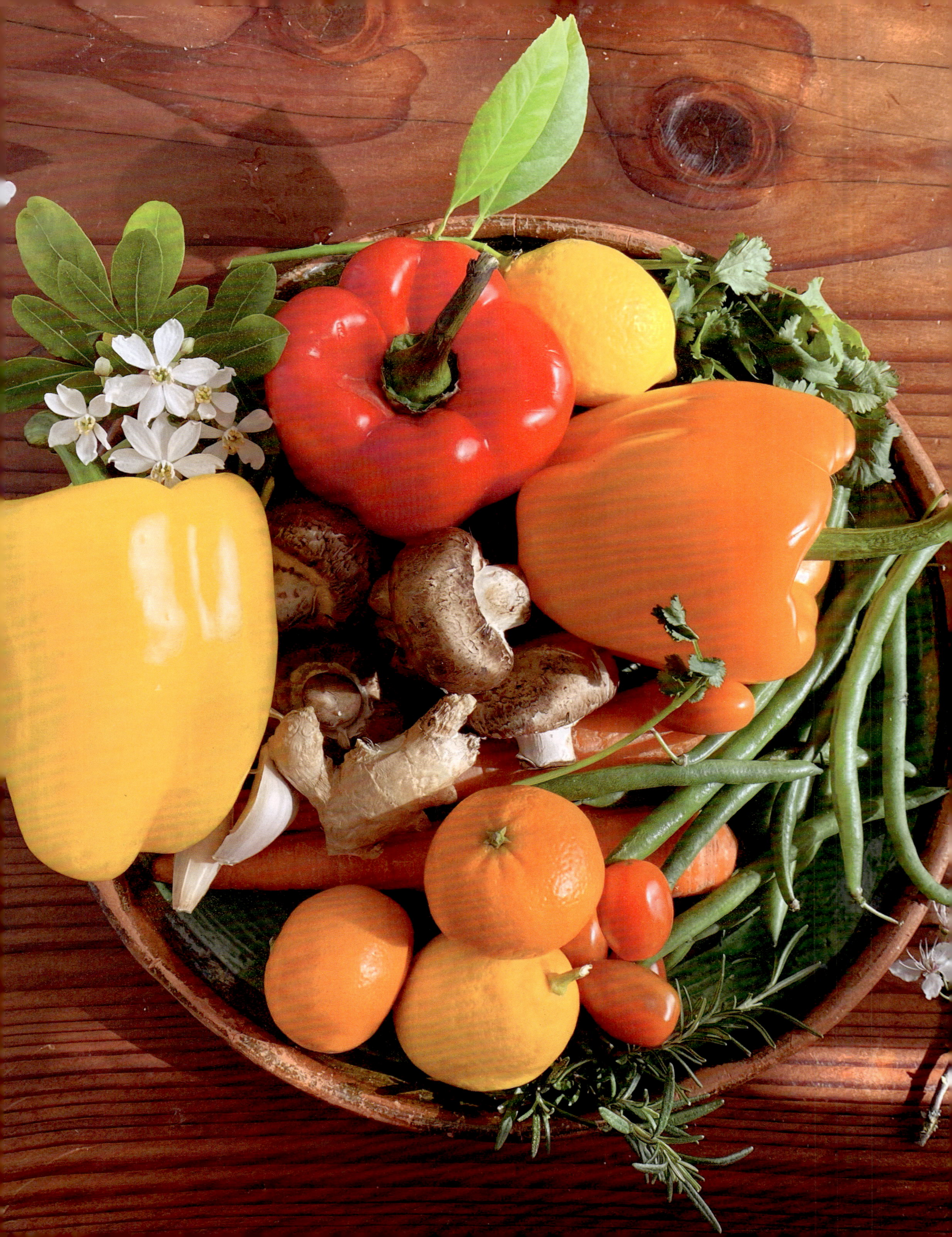

NUTRITION BASICS

Why Do We Call Food Medicine?

What we eat plays a fundamental role in our long-term health and in our ability to prevent and heal illnesses. Increasingly, scientists, researchers and health providers are recognizing the link between eating habits and health.

For tens of thousands of years, humans and our pre-human ancestors evolved interdependently with the plants, fungi and animals found in our immediate environments. We learned how to make foods digestible through cooking, grinding, pressing, filtering, salting and various forms of fermentation. Beyond that, foods were enjoyed in their whole form. Only in the past hundred years have highly-processed and chemically-created foods become abundant in our food landscape. In our busy lives, it can be tempting to turn to "convenience" and take-out foods, but what is time-saving now can compromise our health in the long term.

There is no one explanation for the epidemic of disease that we see happening all around us. Both individual and systemic considerations factor in. Longer life spans, stress, lack of exercise, systemic racism and inequality, industrial agriculture, and pollution in our environment all have a part to play. But the radical change in our eating habits and the stress this puts on our bodies is clearly one of the keys.

The foods available to us today range widely in their effect on our health — from strongly supportive to virtually toxic. When we eat things that our body doesn't recognize (chemically created "low fat" foods or artificial sweeteners, for example), or too much of something that our body isn't used to from an evolutionary perspective (such as refined white sugar), it disturbs our body's balance. Valuable energy is spent trying to process and eliminate these foods, depleting the nutrients and phytochemicals we need for healthy functioning, while providing little or none of those nutrients themselves.

Eating a plant-forward, whole foods and organic diet is the foundation for long-term health — this is why we call these foods "medicine."

This doesn't mean that you have to stick to organic brown rice and collard greens to be healthy! Our bodies are amazingly resilient and have the capacity to process some amount of refined sugars, alcohol, preservatives and so on. If you are basically healthy, sticking to the 80/20 rule will probably work for you — 80 percent of your food choices coming from organic, plant-forward whole foods and 20 percent not quite that nutrient-dense. If you are not at optimum health, however, we encourage you to eliminate most, if not all, of those foods that don't actively support your body. This includes all processed and refined foods, sugar in all its forms, alcohol, and foods containing chemical preservatives.

As you'll discover in the recipes that follow, eating for health doesn't mean that you have to sacrifice taste. We believe food must be beautiful, delicious and nutritious in order to be truly nourishing.

Beyond the Physical Food-Health Connection

There is another way of looking at the food we eat that has nothing to do with how nutritious it is, but might contribute just as much to our wholeness and long-term vitality. Food is our most fundamental connection to both ourselves and the world around us.

When we eat, we take in the energy of the cosmos formed over 14 billion years into the immense complexity of the plant and animal kingdoms... and that energy becomes us. Human existence stands on the evolutionary shoulders of the plants, beginning with the single-celled organisms that figured out how to take sunlight and turn it into energy. This giant leap—what we call photosynthesis—changed the oxygen content of Earth's atmosphere and ultimately allowed for the development of mammals and eventually the human species.

Our eating habits and their effect on our health

In 2017, 11 million deaths worldwide were attributed to dietary risk factors

About one-half of all American adults - 117 million individuals - have one or more preventable chronic diseases, many of which are related to poor quality eating patterns and physical inactivity

More than two-thirds of all adults, and one-third of all children in the United States are now considered to be overweight or obese

Added sugars account for almost 270 calories, or more than 13% of daily calorie consumption in the U.S.

Plants continue to be the only organisms that can grow directly from the combination of water and sunlight. All other species are dependent on them in some form for their existence—and we humans are ultimately the most dependent.

For the past four or five hundred years, we have held the false and damaging notions of human separateness and superiority. As scientific understanding broadens, we have come to realize our absolute connection and dependence on all species.

When we realize that we are literally given life through the gifts of the plant worlds, we come to food from a new and deeply grateful place. We understand that human life is possible because of the enormous success of plants over millions of years. When we walk through a farmers' market, we are touched by the abundance and generosity of the earth. When we sit down to eat, we understand that the food on our plate is the result of billions of years of the universe's evolution, and that we, just like the plants and animals, are intricately interwoven into that reality.

What we eat becomes us. When we eat with the awareness that food is a gift, we locate ourselves in the immense mystery of the universe. Gratitude springs naturally from this place and our lives are deepened and enriched by the knowledge that we, too, have a place at the table. Eating with mindfulness, being aware of the food on our plates, in our mouths and feeding our bodies, inspires us to chew well, eat slowly, and choose our foods carefully.

The Basics: Plant-Forward, Whole Foods, Organic

If you pay attention to the news, it might seem like you need a Ph.D. to figure out how to eat. We'll explore some of the details in the sections that follow, but if you remember this simple phrase you'll be at least 90 percent of the way there: *plant-forward, whole foods, organic*.

Plant-Forward Is Key

While no single nutrient or food can protect against diseases, plant foods contain the minerals, vitamins and phytochemicals that seem to interact to provide extra support for good health. The American Institute of Cancer Research recommends that at least two-thirds of your plate be filled with vegetables, fruits, whole grains and legumes — the plant foods.

A second benefit of a plant-forward eating style is that it helps protect against weight gain, which may be a contributing factor for many health conditions. Many plant foods are nutrient dense, but low-calorie foods.

The best way to do this is to eat a wide variety of colorful vegetables, fruits, whole grains and legumes from the following categories:

- cruciferous vegetables such as broccoli, cauliflower, Brussels sprouts, arugula, kale, collard greens, kohlrabi and cabbage;
- dark leafy greens like kale, chard, collard greens, romaine lettuce and bok choy;
- deep orange and red vegetables like butternut and other winter squashes, yams, tomatoes, and red, yellow and orange bell peppers;
- fruits such as blueberries, red grapes, strawberries and raspberries, and citrus fruits such as oranges, lemons, limes and grapefruit;
- whole grains such as brown rice, millet, quinoa, barley, buckwheat, oats and amaranth;
- legumes such as lentils, split peas, adzuki beans, navy beans, black beans, cannellini beans, kidney beans and garbanzo beans

Eat the rainbow every day, and you'll wind up nourishing yourself with a broad range of the nutrients you need to thrive.

The Whole Is Greater than the Sum of the Parts

An enormous amount of time and energy has been spent trying to identify specific nutrients that can protect against disease. Today, scientists are starting to question this approach. The chemical constituents of plants are extremely complex. Garden thyme, for example, contains 38 different antioxidants that we know of. We are a long way from understanding how these components work together to produce a certain result, but we are beginning to realize that the whole is greater than the sum of the parts.

Eating foods that are as close to their whole state as possible provides the greatest potential for capturing this synergistic effect.

Organic Food: Better for Us, Our Communities and the Planet

Organic food not only is more nutritious, it provides economic, environmental and social benefits. In the California Certified Organic Farmers (CCOF) 2019 Benefits Report[2], they provide impactful evidence for the benefits of supporting our organic farmers. CCOF's research finds organic vegetables to be higher in antioxidants, vitamins, minerals and phytochemicals (non-nutritive plant chemicals that can positively affect health through antioxidant functions). Organic pasture raised meat and dairy have more favorable fatty acids.

Purchasing organic foods also strengthens our local food communities. Organic growers receive a premium price, which supports the next generation of farmers to establish viable businesses. This is especially important as the average age of an America farmer is now 58 years old. Areas with thriving organic farm and food businesses also demonstrate lower rates of poverty. And purchasing organic food from local farmers returns more dollars to the local economy.

Organic agriculture is also a big win for the environment. Pasture raised livestock—animals raised and fed on grass pasture—uses less water and can contribute to sustainable management of grass lands, sequestering carbon to reverse global warming.[3]

From the farm workers to consumers, and the people and animals living downwind of farms, removing pesticides and herbicides benefits us all. Exposure to pesticides is most damaging to children because of their lower body weight and because they are in the early stages of physiological development. Beyond that, pesticide and herbicide use has enormous negative consequences on the health of the water and air on which all life on our planet depends. If the planet isn't healthy, our long-term health suffers as well. Pesticides have been linked to diseases from cancer to Parkinson's.[4] For the sake of all of us we encourage you to purchase organic foods whenever possible.

Making the change to healthier eating habits is a journey. Start with any of the small steps outlined in this chapter. If you keep these concepts in mind, and slowly but surely move your way of eating in this direction, you'll be on your way to better health.

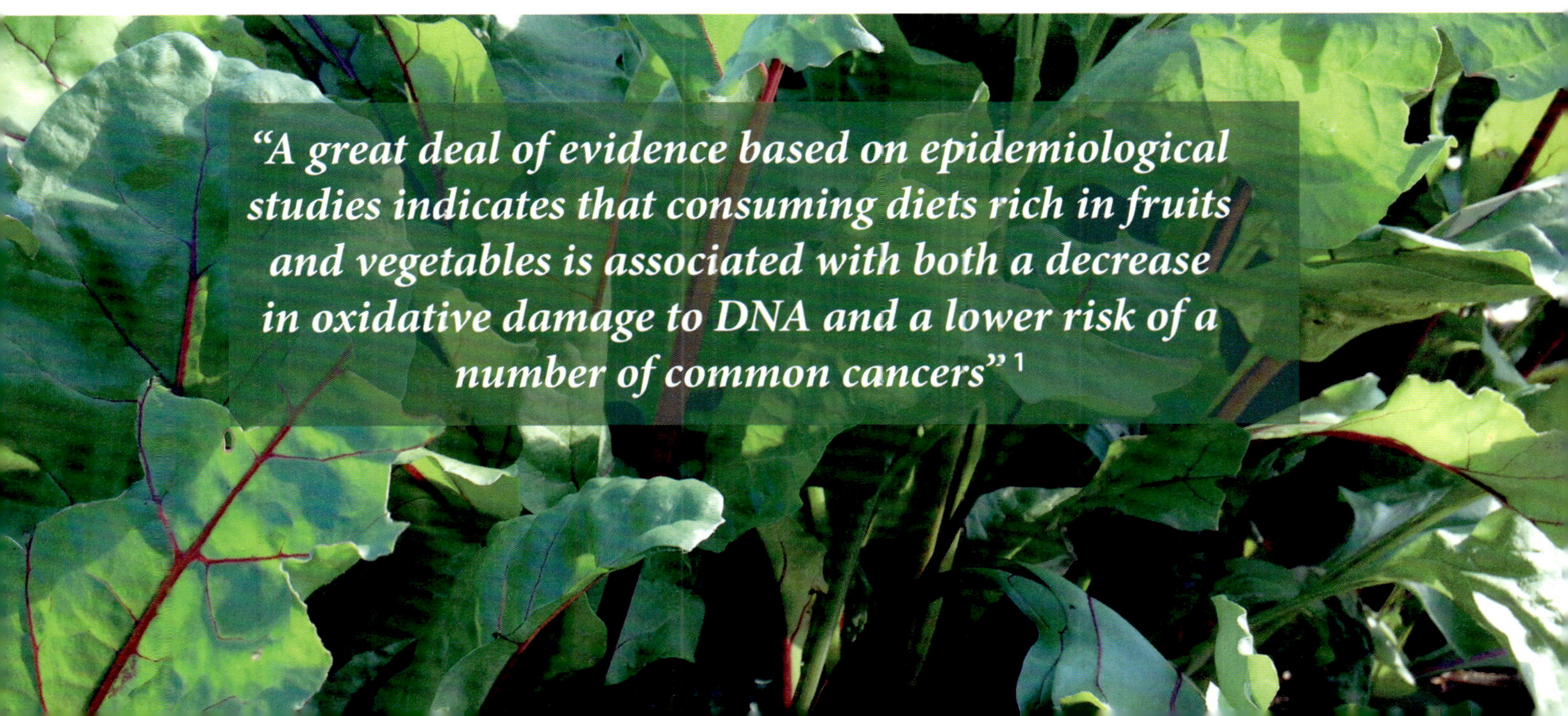

> ***"A great deal of evidence based on epidemiological studies indicates that consuming diets rich in fruits and vegetables is associated with both a decrease in oxidative damage to DNA and a lower risk of a number of common cancers"*** [1]

Nourish Yourself During Illness with Almost No Cooking

Supporting our body through what we eat is relatively simple when we are healthy, but it becomes a bigger and more important challenge when we are dealing with an illness. Illness changes how our energy is used, affects our appetite and ability to eat, and adds nutritional demands. When we are healing from a serious illness, every bite counts.

During a serious illness, the loss of vital energy may be one of the most difficult obstacles we face. Our store of energy is what allows us to do the physical, emotional and mental activities we aspire to during our waking day. Pain associated with illness can further deplete our reserves as the body seeks to repair itself.

How can you feed yourself well during those times — days, weeks or perhaps longer — when you have absolutely no energy? If you have enough money and a good quality grocery store in your neighborhood, you may be able to purchase a healthy array of ready-to-eat prepared foods. If you are blessed with friends and family nearby, they may be able to help by cooking some or all of your meals for you.

If you are like many of our clients, however, you may have little extra money, energy or support.

Building your physical energy takes time. Adopting a few new daily habits can help. Remember:

- When your appetite is low, take small meals and focus on foods that pack a nutritional punch.
- Drink often. Include broths and teas that nourish the body with minerals and helpful herbs along with plenty of pure water.
- Add condiments to your meals such as nuts and seeds, nutritional yeast, goji berries and sea vegetables.

See the Basic Weekly Plan on the next page for suggestions to get the most nourishment with the least amount of work if you are ill and fending for yourself.

Healthy vegetables in the Meals 4 Health and Healing kitchen.

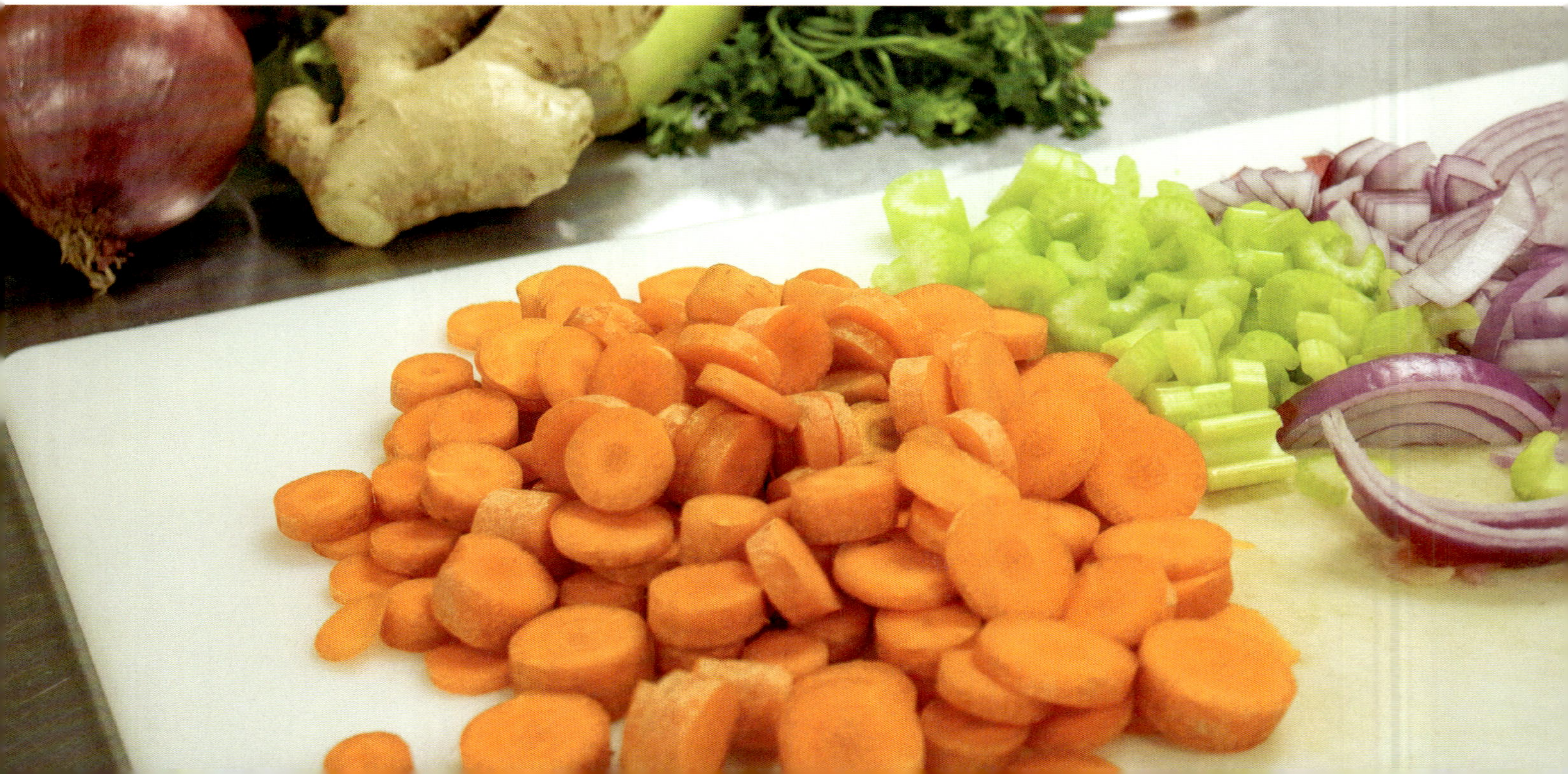

Basic Weekly Plan

1 Make a batch of Healing Vegetable and/or Chicken Broth. Broth requires almost no chopping — most vegetables can be simply cut in two or three pieces and covered with water. It cooks unattended and you have a high-quality source of nutrition that you can sip either warm or cold. Healing Vegetable Broth (page 106) is both tasty and rich in potassium. Healing Chicken Broth (page 108) includes organic bones that are cooked with vinegar or lemon juice to help draw out the marrow, creating a broth that is rich in minerals and protein yet very easy to digest.

2 Cook 2 cups of a grain of your choice following the instructions on pages 52 to 53. Add a piece of kombu (see Sea Vegetables, page 41) to add minerals and make the grain even easier to digest. This will give you about 5 cups of a whole grain enhanced with the nutrients from the broth and sea vegetable. If you use a chicken broth, you'll have some added protein. Making the grain will take five minutes or less to start and then will cook virtually unattended for 15 to 40 minutes (depending on the grain you choose). A rice cooker with a timer will allow you to walk away and be assured that your grain will not burn.

3 Make a batch of overnight oats. Pour an equal amount of plain whole milk, non-dairy milk, kefir, or yogurt over some regular rolled oats and put it in the refrigerator. Let it sit overnight and then eat small amounts with nuts, seeds and/or a bit of fruit. Adding a mashed banana or a bit of unsweetened applesauce will sweeten the oats without sugar.

4 Add a few vegetables. Here's a list of cooked and raw vegetables that require almost no preparation:

- Baked sweet potatoes, yams or regular potatoes
- Baked acorn, butternut or other winter squash
- Raw carrots, celery, cherry tomatoes, tiny asparagus spears, red, yellow or orange sweet peppers, cucumbers, romaine lettuce, spinach, arugula, peeled kohlrabi or jicama bulb, fennel bulbs and radishes.

5 Bake fish or chicken in the oven just until it is cooked through. Cool slightly, refrigerate and use daily, adding to salads, soups or cooked vegetables.

If you have a bit more energy, you might include the following:

6 Make a miso soup using one of our Healing Broths or a purchased broth as a base. Add some greens, or other vegetables you have on hand. Cook the vegetables in the broth until they are tender, take it off the heat and stir in miso to taste. Including a bit of sea vegetable such as arame, wakame, sea palm or crumbled nori, will add even more nutrition.

7 Steam or roast 3 to 5 cups of vegetables and put them in smaller containers to heat as you like.

8 Make a soup or stew in a crockpot. Here are three suggestions for simplicity, balanced nutrition and digestibility:

- Minestrone Barley Soup, page 126
- Curried Red Lentil Soup, page 120
- Sancocho Columbian Chicken Stew, page 131

9 Make "planned overs." Prepare additional amounts of basic ingredients that can be added to different meals. Prepare extra beans or grains to use in soups or salads. Hard boil a few eggs and add them to your meals. Roasting a whole chicken is less expensive than buying specific parts and you can use it for several meals. Puréed soups and stews freeze well in individual portions.

Understanding Sweeteners

Humans are born with the desire for sweet flavors. Mother's milk is sweet and it is the natural sugars in the milk that support the growth and development of the young child. Sweetness comes in many forms, and some are significantly better for our bodies than others. How we eat sweet foods also makes a difference in how we process them and hence their impact on our health.

The most important recommendation is to eat whole rather than refined foods. Whole grains, legumes, fruits and vegetables contain carbohydrates that provide a balance of whole sugars, fiber and, in some cases, protein. The complex nature of these foods means that we digest them without a rapid rise in blood sugar. While most people don't think of these foods as sweet, chewing them thoroughly will release their natural sugars. Many people discover that as they eat more whole foods, they begin to lose their desire for refined sweet treats.

Processed sugars like high fructose corn syrup and refined white sugar create a strain on the liver. The body cannot function correctly with excess sugar in the blood stream. The pancreas produces insulin to store the sugar in the body's tissues. Eating sugar frequently leads to exhaustion of the pancreas and excess sugar in the blood, damaging many cells. A diet high in sugar leads to an inflammatory response in the body and an aggravation of many disease processes. Due in part to excess consumption

Revive & Thrive client Tammy and her daughter with their healthy meals.

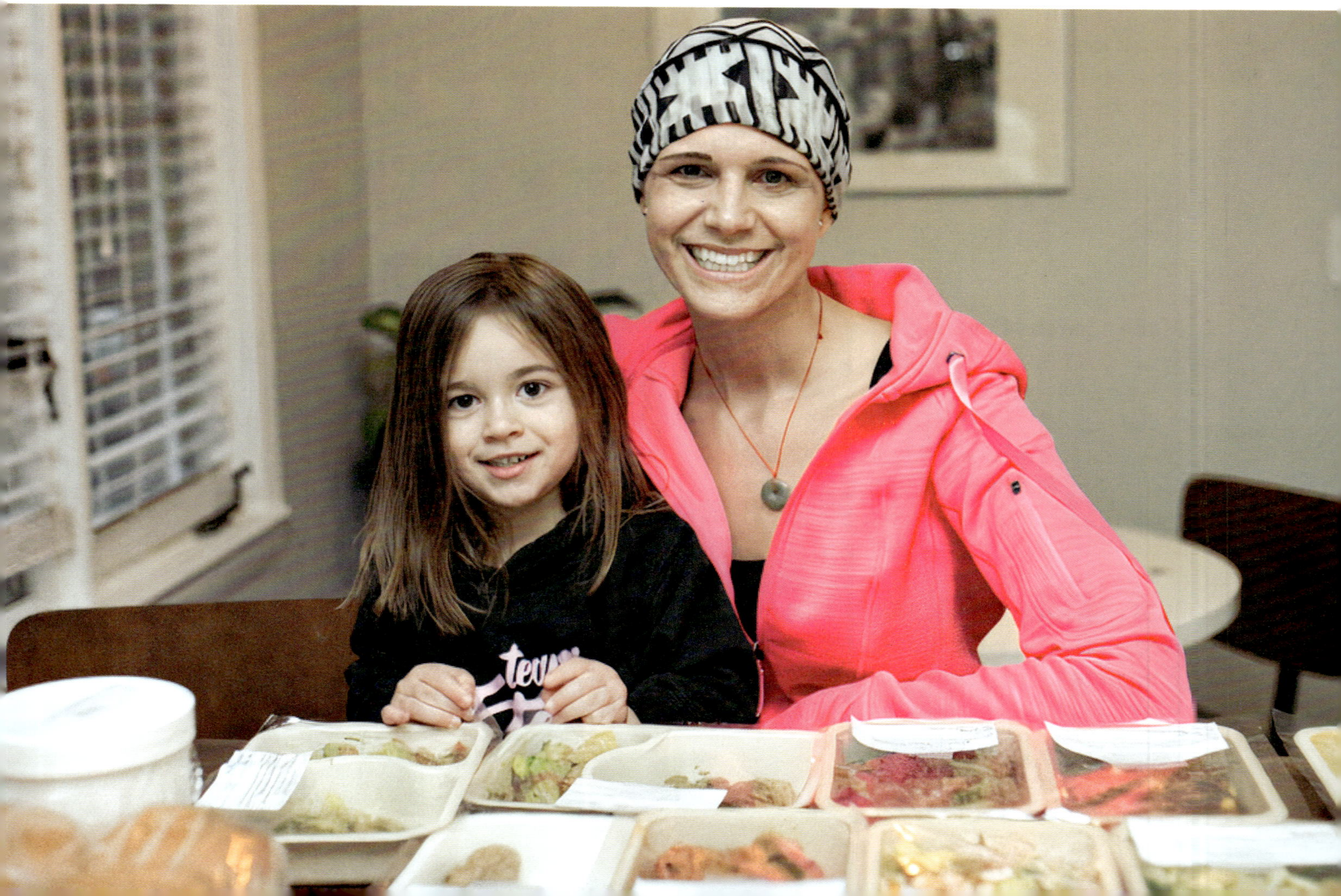

of high-calorie, low-fiber fast foods, many people have metabolic illness, a disorder that frequently leads to diabetes. According to some research, only 12% of people in the United States have healthy metabolisms, while 88% of the population suffers from metabolic illness.[5]

Making Healthy Choices

Excess blood sugar levels are implicated in a wide range of disease processes including diabetes, heart disease and cancer. While everyone benefits from reducing the amount of processed sugars and simple carbohydrates they eat, for those who are ill this may be critical.

Sugar is habit forming. Notice how and when you look for something sweet to eat. If you eat less refined sweeteners, your taste buds will adapt and subtle sweetness from berries and sweet vegetables will taste much more satisfying. Notice how you feel when you eat less refined sweeteners.

Here are some suggestions to keep your blood sugar in balance and make healthier choices for sweet treats:

1 Avoid refined sugars including white and brown sugar, organic cane sugar, fructose, and all forms of corn syrup. Be aware that corn syrup is lurking in many processed foods. If you purchase prepared or processed foods, read the labels carefully. Sugar has dozens of names you'll find on food labels!

2 Stick with whole fruits. Whole fruits include fiber which slows the release of sugars into the blood. Fruits also include a wide range of vitamins and minerals. Berries are excellent as they are low in sugar, but high in fiber and antioxidants.

3 Experiment with stevia. Stevia is an herb that has been used as a sweetener by the Guarani Indians of Paraguay for hundreds of years. The leaves of the stevia plant can be 30 times sweeter than sugar yet the body does not metabolize the glycosides from the stevia leaf so there is no impact on blood glucose levels.

4 Use sweeteners that are minimally processed and made from whole foods *in very small quantities*. If you are going to use a refined sweetener, choose Barbados molasses, sorghum molasses, maple syrup, honey, barley malt syrup, palm syrup, coconut palm sugars or date sugar. These sweeteners are less processed than other forms of sugar and include minerals, enzymes, vitamins and fiber. Because they are somewhat more complex, they are processed more slowly and hence keep insulin levels more stable.

5 Avoid artificial sweeteners such as saccharin, neotame, sucralose, aspartame, and acesulfame, as they are chemicals that may have negative health risks. Avoid agave as it is a source of concentrated fructose and is a highly processed sugar.

Making Sense of Dietary Fats

Fats are essential to maintaining good health. Every cell in our body is surrounded by a cell membrane composed of fat molecules. When the fat molecules are healthy and intact, we can utilize nutrients more effectively and cell communication is more efficient. Fats are the carriers of the fat-soluble vitamins A, D, E, and K. They support the health of our bones, eyes, hair, weight management, nervous system, blood, immune system, and brain function. In fact, over 65 percent of the brain is composed of fats! The hormones and hormone-like substances that are created from fats regulate many body systems including the endocrine system.

Our body's first choice of energy to burn is fats as they offer more calories per gram than protein or carbohydrates. Fats satiate our appetites and help us to moderate the digestion of sugars. How do we know which fats are healthy and which fats we should avoid?

Most processed and fast foods are made with fats that have themselves been highly processed, often using chemicals and high heat that are damaging. When fats used as cooking oils — like safflower oil, canola or other vegetable oils — are processed with heat they become oxidized, causing rancidity. This removes the vitamin E and changes the composition of the fat to a form that our cells do not recognize. One of the most important steps you can take in improving your health is to avoid processed and fast foods, and refined or heat-processed oils. These polyunsaturated plant oils include: canola, corn, cottonseed, safflower, soy and sunflower oils. These oils are often extracted with chemical solvents and high heat, and are then bleached and scented to remove discoloration and a rancid smell.

Fats to Avoid

- Hydrogenated or partially-hydrogenated fats and trans-fats.
- Fried foods from most restaurants and all foods fried at high temperatures. Sautéing foods at a medium heat with coconut oil, ghee or olive oil is fine.
- Most polyunsaturated fats, especially refined vegetable oils such as canola oil, sunflower oil, safflower oil, peanut oil, soy oil and corn oil.
- Excessive consumption of saturated fats such as butter, heavy cream, lard and animal fats.

Fats to Include

Include these three types of healthy fats in your daily choices:

- Monounsaturated fats such as cold-pressed olive oil or sesame oil, nuts and avocados.
- Polyunsaturated fats (omega-3 and 6's) from fresh cold-water fish, fish oils, flax and hemp oils, and olive oil. These fats are the most unstable and are damaged by heating or processing. Be sure to choose cold-pressed oil. Refrigerate nuts and seeds, hemp and flax oils. Eat them raw or freshly ground. The exception is chia seeds which are very stable and do not need to be refrigerated.
- A small amount of high-quality saturated fats including organic butter and cream, organic whole milk products, organic cheese, coconut oil, meat fats and clarified butter or ghee.

Twinkle (right), and the other hens at the Ceres garden produce pastured organic eggs - a great source of healthy dietary fat.

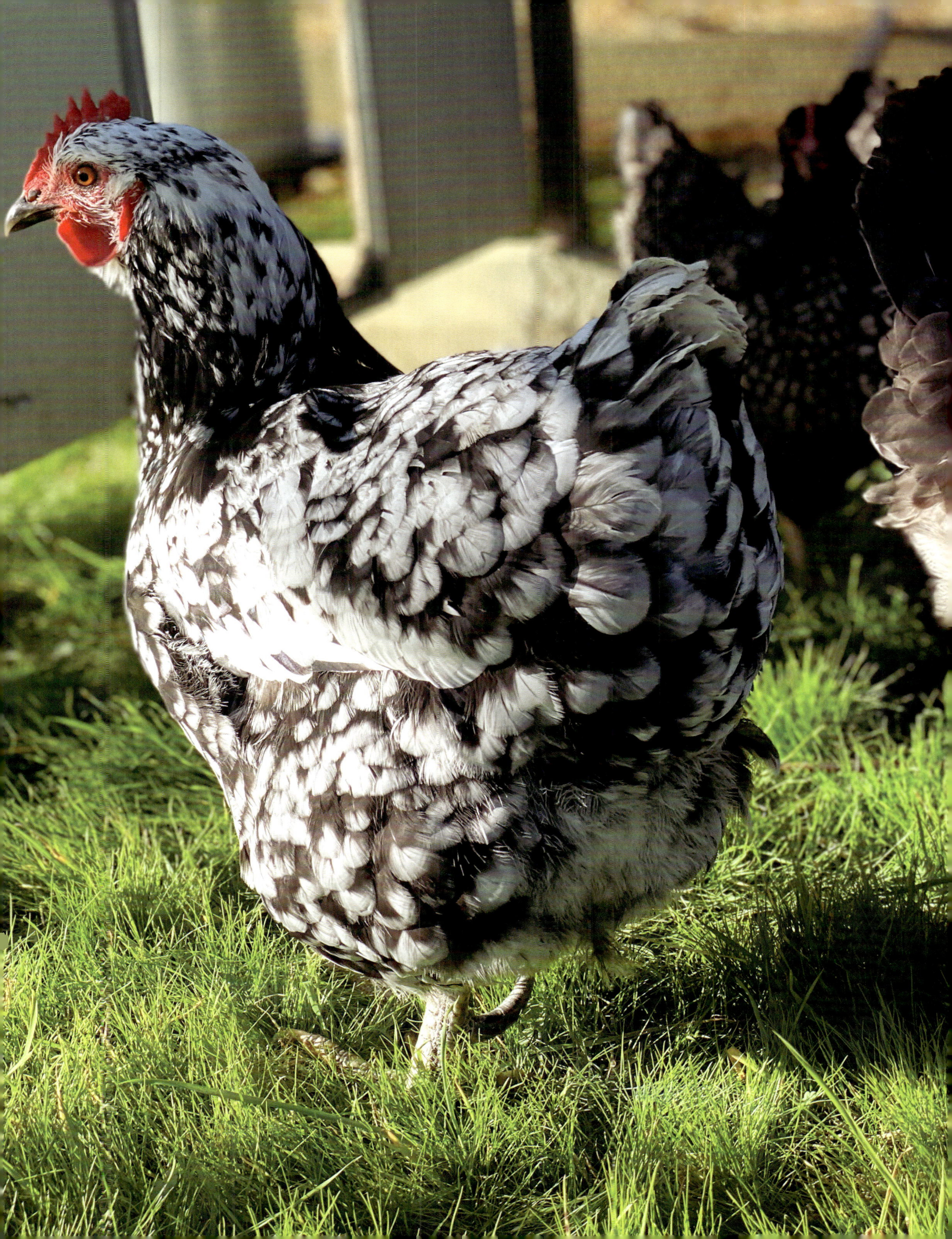

We all need to include healthy dietary fats. Eat some of these foods each day:

- Nuts such as almonds, walnuts, Brazil nuts, pecans and cashews
- Seeds including sunflower, sesame, pumpkin, flax, chia and hemp
- Avocados
- Organic whole dairy: butter, milk, yogurt, kefir and cheese
- Organic eggs
- Sustainably caught cold-water fish, high in omega-3 fatty acids.
- Organic coconut products: coconut milk, oil, meat and butter
- Cold-pressed organic olive oil, sesame oil, coconut oil, ghee, hemp oil and flax oil

Choosing Animal Foods Rich in Good Quality Fats

Wild caught fish, especially cold-water fatty fish, such as Salmon, Mackerel, Anchovies, Sardines and Herring (SMASH fish) are high in omega-3 fatty acids, which have been shown to reduce inflammation. There are 3 main types of these fatty acids. Two are found primarily in fatty fish: eicosapentaenoic acid (EPA) and docosahexaenoic acid (DHA). The third type of omega-3, alpha-linolenic acid (ALA), is found in plant foods, including walnuts, hemp hearts, chia and flax seeds. We are not able to easily convert ALA into EPA and DHA, which are the forms that function as anti-inflammatories in our bodies. Thus while some plant foods do have omega-3 fatty acids, the conversion rate is so low that the anti-inflammatory properties are negligible. The American Heart Association recommends eating one to two servings of seafood per week to reduce your risk of some heart problems.

What Kind of Fat for What Use?

- Oils like flax and hemp are best when used for salad dressings, but should not be heated.
- Olive oil is also most nourishing when unheated. If used for cooking, keep the heat low to medium. Do not let the oil reach the smoking point as this indicates that the oil is burning, changing the molecular structure and releasing free radicals which have been positively linked to cancer and other disease processes.
- Sesame oil is an excellent choice for cooking at medium heats. It has a lovely fragrance and a nutty flavor and also makes delicious salad dressings and marinades.
- For cooking at high heat, choose either coconut oil or ghee, a clarified butter which has a light, lovely taste. Neither of these oils needs to be refrigerated (unless the temperature is very warm) as they stay solid at room temperature and are very stable fats. Use them for frying, sautéing and baking, but note that coconut oil will add a coconut flavor to your dish.

Remember that fats need to be cared for so they don't go rancid. Store nuts, seeds and liquid oils in glass containers in the refrigerator or freezer.

Your body needs fats for energy and to maintain health. Replacing processed and trans-fats with the fats found in organic whole foods such as fish, coconut, avocado and nuts is an important step in building a foundation of health.

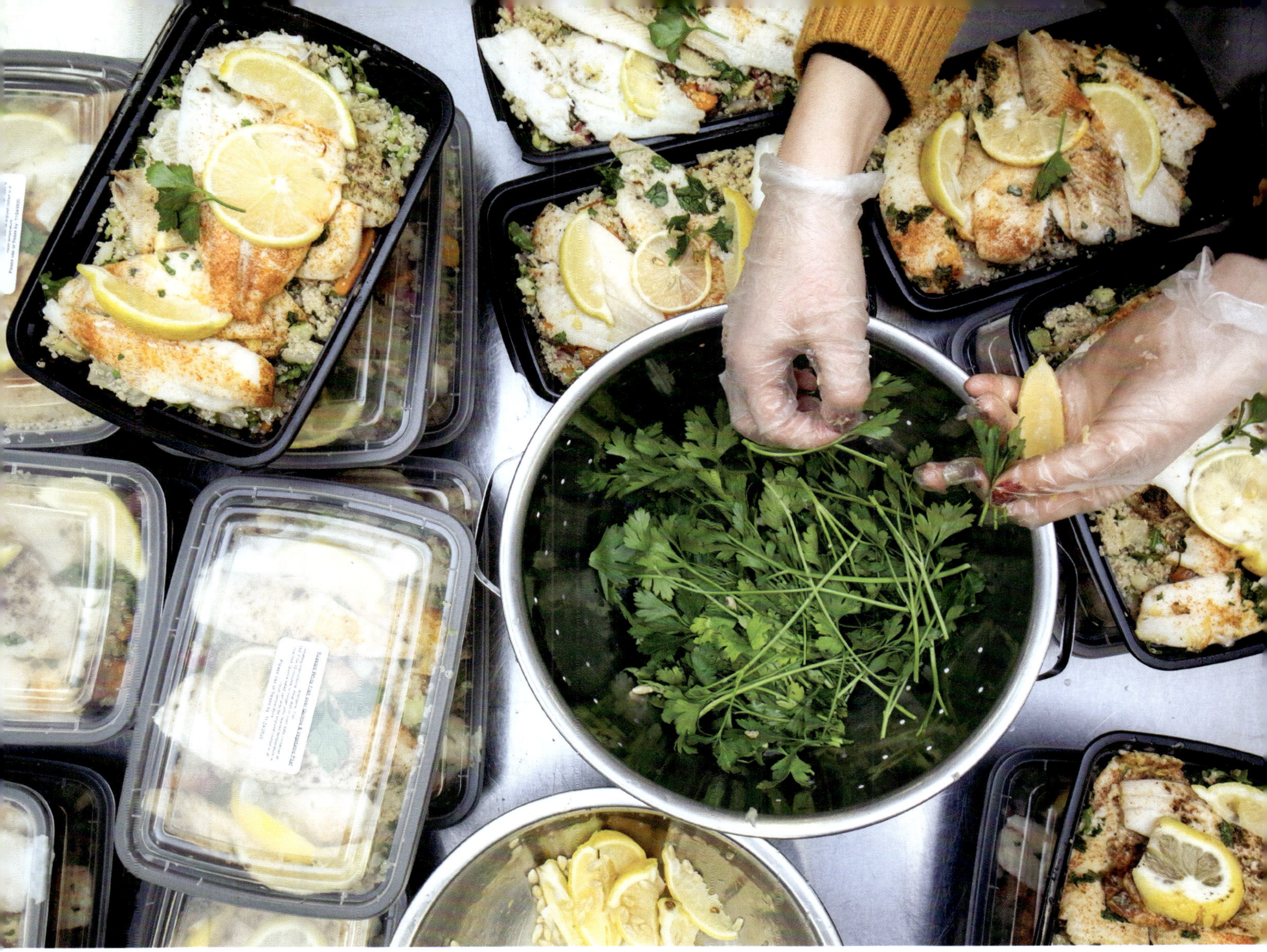

Fish from Healing Meals Community Project: an excellent source of nutrition.

Nutrient-Dense Sea Vegetables

Sea vegetables provide a broad range of minerals that are readily available to our bodies. Sea vegetables are an excellent source of iodine and vitamin K, a very good source of the B vitamin folate and magnesium, and a good source of iron, calcium, and the B vitamins riboflavin and pantothenic acid.

Incorporating sea vegetables into your diet is easier than you might think. Here are our favorite suggestions:

1 Whenever you cook grains, beans or soup stock, add a large piece of kombu. The minerals from the kombu will enhance the nutrient content of the dish and also help make the beans or grains more digestible and less gas producing.

2 Keep a container of dulse flakes on the dinner table and sprinkle them on food instead of table salt. Grind toasted wild nori or toasted dulse or dulse flakes with toasted sesame seeds and sea salt to make gomasio, a traditional Japanese seasoning high in nutrients.

3 Experiment with arame, a mild tasting, tender sea vegetable that looks like thin brown noodles. Easily rehydrated, it can be added to rice dishes, vegetable stir fries, rice noodles, and many other dishes.

4 Create a nutrient-rich salad with sea palm, a delicate sea vegetable that can also be enjoyed toasted as a snack.

5 Use nori sea vegetable sheets to wrap steamed vegetables instead of a tortilla. Or make nori rolls with rice and vegetables.

Preparing Delicious Healthy Food with a Limited Budget

Eating seasonally will help keep the price of vegetables lowest, while maximizing the vitality and nutrients in your meals. If you are able to join a garden project, either by purchasing a share in a "community supported agriculture" farm, tending a plot in a neighborhood garden or beginning a small home garden, you will have the enhanced pleasure of connecting to the ecosystem in your area.

Local farmers' markets often will provide produce more affordably, as the money goes directly to the growers. Many communities also offer Market Match—which doubles the value of SNAP (Supplemental Nutrition Assistance Program) benefits when spent at a farmers' market—or accept payment from SNAP to make fresh produce more accessible.

Frozen vegetables can be an excellent choice for capturing produce at its peak for a more reasonable price, especially if there are sales. Be careful with canned produce as there can be added salt or preservatives.

Canned fish is often less expensive than fresh fish and is nutrient rich. When purchasing canned tuna, choose "skip jack", which is from smaller fish and is lower in mercury toxicity. Try a can of sardines over a green salad.

Delicious, affordable dishes, high in protein and fiber, can be made with a base of grains and beans. These foods are the foundation of many traditional meals: burritos, tofu and rice stir fries, minestrone soup, rice with dhal, hummus and pita bread, pasta with cannellini beans, corn bread with bean chili, and many others. When making recipes with meat, experiment with using half as much meat, while adding additional portions of beans, vegetables, or mushrooms.

Take time before you go shopping to plan a few meals to help guide your purchases toward healthy choices. Avoid shopping when you are hungry and may have a tendency to purchase processed food snacks. These snacks are often far more expensive than the healthy ingredients for cooking simple meals.

Learn several recipes that are adaptable to a variety of vegetables, such as a "rainbow frittata" or a "seasonal vegetable stir fry". You can use these recipes when you have a mix of extra vegetables. Often the most creative and delicious recipes are those that we make with leftover ingredients. Be creative and resourceful, and make use of what is around you. You may find people who can teach you about local wild vegetables, berries or nuts to sustainably harvest, or perhaps there are areas nearby to fish or hunt.

Mindfully eating your meals, chewing well and keeping your portion sizes smaller will help you manage your budget and your wellbeing.

References

1. Institute of Medicine (US) Panel on Dietary Antioxidants and Related Compounds. "Dietary Reference Intakes for Vitamin C, Vitamin E, Selenium, and Carotinoids." Washington DC: *National Academies Press (US);* 2000. Available from: https://www.ncbi.nlm.nih.gov/books/NBK225471

2. California Certified Organic Farmers. 2019. "Roadmap to an Organic California: Benefits Report."Available from: https://www.ccof.org/page/roadmap-organic-california

3. Teague, W. R., Apfelbaum, S., Lal, R., Kreuter, U. P., Rowntree, J., Davies, C. A....& Wang, F. 2016. "The role of ruminants in reducing agriculture's carbon footprint in North America." *Journal of Soil and Water Conservation* 71(2), 156-164.

4. Nicolopoulou-Stamati, P., Maipas, S., Kotampasi, C., Stamatis, P., and Hens, L. "Chemical Pesticides and Human Health: The Urgent Need for a New Concept in Agriculture." *Frontiers in Public Health.* 2016; 4: 148. Available at: https://www.ncbi.nlm.nih.gov/pmc/articles/PMC4947579/

5. Saklayen, M. G. 2018. "The Global Epidemic of the Metabolic Syndrome." *Current Hypertension Reports* 20(2), 12. Available at: https://link.springer.com/article/10.1007%2Fs11906-018-0812-z

Packaged meals for Revive & Thrive clients await delivery.

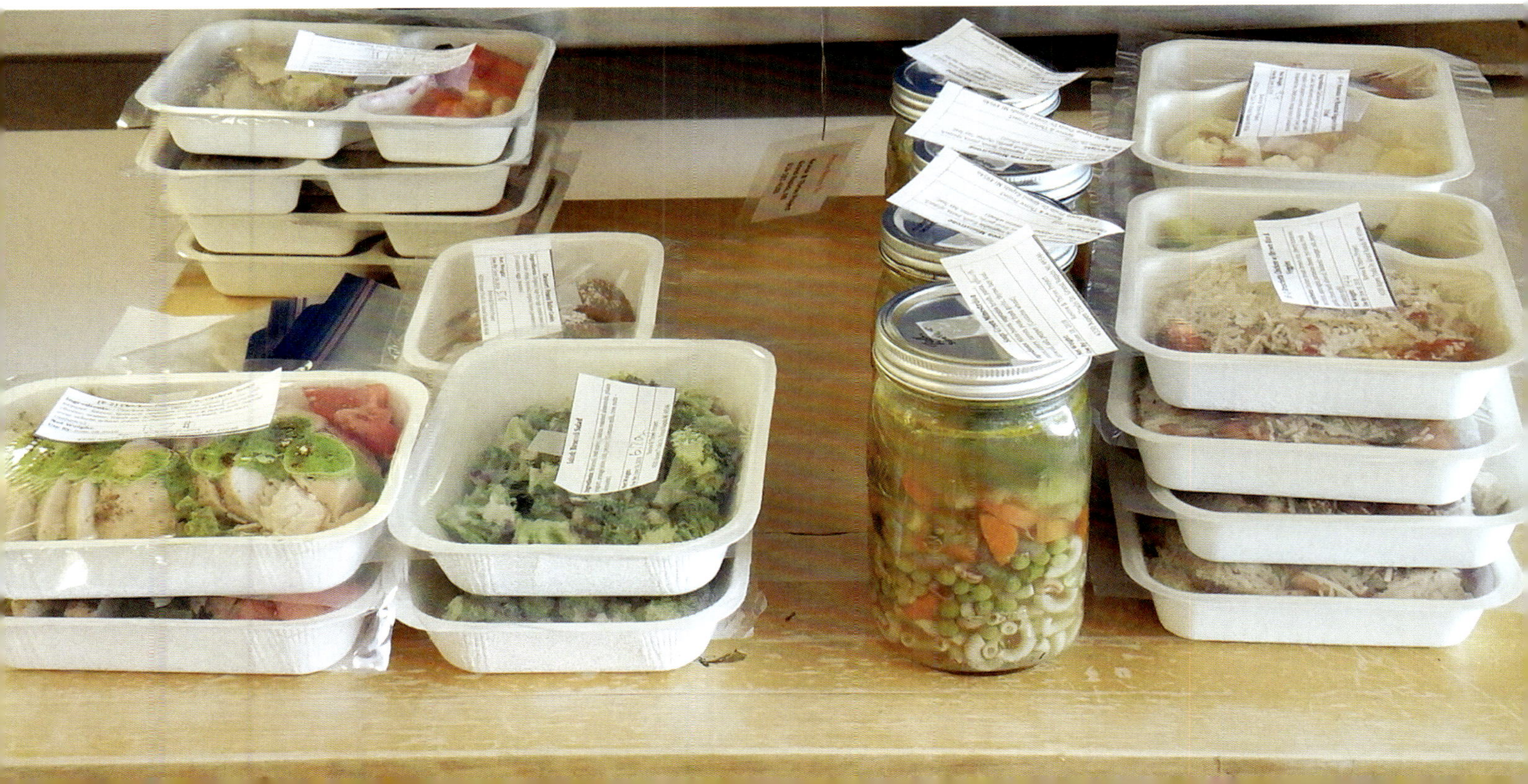

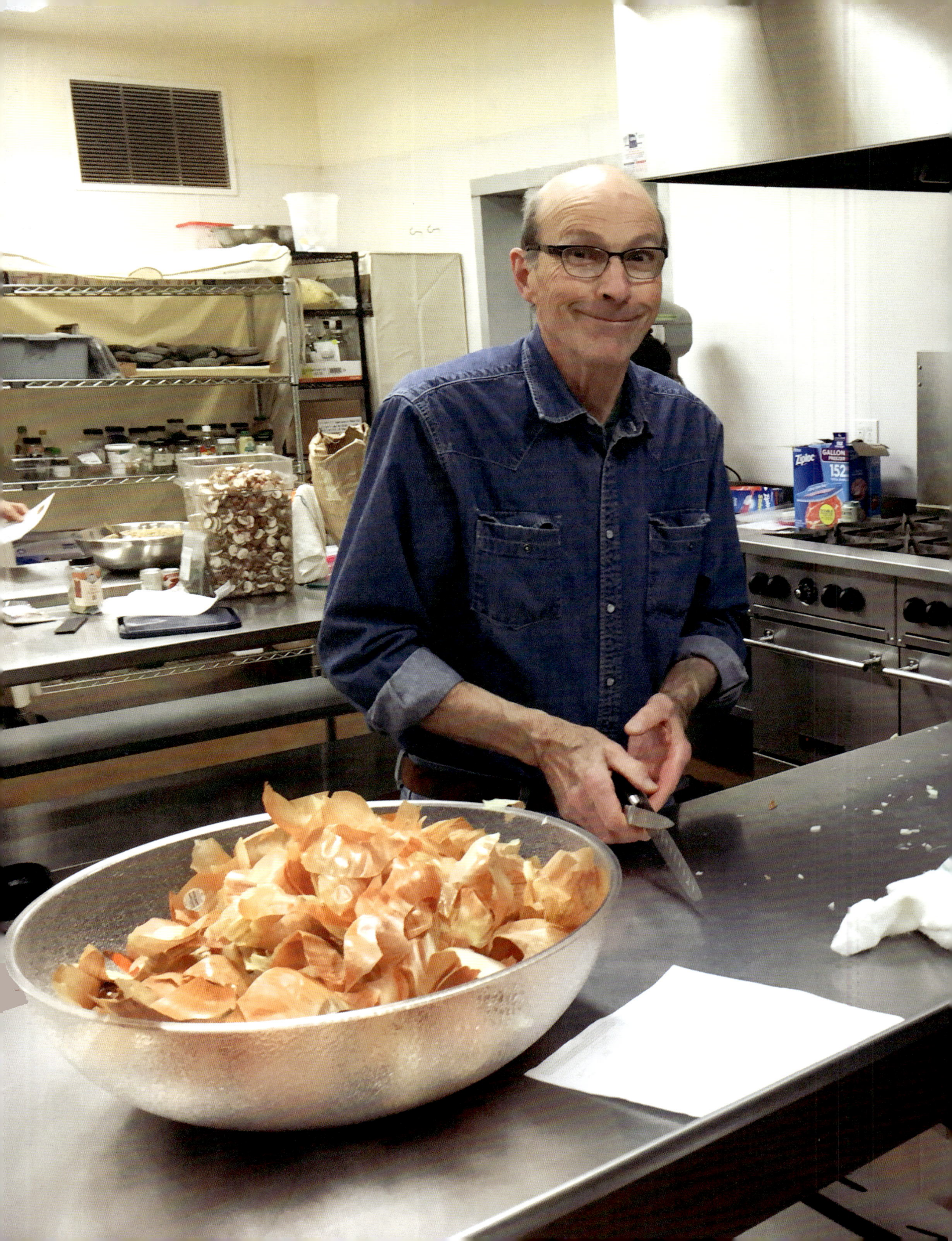
Ziploc
GALLON
152

COOKING BASICS

Cooking Basics

Making Cooking Fun and Manageable

Creating nutritious meals doesn't need to feel like a chore, nor does it need to take a huge amount of your time.

Preparing food is akin to painting with a pallet of flavors, colors, aromas and textures. Thinking of your meals as your art will awaken your creativity and help make the entire process more satisfying.

When you shop, let yourself be drawn to the colors and textures of the produce. When you cook, let your senses come alive to the sounds, the smells and the tastes. When you eat, let your whole being absorb the beauty and nourishment of your food.

Let go of thinking that there is a right way to cook and the entire process can become a time to relax, slow down and be present.

Our lives are often full of busyness and we rush through our days packing in as many tasks as possible.

The good news is that you can't hurry food! The onions will take as long as they need to caramelize into a golden sweetness. The broccoli will be crisp tender when it's good and ready. Cooking can slow us down again to a more natural pace, allowing our bodies and our beings to settle and let go. Creating an hour a day to cook can be one of the best gifts you can give yourself. Not only do you end up with nourishing meals, but your spirit will be nourished as well.

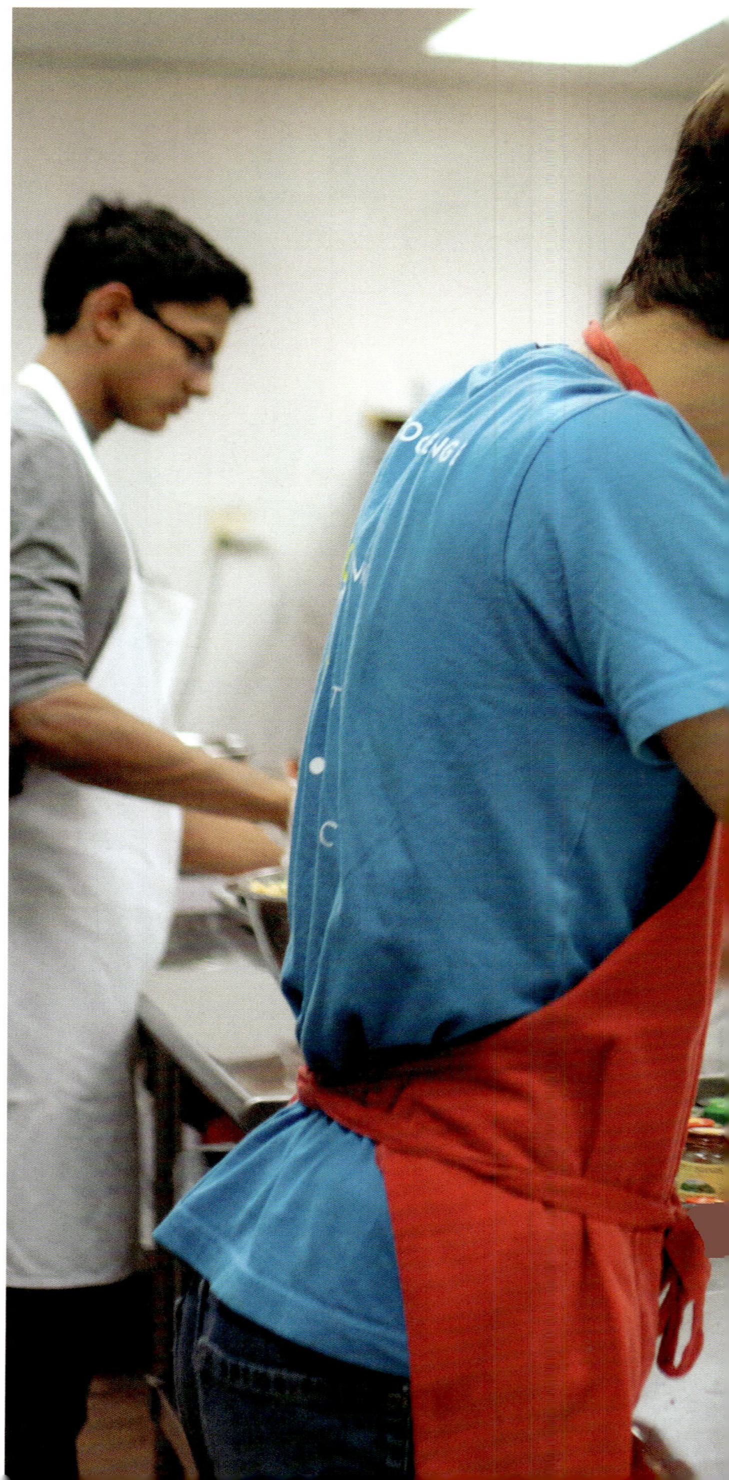

In the kitchen, anything goes. If you've grown up cooking with recipes, this idea can be both liberating and a bit unnerving. In the pages that follow, we'll show you that with a few basic skills in your tool kit you can learn to trust your own instincts in the kitchen and cook to please your own body and sensibility from day to day.

Ultimately, our hope is that your entire relationship with food becomes a source of nourishment in your life — from consciously gathering produce in a local market or in your garden, to preparing it with love in your kitchen, and finally eating it with gratitude alone or surrounded by friends and family.

Previous page: "Onion-chopping George" from Positive Community Kitchen.
Below: Cooking together at Fox Valley is creative, fun and nourishing.

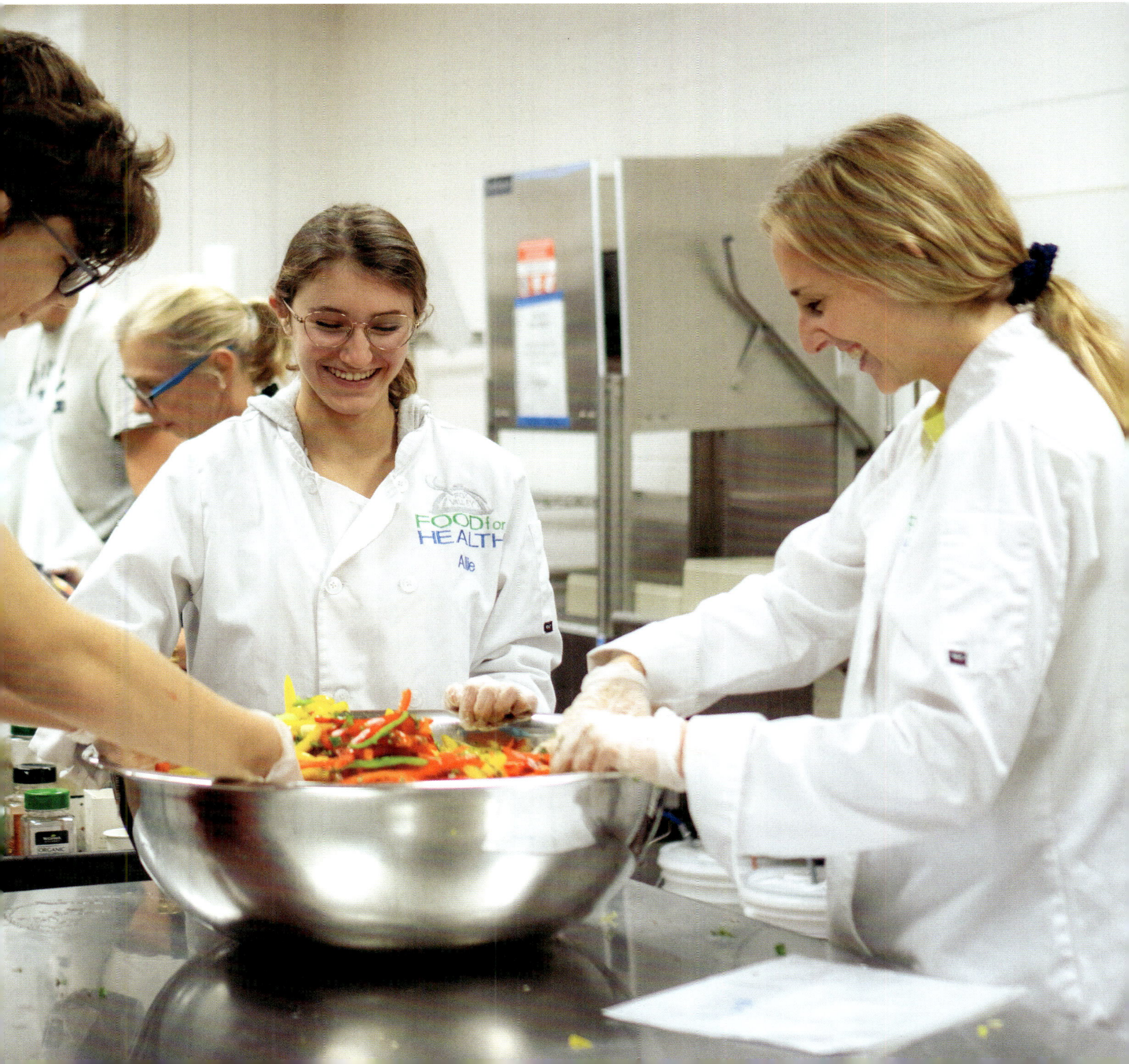

Keeping it Simple

Thinking about cooking can seem overwhelming if it isn't already part of your life. The tasks—planning, shopping, chopping, cooking and cleaning up—when taken together can feel daunting and you may be tempted to stop before you even start. In this section, we help you break down the tasks into manageable steps that can happen at different times in your week or day.

Plan

Plan a simple menu for the week with some easy breakfast foods, two lunch items, two dinner ideas and several things you can snack on. For example, you might want to cook a grain with some dried fruit for breakfast and also make sure you have ingredients on hand for a breakfast smoothie. Lunch items might include a soup or stew plus a purchased hummus and two or three different steamed or roasted vegetables. For dinner, you might make a casserole that you can freeze half of for another week, two roasted chicken breasts or some tempeh treats, and a dish of sautéed greens.

Check your pantry and create a shopping list

Keeping a pantry stocked with the basics will keep your weekly shopping simpler and give you more options on a day-to-day basis. Once you've checked your pantry, make a shopping list for the week. Remember, shopping is a great job for a friend or family member who wants to help.

Organize a cooking day with a friend or family member

Cooking with someone else makes the whole process both more fun and more manageable. You can have a friend help you cook for yourself or cook with someone else who also needs meals and share the results of your day. Cook as many meals as you can. Remember, if you get through the cooking in one afternoon you won't have to cook the rest of the week. Before you get started, read through the recipes you plan to make and figure out what will take the longest. Start with those tasks first, along with things like cooking a pot of rice — which takes just a minute to start and can cook unattended as you work on other things.

If you cannot cook with others, reserve your energy by breaking up the cooking tasks

If you are cooking alone and your energy is at a low ebb, do your cooking in discrete chunks throughout the day or over several days. Here are some ideas:

- Most vegetables can be prepared ahead of time and then stored in the refrigerator until you are ready to cook. If you chop potatoes, store them in cold water to prevent browning. If you need onions for three different dishes, prepare the entire amount at once. Use a food processor for jobs like chopping onions, shredding carrots, and making pestos.
- Roast, steam or sauté vegetables in advance for use in several dishes or simply

to have ready to eat. Vegetables can be stored for later use in glass containers, like the ones that Pyrex now makes with plastic lids.

- Make two quarts of broth in a slow cooker. Include the tops and peelings of the vegetables you have prepared along with some coarsely chopped whole vegetables. (See page 106 for our Healing Vegetable Broth recipe or page 108 for our Healing Chicken Broth recipe.) The next day make one or two different grains for the week using your broth instead of water.

- Use your slow cooker again and make a soup using the rest of your broth. A recipe that makes six to eight cups will give you one cup of soup each day.

- Soak beans overnight (see page 54) to reduce their cooking time.

- Clean up as you go and know that if you are too tired, the dishes can wait!

Slow cook and freeze to save time and energy

- Many stews, chilies and soups can be made without any attention on your part using a slow cooker. Put in the ingredients, turn it on low and head off to work or to bed. You'll return home or wake up to a lovely aroma.

- Freeze half of whatever you make. This allows you to have some soup and a few main dishes in the freezer — giving you more variety in the weeks to come as well as some options for those days when you just don't have the energy to cook.

Keep a few simple snacks on hand

Keeping a variety of healthy snacks on hand can be a great help when you don't feel like a meal but know you need to eat.

- Cut up raw vegetables such as jicama, red bell peppers or carrots and store them in the fridge; steam cauliflower; roast acorn squash halves. Many stores carry washed, chopped vegetables that are ready to eat.

- Cut up fruit, dip it in some water with a bit of lemon juice to keep it from browning, and store it covered in the fridge.

- Make or purchase hummus, avocado dip and nut butters.

- Freeze a smoothie in Popsicle molds for a nourishing and refreshing treat.

Remember, these are just suggestions. Do as much or as little as you have the energy for. Ask for help from friends or family members, or find a cooking buddy to help make the process more enjoyable. If you haven't cooked much, making this a regular part of your life will take time. Start simply and celebrate your accomplishments. Change takes time, but even small changes can reap big rewards physically and emotionally.

Kitchen Tools

Having the right tool for the job will make your cooking experience both more pleasant and more efficient. The best way to discover what you need is to start cooking. As you work in the kitchen, make a list of the things you wish you had. This way, you will slowly gather the tools that you'll actually use.

Here are a few suggestions of things we think are especially useful, or that we know you will need for the recipes that follow.

Knives & Knife Sharpeners

There is nothing as important as having a good quality, sharp knife. Experiment and find what works for you. Many chefs have a whole set of different knives for different jobs. If you are just starting to cook, we recommend getting a basic knife that you can use for most jobs, plus a knife for mincing herbs, and a paring knife for small jobs.

Invest in a good knife sharpener and sharpen your knife every time you begin cooking. There are

The right tool for the job makes the cooking experience pleasant and more efficient.

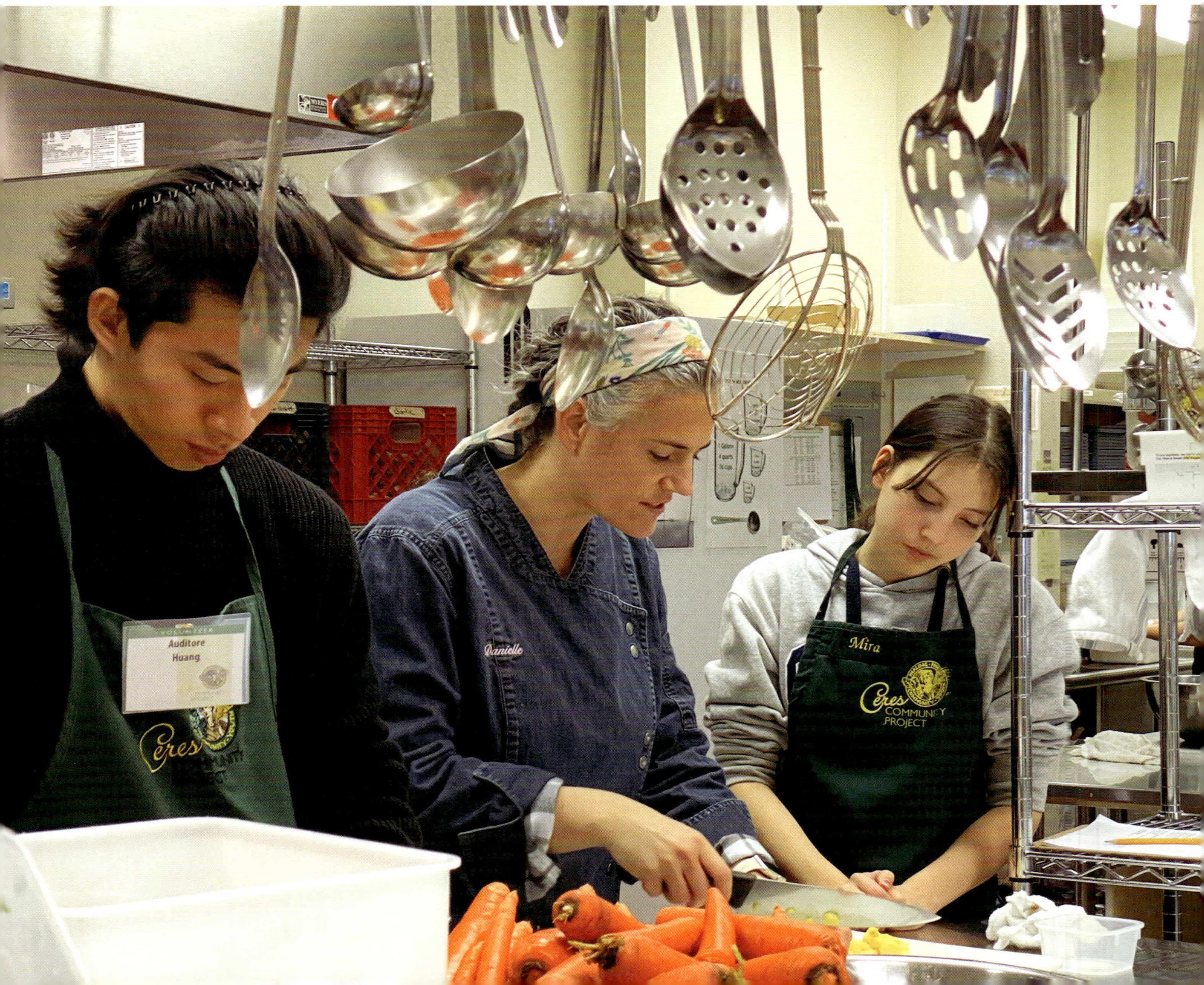

many good table top knife sharpeners available that will sharpen your knife simply by drawing it through the middle. No special skills are needed and you can leave it sitting on your counter to remind you to sharpen your knives regularly.

Handy Utensils

Here are the utensils we use most often:

- Long-handled wooden spoon
- Rubber spatula —a few in different sizes
- Whisk— again, in a few different sizes
- Metal spatula
- Good quality peeler
- Microplane for zesting oranges lemons and limes (this looks like a ruler and has small grating holes on it that allow you to zest the skin of citrus fruit without getting the white, bitter pith).

Spider

A spider has a long handle with a mesh "basket" on the end. You can find them at good culinary stores. A spider is a great tool to have on hand for blanching vegetables. It will allow you to scoop out whatever you are cooking so you can re-use the water for another vegetable.

Fine Mesh Strainer and Colander

If you plan to eat quinoa, you'll need a fine mesh strainer in order to rinse the tiny grains before soaking. Of course, there are many other uses for this tool! Add a larger colander for draining vegetables and pastas and you should be able to handle every rinsing and draining job in your kitchen.

Immersion Blender

This is one of the handiest tools as it allows you to blend soups and sauces easily while they are hot. You can leave whatever you are blending right in the bowl or pot, minimizing the number of dishes you will have to wash.

Spice Grinder

A good quality coffee or spice grinder is essential for finely grinding things like flax and sesame seeds.

Food Processor

If you are cooking for one or two, a mini food processor is a great choice. You can easily chop small amounts of vegetables or nuts, make a pesto, or blend together a salad dressing. It doesn't take up much room and is quick and easy to clean.

If you like to make larger batches of things, or want to use the processor for grating and chopping vegetables, you'll want a regular size one. These are also wonderful for making hummus and other vegetable dips and spreads.

Rice Cooker

These come in a variety of sizes and will let you cook almost any grain totally unattended. You can also add seasonings, chopped onions, minced garlic or ginger, coconut milk, etc. and create an instant pilaf. Try to avoid the Teflon coated cookers, as Teflon has been found to leach into the food.

Slow Cooker

This old stand-by is enormously helpful when you have limited time and energy. Put all your ingredients in the slow cooker, turn it on low and let it cook overnight or all day. You can make enough of a nourishing soup or stew to feed yourself for most of a week with just a few minutes of chopping and measuring.

High-Powered Blenders

If you have the resources, we encourage you to invest in a Blendtec or Vitamix. Nothing beats this all-in-one tool for juicing, smoothies, sauces, grinding nuts and making nut butters, and puréeing soups to a velvety texture.

Whole Grains

Grains are an excellent source of fiber, protein, vitamins and minerals and have, for thousands of years, been the staple food for most cultures.

The health benefits of grains are greatly improved by a few simple steps: soaking grains before cooking, and cooking them with a sea vegetable such as kombu. Soaking grains overnight with lemon juice or apple cider vinegar, then discarding the soaking water, accomplishes two important things — it removes the phytic acid which inhibits the absorption of zinc, calcium, iron and other essential minerals, and it transforms the grains from acidic to alkaline-forming. Cooking grains with kombu enhances the mineral content of the grains and further strengthens their alkaline effect.

Grains vary in their protein, vitamin and mineral content. To get the best nutrition, include a good variety of grains in your diet.

Following are some basic guidelines to get you started. Experiment and discover what works best for you. Increasing the amount of liquid will give you a softer grain as will increasing the cooking time.

Consider investing in a small rice cooker and you'll make grain cooking that much simpler — you just add the soaked, rinsed grain, liquid and kombu or sea salt and turn it on. Please note that the ratios of grain to liquid that follow are based on soaking your grain for at least four hours and preferably overnight. If the grain is not soaked, you will need to increase the amount of liquid.

Brown Rice, Whole Oats, Kamut and Wheat Berries

1 cup grain
1 Tbsp apple cider vinegar or lemon juice
3 cups water for soaking
1½ cups stock or water
2" piece of kombu seaweed (discard after use)
or ¼ tsp sea salt

Rinse the grain and then place in a bowl. Mix the apple cider vinegar with the soaking water and pour in bowl to cover the grain. Let soak overnight. Drain, discarding the soaking water, and rinse well.

Place the grain in a pot with the water and the kombu. Bring to a boil, reduce the heat to low and cover. Cook for 25 to 35 minutes, or until the water is absorbed and the grain is tender. Experiment with the amount of water to get the consistency that you want. More water will yield a softer grain. If the grain is not tender and all of the water has been absorbed, add ¼ cup of water per cup of grain, cover and continue to cook for another 5 minutes, then re-check and repeat if necessary.

Barley and Wild Rice

1 cup grain
1 Tbsp apple cider vinegar or lemon juice
3 cups water for soaking
4 cups water or stock
2" piece of kombu seaweed (discard after use)
or ¼ tsp sea salt

Rinse the grain and then place in a bowl. Mix the apple cider vinegar with the soaking water and pour in bowl to cover the grain. Let soak overnight. Drain, discarding the soaking water, and rinse well.

Rinse wild rice or soaked barley and then place in a pot with the water and sea salt or kombu. Bring to a boil, cover and reduce the heat to low. Cook until the grain is tender, 25 to 30 minutes for barley and 35 to 40 minutes for wild rice. Drain excess water.

Quinoa

1 cup quinoa
1 Tbsp apple cider vinegar or lemon juice
3 cups water for soaking
¾ cup water or stock
2" piece of kombu seaweed (discard after use)
or ¼ tsp sea salt

Rinse the quinoa well using a fine mesh strainer, then place in a bowl. Mix the apple cider vinegar with the soaking water and pour in bowl to cover the grain. Let soak overnight. Drain, discarding the soaking water, and rinse well.

Rinse again, and then place the quinoa, ¾ cup water and kombu in a small pot. Bring to a boil, cover, reduce heat to low, and cook for about 10 minutes or until the water is absorbed and the quinoa is tender.

Millet

1 cup millet
1 Tbsp apple cider vinegar or lemon juice
3 cups water for soaking
2 cups water or stock
2" piece of kombu seaweed (discard after use)
or ¼ tsp sea salt

Rinse the grain and then place in a bowl. Mix the apple cider vinegar with the soaking water and pour in bowl to cover the grain. Let soak overnight. Drain, discarding the soaking water, and rinse well.

Place the millet in a saucepan and toast over medium heat, stirring constantly, until the millet begins to have a nutty, toasted aroma. While the millet is toasting, bring two cups of water or stock to a simmer. Carefully add the hot water to the toasted millet along with the kombu or sea salt. Cover, reduce heat to low, and cook until the water is absorbed and the millet is tender, 20 to 25 minutes.

If you are making a salad with the millet, turn the grain out onto a cooking sheet and spread it out to cool. Once the millet is cool, use your fingers to separate the grains. It will resemble couscous.

To make millet porridge increase the water by 1 cup and cook slightly longer.

Beans and Peas

Legumes—or beans as we call them—are a wonderful source of protein, vitamins and minerals. Like grains, it is essential to pre-soak beans before cooking. This not only greatly reduces cooking times, but also makes beans more alkaline by neutralizing phytic acid. Again, like grains, we recommend adding a bit of kombu to your cooking pot. Kombu helps make beans more digestible, reduces their gas-producing tendency, and adds valuable nutrients.

We recommend pre-soaking all beans and peas. Rinse them well, then place in a pot, cover with at least three times as much water as beans and soak overnight or longer (*see Bean Soaking Guidelines below*). Drain the beans, then place in a pot with water, covering by at least one inch. Add a generous piece of kombu and bring the beans to a boil. Reduce the heat to a simmer, partially cover, and cook until the beans are tender. Discard the kombu.
Bean cooking times vary widely based on the freshness of the beans, altitude, and how long the beans were soaked.

1 cup of dry beans will yield about 2¼ to 3 cups of cooked beans. Beans freeze well so consider cooking a larger amount than you need and freezing the left-overs for future use.

Bean Soaking Guidelines

Lentils, Split Peas	10-12 hours
Aduki, Navy, Lima	24 hours
Black, Kidney, Mung	24 hours
Chickpeas	24-48 hours

For each cup of beans add 1 tablespoon of organic raw apple cider vinegar and 3 cups warm water.

Bean Cooking Times

Lentils	8-20 minutes for salads, up to 35 minutes for very soft
Split Peas,	
Aduki, Mung	45-60 minutes
Black	60-90 minutes
Kidney, Navy, Pinto	
Chickpeas	90-120 minutes

Most other beans will be tender in 30 minutes to 1 hour. To test beans, remove one from the pot and let it cool for a few minutes, then taste. The beans should be soft with no starchy taste.

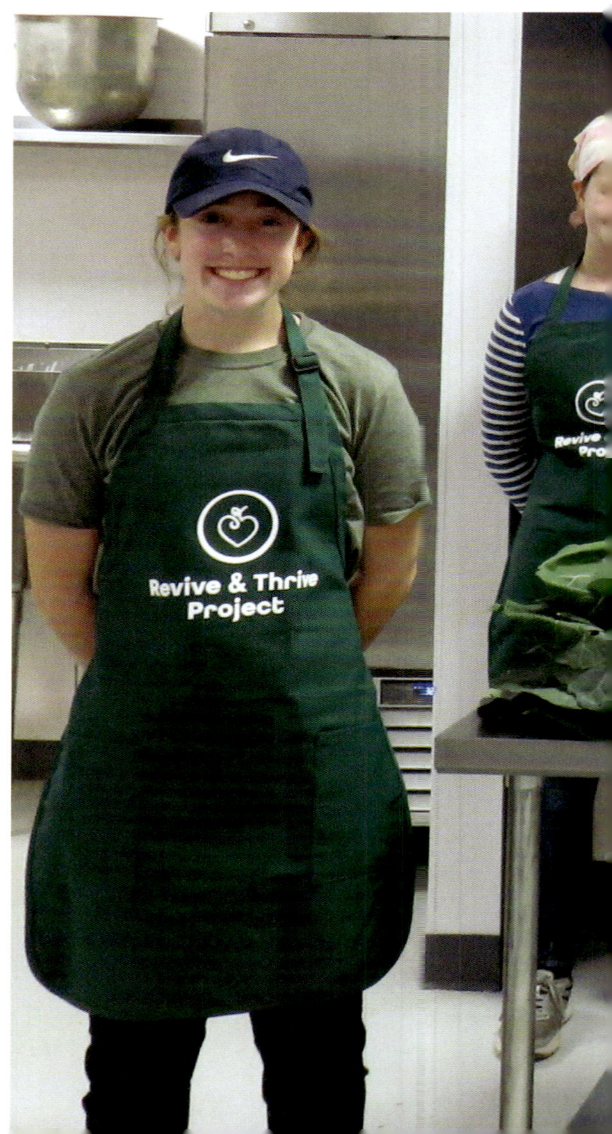

Vegetables

There are an infinite number of ways to prepare vegetables, but if you understand the three techniques that follow, you'll have the basics for experimenting on your own.

Blanching and Steaming Vegetables

Blanching is a technique for cooking vegetables quickly in boiling water just until their color brightens and they no longer taste raw. You can also accomplish this same result by steaming vegetables in a steamer basket over boiling water. Blanching and steaming are great techniques for taking the raw edge off vegetables such as broccoli or even carrots, that you might want to eat cold or add to a vegetable salad. It's also the one method of vegetable preparation that involves no added oil.

Bring a pot of water to a boil with a bit of salt. The size of the pot and amount of salt depends on the quantity of vegetables you need to blanch. If you only have a few cups, fill a two-quart saucepan about ¾ full and add ¼ teaspoon of salt. When the water is boiling, add one kind of vegetable. As soon as its color brightens and it tastes just barely tender, use a spider or small wire mesh colander to remove

Ready for action! The team at Revive & Thrive with an array of fresh vegetables.

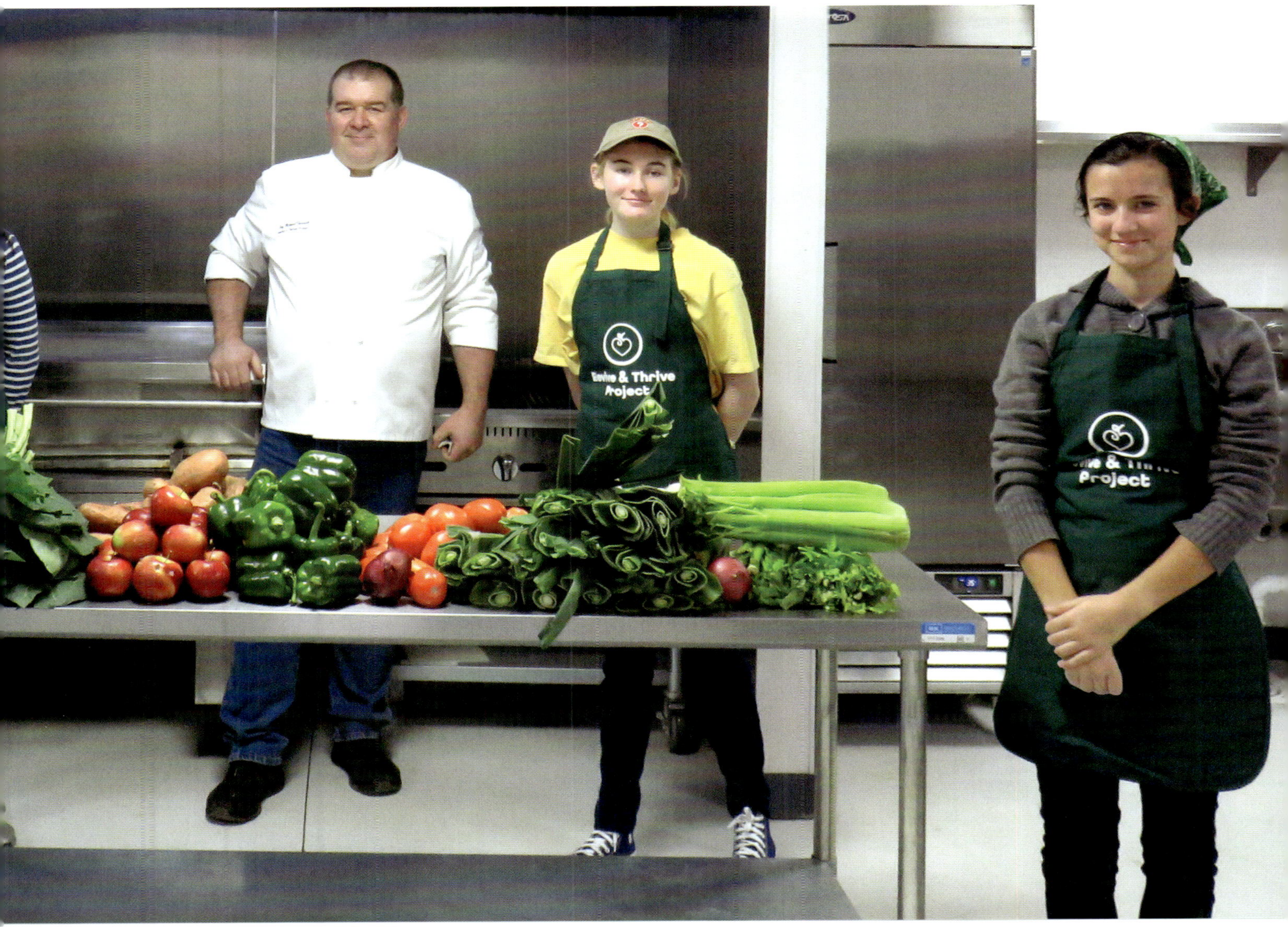

A Note about Nuts

Many of the recipes that follow call for nuts or seeds. Like grains and beans, nuts contain enzyme inhibitors that can restrict our ability to digest the nutrients they contain. Soaking nuts and seeds in water, then drying in a low oven or dehydrator, neutralizes the enzyme inhibitors and makes their nutrients more readily available.

Soak 2 cups nuts or seeds in filtered water to cover according to the soaking guidelines below. The next day, drain and rinse the nuts or seeds and spread them on a baking sheet in a warm oven (not more than 150˚) or place them in a dehydrator. Cook or dehydrate until they are completely dry and crisp. This will take 6 to 12 hours in your oven, 1 to 3 days in a dehydrator.

For cashews, avoid soaking for longer than 6 hours. After soaking, immediately roast for 12 to 24 hours in a 200° to 250° oven. Stir occasionally until crisp.

How to Toast Dried Nuts or Seeds

Preheat your oven to 350˚. Place the nuts in a small baking pan. Roast them until they are fragrant and starting to brown. This will take anywhere from 6 to 12 minutes depending on the nuts and your oven. Watch carefully, though, as nuts can burn quickly! You can also toast nuts in a heavy-bottomed skillet over low heat, stirring the nuts often. This will take 6 to 10 minutes. Don't try to hurry things— you want to toast the nuts all the way through, not simply get them brown on the outside.

Nut and Seed Soaking Guidelines

Nuts
Soak nuts in warm water to cover with 1½ teaspoons sea salt per 2 cups of nuts

Walnuts & Pecans	4-8 hours
Almonds	12-18 hours
Cashews	No more than 6 hours

Seeds
Soak seeds in water to cover with 1 teaspoon salt per cup of seeds.

Sesame	2 hours
Sunflower, Pumpkin	4-6 hours

Positive Community Kitchen volunteers packaging nuts.

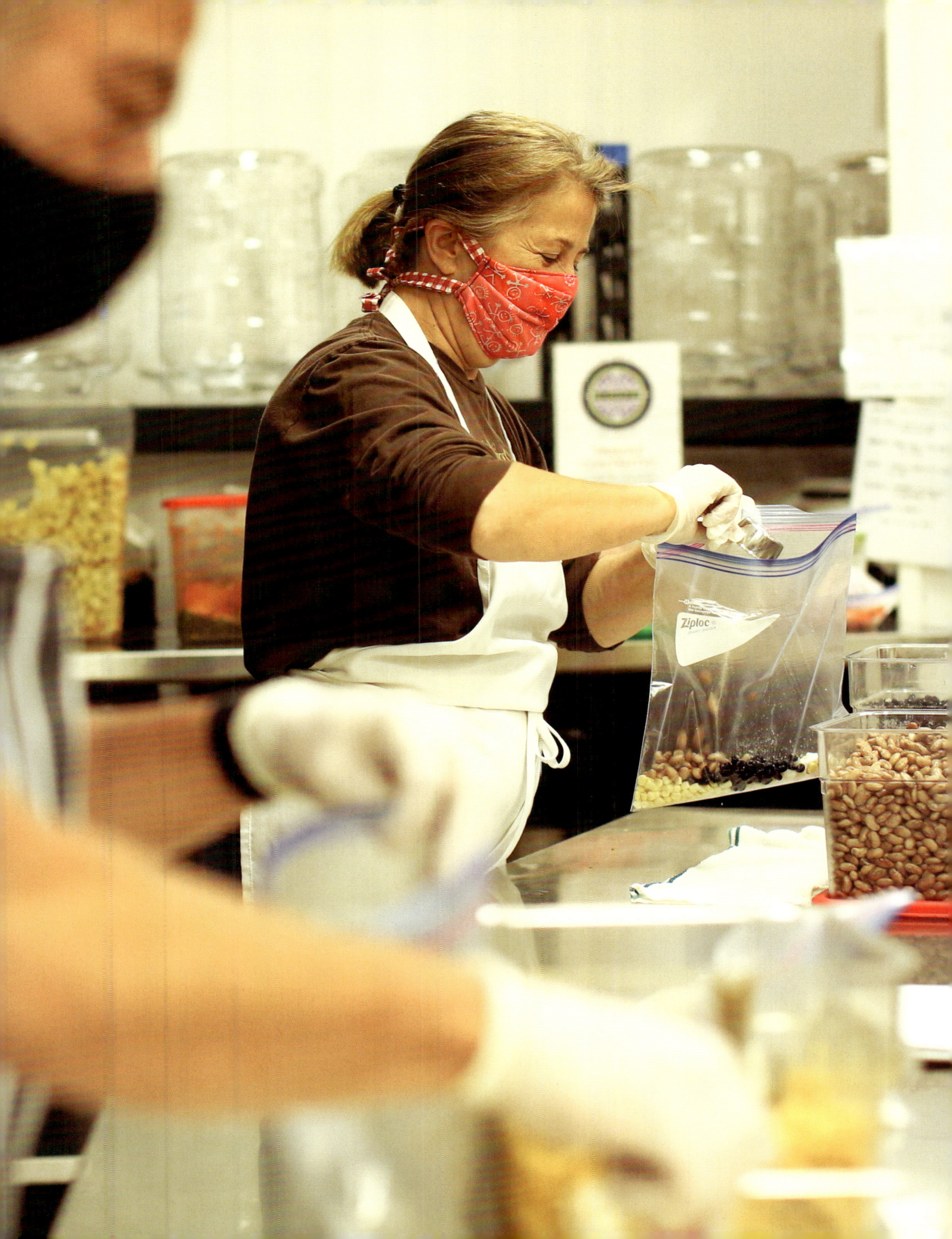
Ziploc

Fermenting Basics

Our ancestors have used the simple process of lacto-fermentation for thousands of years as a means of preserving foods without refrigeration or canning. Today we understand that beyond preserving foods, fermentation enhances their nutritional value. Eating small amounts of fermented foods on a daily basis helps to maintain healthy bacteria in the digestive tract. Healthy digestive bacteria are key to the digestion and absorption of the nutrients in our food. Making your own sauerkraut is remarkably simple and extremely satisfying Here are two easy recipes for fermented foods to get you started.

Basic Sauerkraut

5 pounds of cabbage, cored and shredded or chopped (save the outer leaves)
1½ Tbsp sea salt
4 - 6 Tbsp whey (or an additional 1½ Tbsp sea salt)

Optional additions

Small handful of arame sea weed, soaked in hot water, then rinsed
½ - 1 Tbsp finely minced or grated ginger
½ - 1 Tbsp finely minced garlic
2 - 3 Tbsp fresh dill, minced
1 Tbsp caraway seeds or fennel seeds

Mix the cabbage with the salt and whey (if using). Add any optional ingredients. Pound the cabbage with a mallet or massage with your hands for about 10 minutes to release the juices.

Place the cabbage in a large glass jar or crock, pressing down firmly with your fist to pack the cabbage tightly. Liquid should cover the cabbage by at least ½ inch. Place the reserved outer leaves over the shredded cabbage.

Fill a smaller jar with water and place it inside the jar to weigh down the cabbage and keep it below the liquid.

Cover the jars with a towel and leave it at room temperature for at least 4 days and up to two weeks. Check the jar every few days to make sure the cabbage is still below the liquid. Taste the sauerkraut on the 4th day to see if you like it. The sauerkraut is ready if it tastes good to you. When you like it, refrigerate it in a sealed jar, making sure there is water over the sauerkraut. It will keep for 6 months in your refrigerator.

Ginger Carrots

4 cups grated carrots
1 Tbsp freshly grated ginger
1 Tbsp sea salt
4 Tbsp whey
(or an additional 1 Tbsp sea salt)

Follow the directions for Basic Sauerkraut.

Tip: *Make sure there is water over the cabbage or other vegetables as this is an anaerobic fermentation. Air will yield mold. If there is foam or some discoloration on the top layer of the sauerkraut just remove it as all the kraut under the water will be fine.*

A Final Word

Remember, great cooking begins with the freshest whole foods you can find. The best recipe in the world can't make up for mealy, flavorless tomatoes or bitter, tough greens. On the other hand, tender young greens out of the garden will be a delight raw or with just a quick sauté in olive oil and a sprinkling of salt and pepper.

Finally, we can't say this enough: Test and taste. Foods are infinitely variable and so are we! A carrot fresh out of the garden will vary in sweetness from a carrot that has been in the food system for a week or two. It might have a higher water content and cook more quickly as well. On top of that, what seems tender to me might not be tender enough for you. Your taste buds are unique — and may vary as well from week to week if you are going through treatment. When you cook, guidelines can be helpful but ultimately, cooking is about being present, paying attention, and learning to please yourself in this moment.

Preserved lemons at the Caring Kitchen Project.

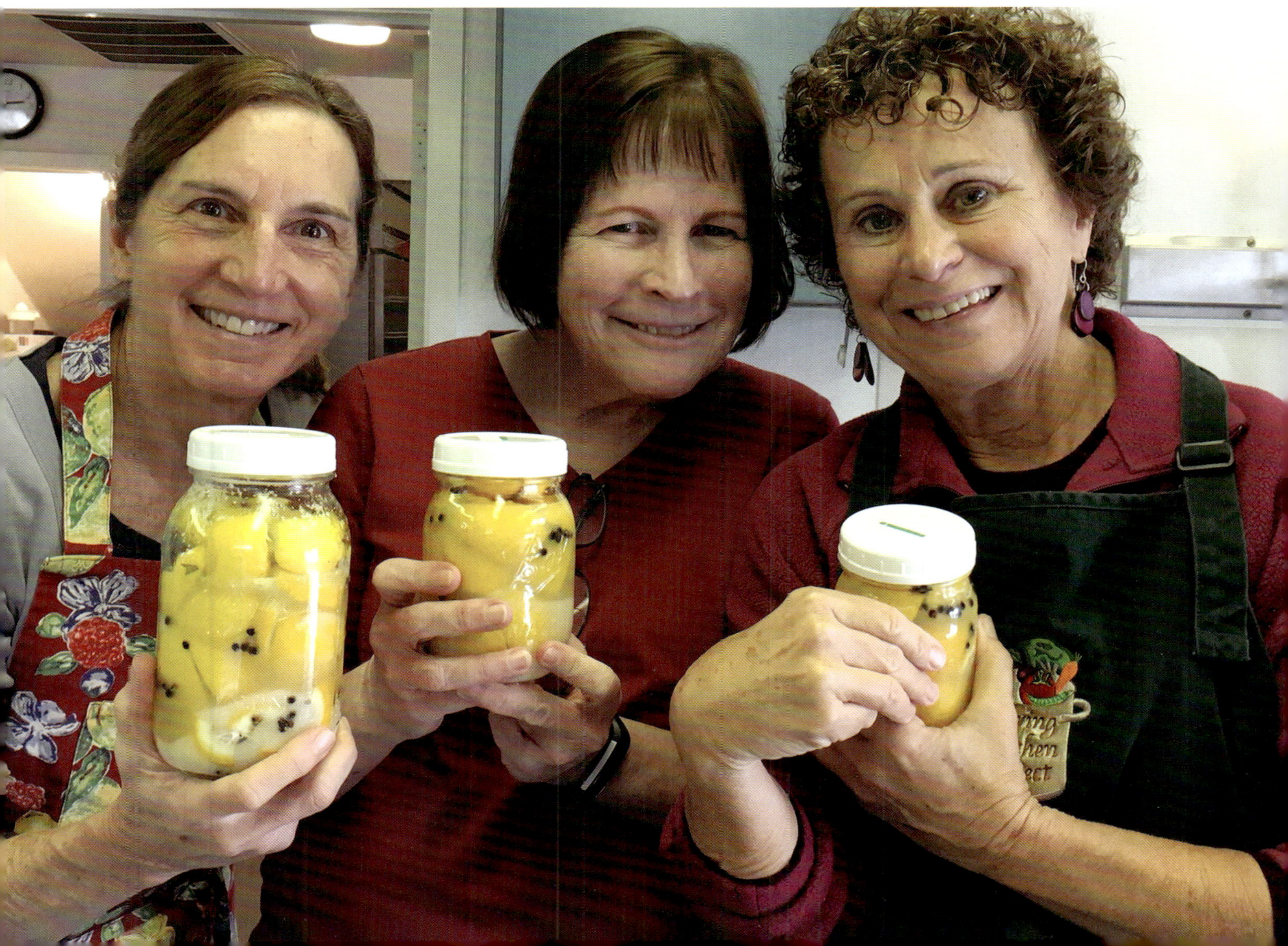

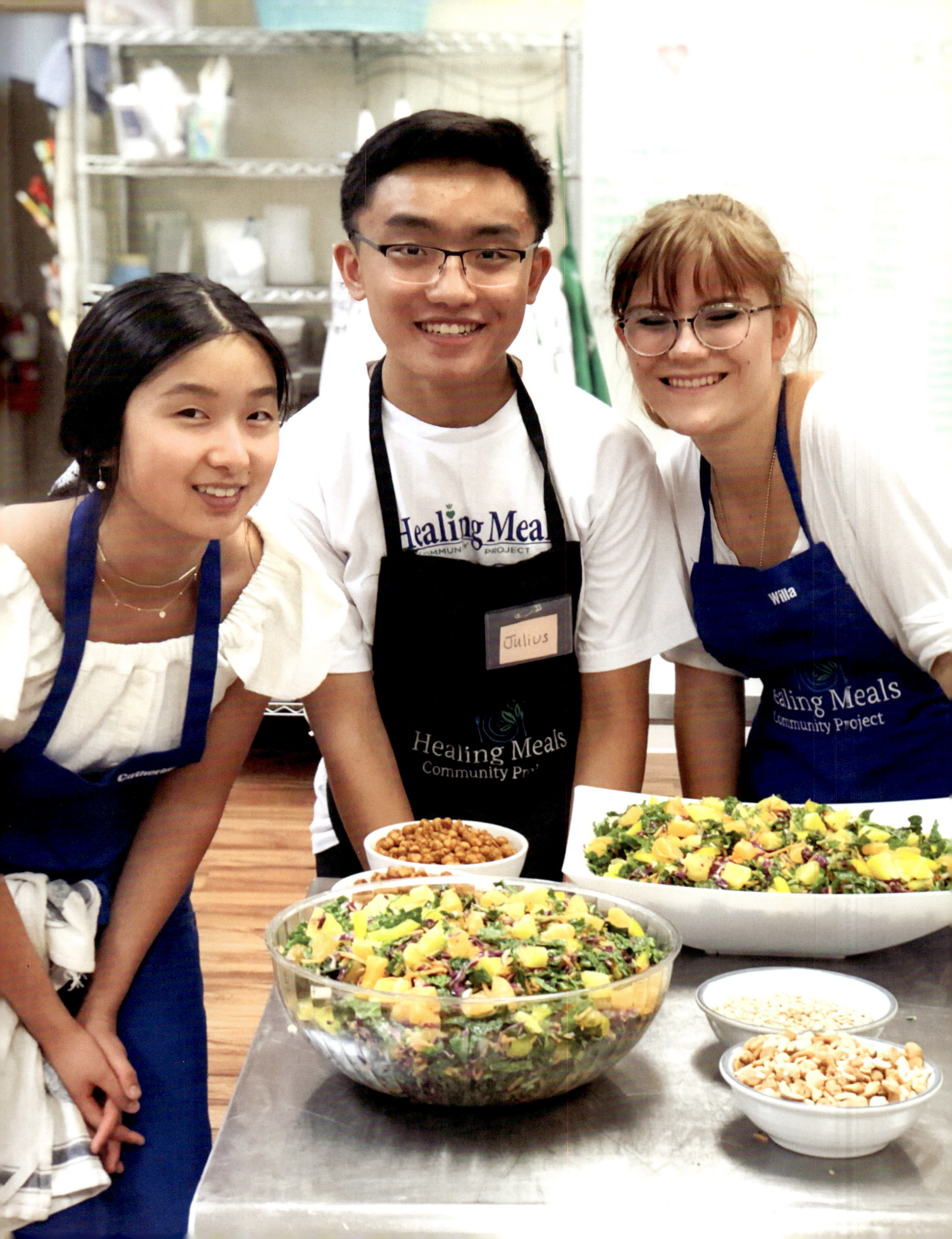
Healing Meals
Julius
Willa

SAUCES & SPREADS

Sriracha Remoulade

"I dedicate my time to Healing Meals because I make a positive impact in the community while working with incredible individuals who are very supportive and caring. Being young and having such great role models makes me want to be a better leader, not just in the kitchen but also in my everyday life"

— Imani, Healing Meals Community Project Youth Volunteer

Serves 8, about 2 cups
Prep time: 5 to10 minutes

Ingredients

1 (15-ounce) can cannellini beans
2 Tbsp lemon juice
3 cloves roasted garlic
1 Tbsp Sriracha
½ tsp ground cumin
¼ cup olive oil, plus more for drizzling
3 sprigs fresh parsley
Salt and ground black pepper to taste
Lemon zest, to garnish

Instructions

Pulse all ingredients except lemon zest in food processor fitted with a metal blade, or blender, until smooth and creamy. Garnish with lemon zest and a drizzle of olive oil.

Nutrition info. *Serving size, 4 Tbsp: 123 calories, 7g fat, 4g protein, 11g carbohydrate,38mg sodium*

Previous page: Teen volunteers from Healing Meals, this page: adult volunteers on the Auerbach farm.

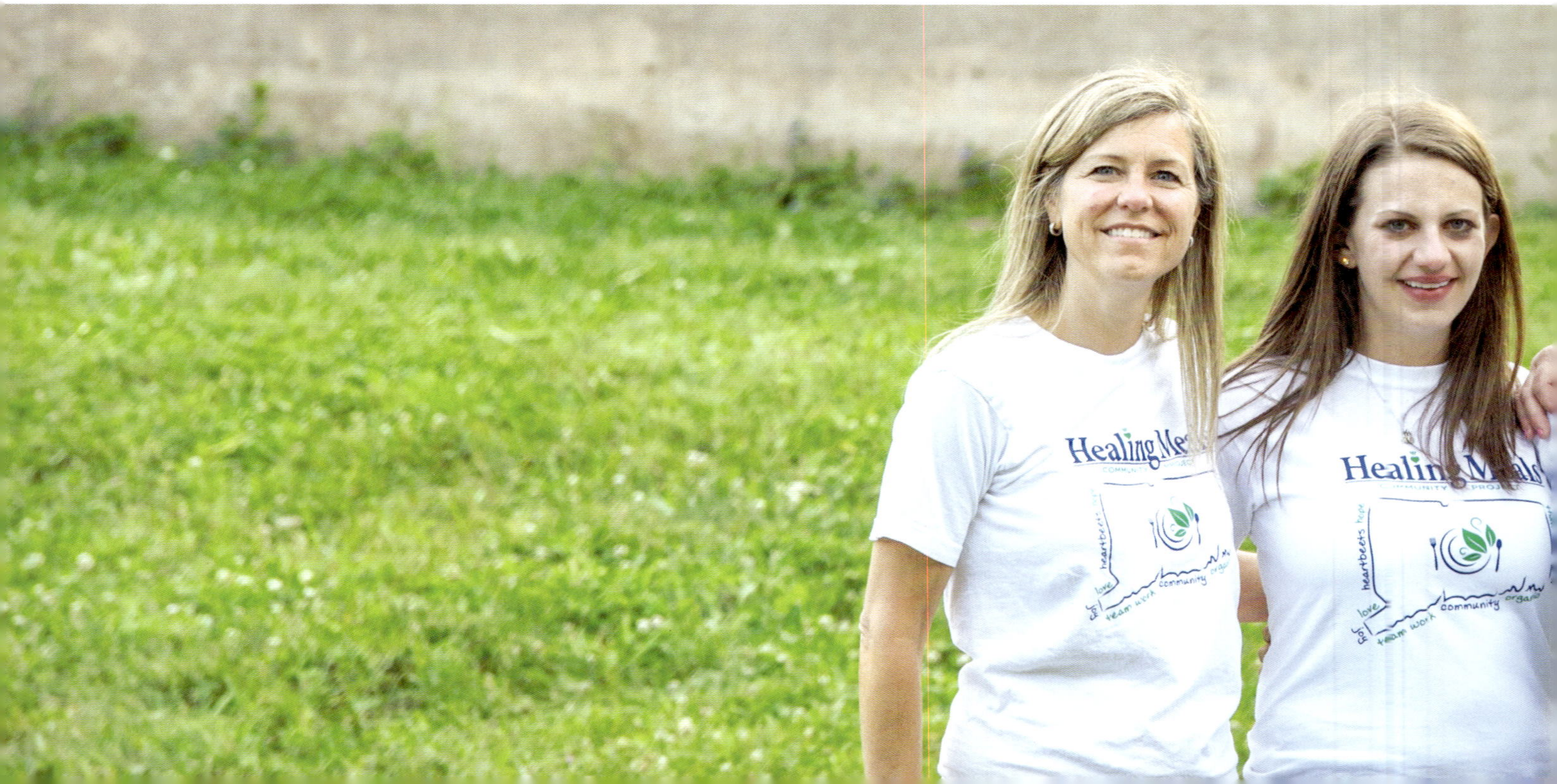

Cumin Lime Vinaigrette

A staff favorite, this zippy dressing is fantastic with a cabbage slaw or any green salad. Drizzle on top of a tostada or as a side with any Mexican-inspired dish.

— The Ceres Community Project Team

Serves 6, about ½ cup
Prep time: 10 minutes
Gluten-free
Dairy-free

Ingredients

2 Tbsp lime juice
2 Tbsp rice wine vinegar
1 Tbsp honey
1 tsp ground cumin
1 tsp minced garlic
¼ tsp salt
¼ tsp pepper
½ cup chopped cilantro
2 Tbsp olive oil

Instructions

Whisk together lime juice, vinegar, honey, cumin, garlic, salt, pepper and cilantro. Drizzle in olive oil, whisking constantly to blend. Or, put all ingredients in a blender and blend until smooth.

Nutrition info. *Serving size, 1 ½ tablespoons: 56 calories, 5g fat, 2g protein, 4g carbohydrate, 87mg sodium*

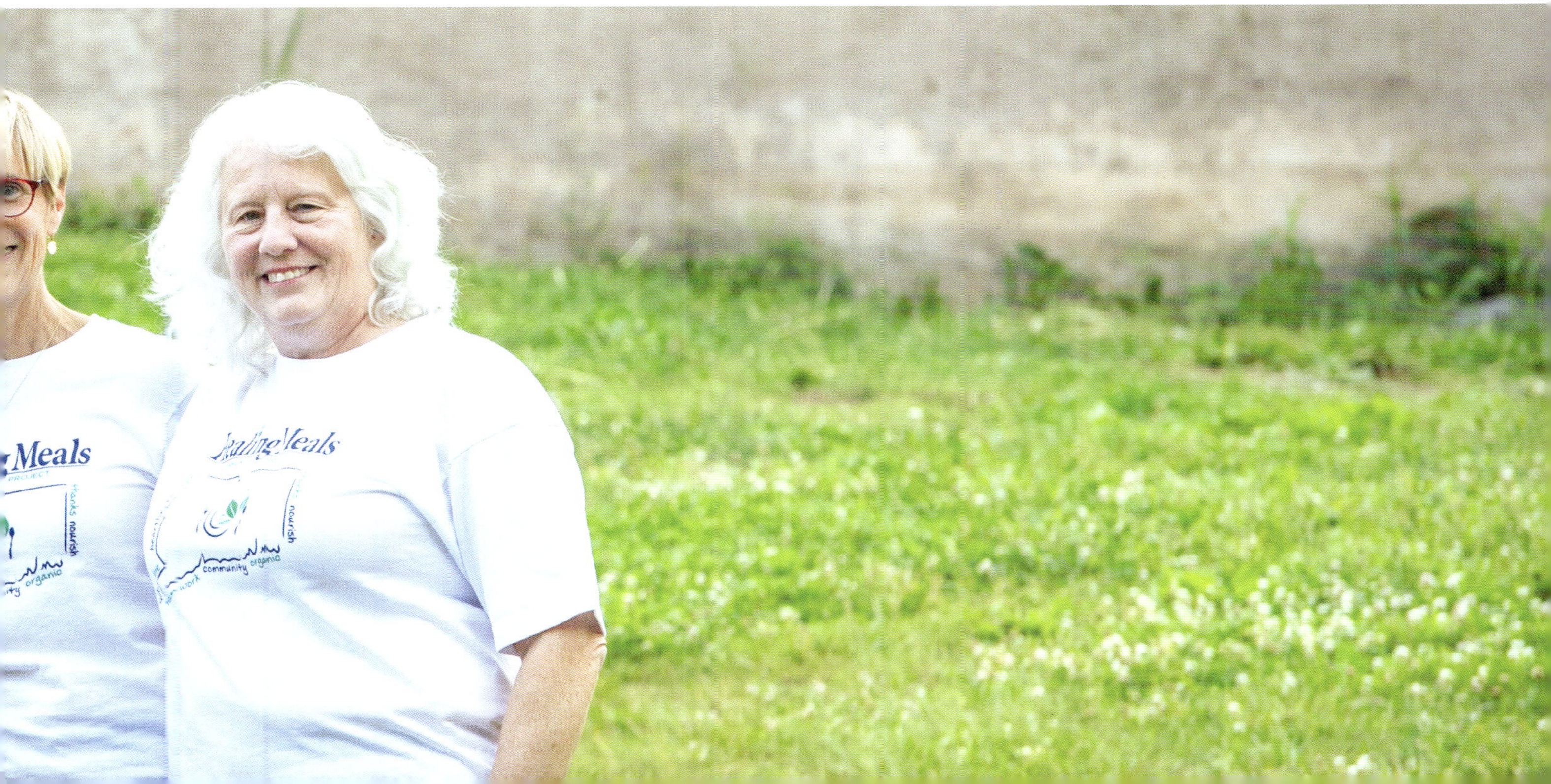

Parsley Spinach Pesto

Picking leaves from herbs in the kitchen with a group of teens is such a great opportunity to converse and connect. We love to combine all the fresh green herbs from the garden to make pesto. Once, when we were short on herbs, we added spinach. Delicious on pasta, veggies, or on the side with a veggie frittata.

— The Caring Kitchen Project Team

Yields 3 cups
Prep time: 40 minutes
Vegan
Gluten-free

Ingredients

1 whole bulb garlic
Olive oil and salt, for roasting

½ cup whole almonds
8 cups fresh whole spinach leaves, stemmed and lightly packed
3 cups Italian parsley leaves, stemmed and lightly packed
1 Tbsp lemon zest
¼ cup lemon juice

¼ tsp salt
¾ cup extra-virgin olive oil
Pinch cayenne or powdered red chili pepper

Instructions

Preheat oven to 400° F . Cut the top off of a whole garlic bulb, baste with olive oil, sprinkle with salt, wrap in foil and bake in a shallow oven-proof dish for about 45 minutes. Cool slightly and squeeze out contents of three cloves. Set aside. Reserve the rest of the roasted garlic for another use.

In food processor fitted with the metal blade, chop almonds until fine. Add roasted garlic to almonds and pulse three times.

Add spinach, parsley, lemon juice, zest and salt. Pulse until combined.

Run a rubber spatula around the bottom edges of the processor bowl to make sure all ingredients are evenly blended.

With processor running, drizzle olive oil slowly into the mixture.

Add cayenne or red chili pepper and salt to taste.

NOTE: Pine nuts or walnuts can be substituted for almonds.

Nutrition info. *Serving size, ½ cup: 330 calories, 33g fat, 5g protein, 7g carbohydrate, 125mg sodium*

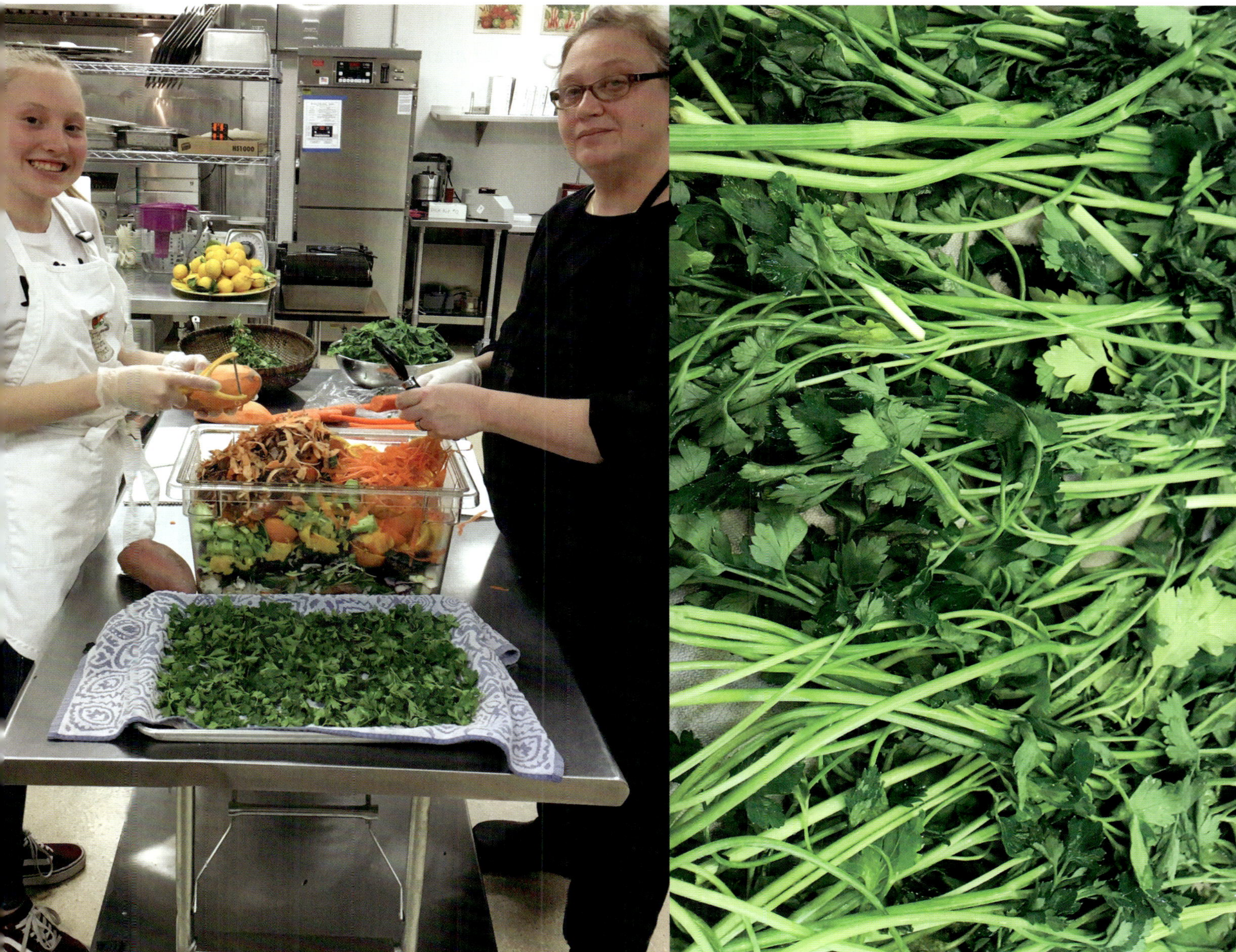

Parsley preparation underway with adult and teen volunteers at the Caring Kitchen Project.

Haydari

This recipe from Det Kærlige Måltid makes a lively and vibrant Middle Eastern spread using feta cheese and roasted red peppers. It's delicious on crusty bread, crackers or with roasted or raw vegetables.

— Det Kærlige Måltid Team

Serves 6
Prep time: 25 minutes
Cooking time: 30 minutes
Gluten-free

Ingredients

¾ pound red bell peppers, 2 large or 3 medium
¼ cup minced parsley
2 garlic cloves, minced
⅓ cup olive oil
½ pound goat or sheep feta cheese, drained well
½ tsp Sriracha sauce, or to taste

Instructions

Preheat oven to 425°F.

Place a baking rack over a baking sheet and set the peppers on the rack.

Bake until blackened (about 25 to 30 minutes). Turn the peppers two or three times while roasting.

Remove peppers from oven and place in a paper bag. Fold down top and place bag on a large plate. Refrigerate for 15 minutes.

Stem, peel and seed peppers. Chop coarsely.

Place the peppers in a food processor fitted with the metal blade. Add the parsley, garlic, olive oil and feta cheese. Process to a chunky spreadable texture. Add Sriracha to taste.

Nutrition info. *Serving size, ½ cup: 283 calories, 27g fat, 6g protein, 6g carbohydrate, 365mg sodium*

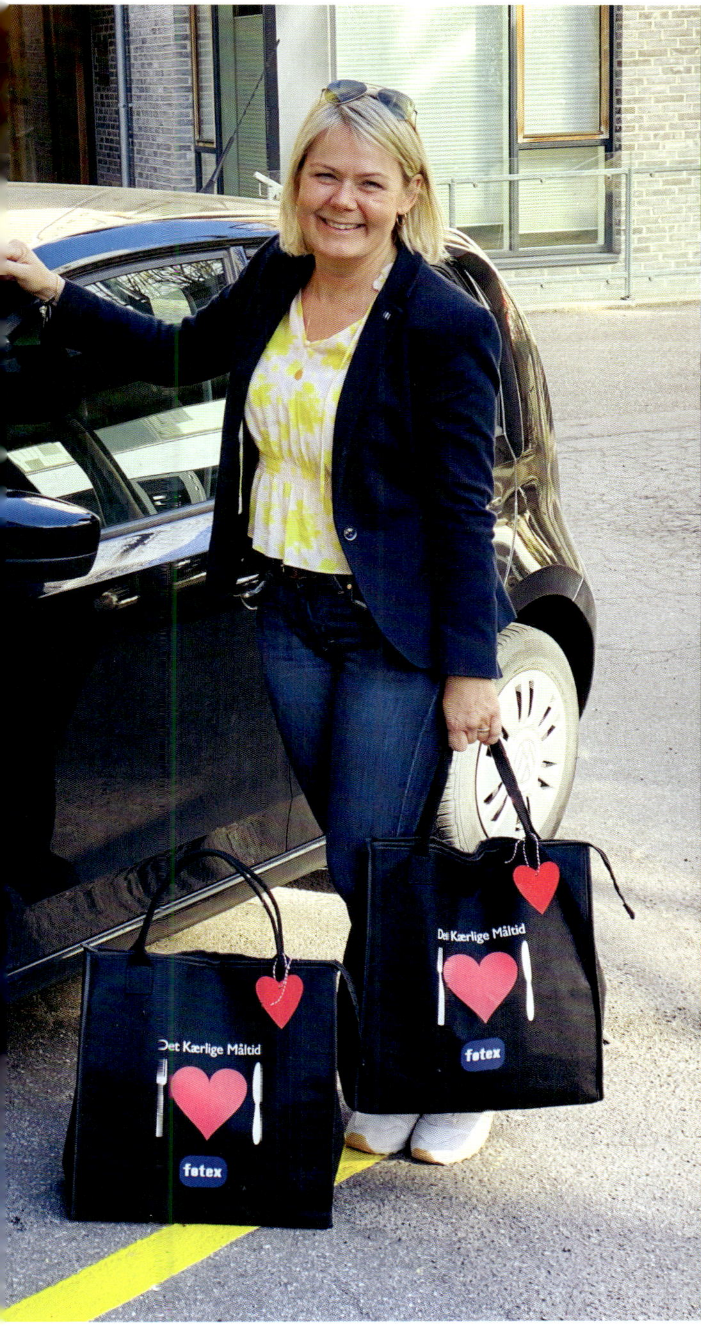

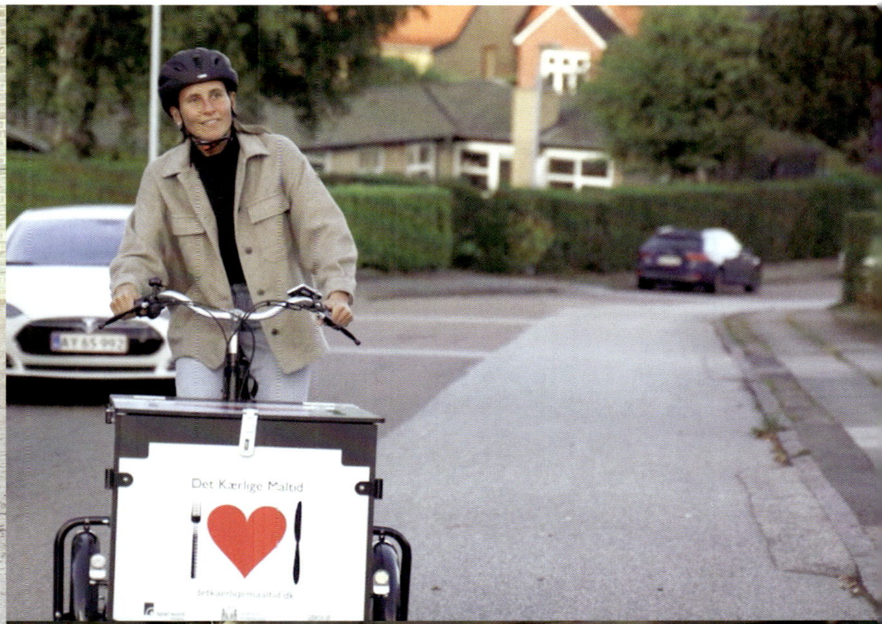

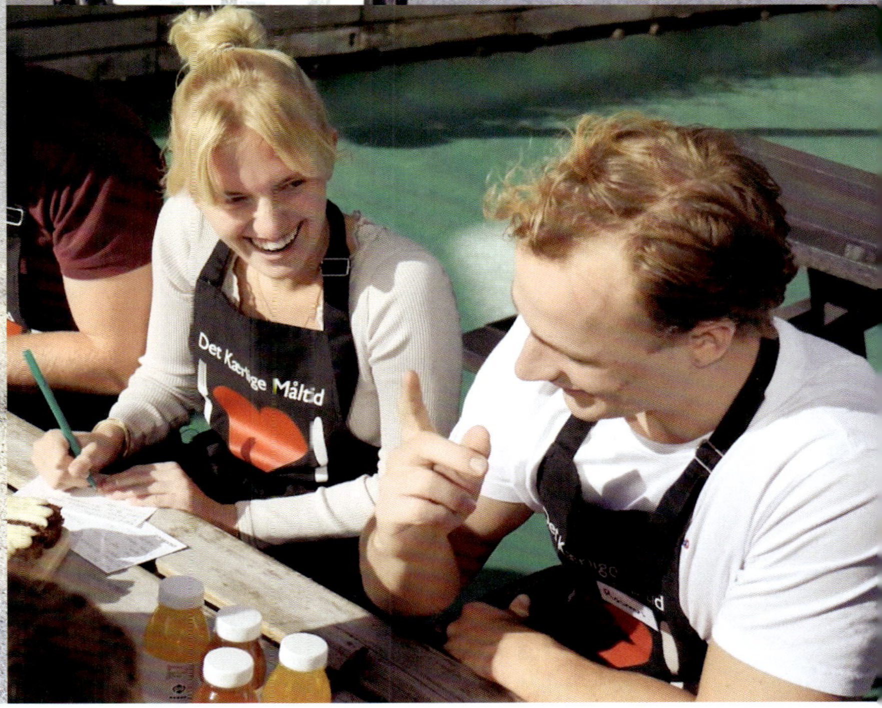

Delivery Angels for Det Kærlige Måltid travel by car and by bike, and below, teens write good wishes cards for clients.

"Peanut" Sauce

We served this crowd pleaser at our annual event. Teens made it on site and served it with our Vegetarian Spring Rolls (page 147). They were wowed to learn how spring roll wrappers worked and that this sauce is peanut free!

— The Positive Community Kitchen Team

Serves 8, about 2 cups
Prep time: 10 minutes
Gluten-free, if using coconut aminos
Dairy-free

Ingredients

⅔ cup sunflower seed butter
⅔ cup coconut milk
5 Tbsp coconut aminos, or soy sauce
2 Tbsp honey
2 Tbsp rice vinegar
1 Tbsp sesame oil
1 ⅛ tsp fresh minced ginger
1 ⅛ tsp minced garlic

Instructions

Process all ingredients in a blender until thoroughly combined and smooth.

Nutrition info. *Serving size, 4 Tbsp: 211 calories, 16g fat, 5g protein, 12g carbohydrate, 336mg sodium*

Chef Nicole gives instructions at Positive Community Kitchen

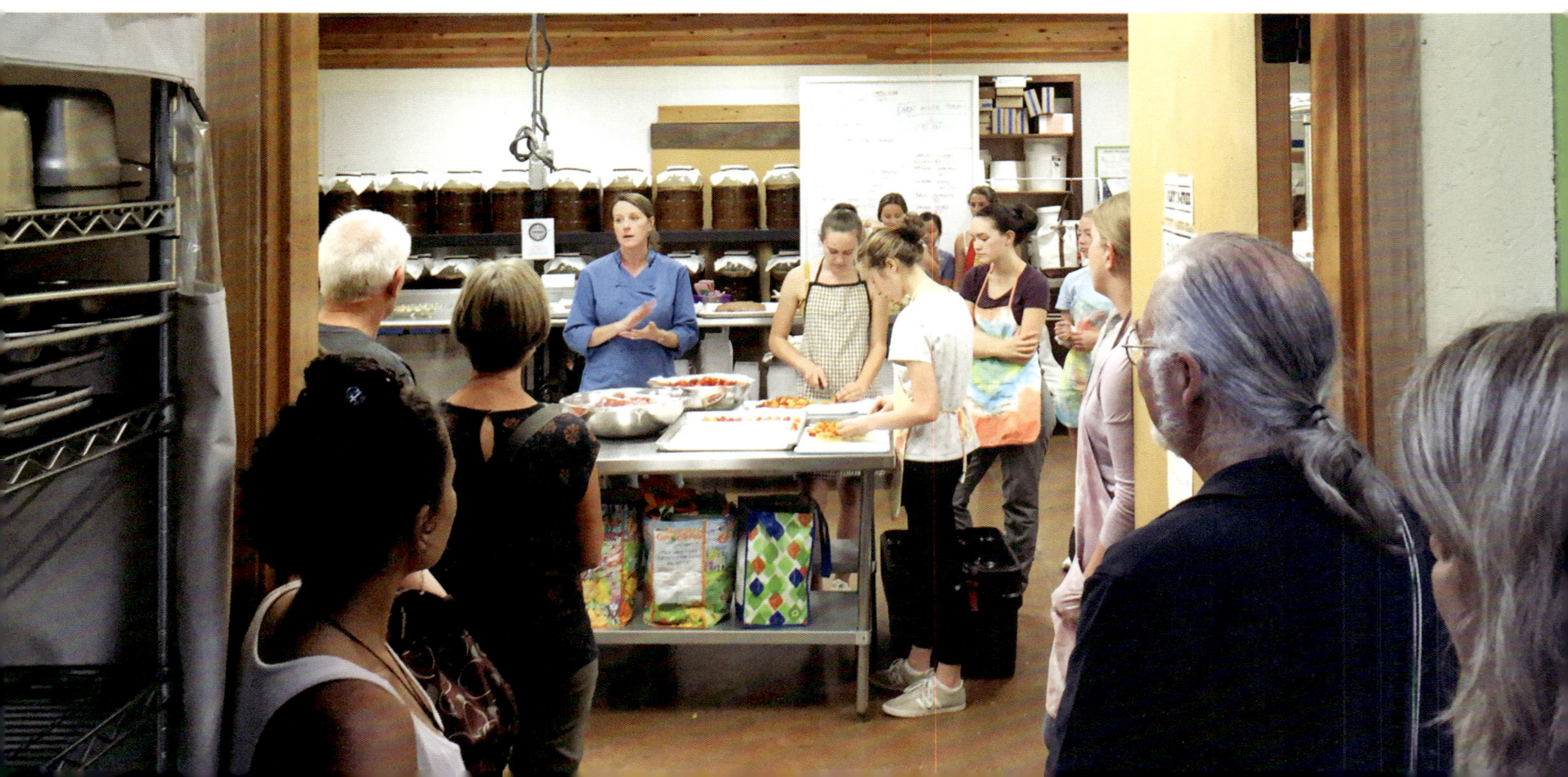

Almond Tamari Sauce

This versatile sauce gets its velvety texture from almond butter, creating a smooth sauce to coat your veggies, mix with rice noodles, or drizzle on poultry or fish. Try it stir-fried with vegetables such as broccoli, cauliflower, carrots, green beans, snap peas, asparagus, or peppers. Add chopped almonds for extra crunch.

— The Caring Kitchen Project Team

Serves 6
Prep time: 15 minutes
Cooking time: 15 minutes
Gluten-free
Dairy-free

Ingredients

½ cup water
3 Tbsp gluten-free soy sauce or tamari
1 Tbsp Chinese rice wine or other sweet white wine
1 Tbsp rice vinegar
1 Tbsp honey
4 tsp toasted sesame oil
¼ tsp cornstarch
1 ½ Tbsp almond butter
1 tsp ginger, grated and squeezed for juice, pulp discarded (or substitute 1 tsp peeled and finely chopped ginger)
⅛ tsp Sriracha or similar hot sauce
3 Tbsp sunflower or grapeseed oil

Instructions

Combine all sauce ingredients in small saucepan. Heat on the stove over low heat, whisking constantly until mixture comes to a simmer. Simmer 1 minute, until smooth and thickened.

Nutrition info. *Serving size, 2 Tbsp: 128 calories, 11g fat, 2g protein, 5g carbohydrate, 460mg sodium*

Roasted Beet Hummus

This is a wonderful recipe to utilize leftover roasted beets. Roasting really enhances the flavor of this hummus. However, if you don't feel like roasting your own beets, you can find packages of pre-cooked beets at the market that would work just fine. Just skip the roasting part of the recipe. The leaves of the beets are delicious and nutritious. They can be sautéed similarly to kale or spinach.

— The Positive Community Kitchen Team

Serves: 8
Prep time: 10 minutes
Cooking time: 30 minutes
Vegan
Gluten-free

Ingredients

2 red beets (2-inch diameter)
3 cloves garlic, minced
1 (14-ounce) can chickpeas, drained and rinsed (or 1 ½ cup cooked)
2 Tbsp tahini paste
1 Tbsp red miso paste, or substitute white miso paste
1 lemon, zested and juiced
1 tsp paprika
⅓ cup olive oil, plus more for drizzling
¼ tsp salt
¼ tsp ground black pepper, or to taste

Instructions

Preheat oven to 425°F. Line a sheet pan with parchment paper or lightly oil.

Remove the stems and leaves from the root of the beet. With a paring knife or vegetable peeler, remove the outer skin of the beet. Dice beet into small ½-inch pieces.

Place beets on prepared sheet pan. Drizzle with a little olive oil and sprinkle with salt and pepper. Roast for 20-30 minutes, until cooked through.

Once beets are cool enough to handle, place them in a food processor fitted with the metal blade or in a blender. Add the garlic and chickpeas. Process until the mixture is broken down into small bits.

Add remaining ingredients and process until smooth, adding more olive oil if needed to reach the consistency you desire.

Taste and season with more salt, pepper or paprika if needed. Serve with crackers, chips, or vegetables.

Nutrition info. *Serving size, 1 serving: 188 calories, 12g fat, 5g protein, 16g carbohydrate, 269mg sodium*

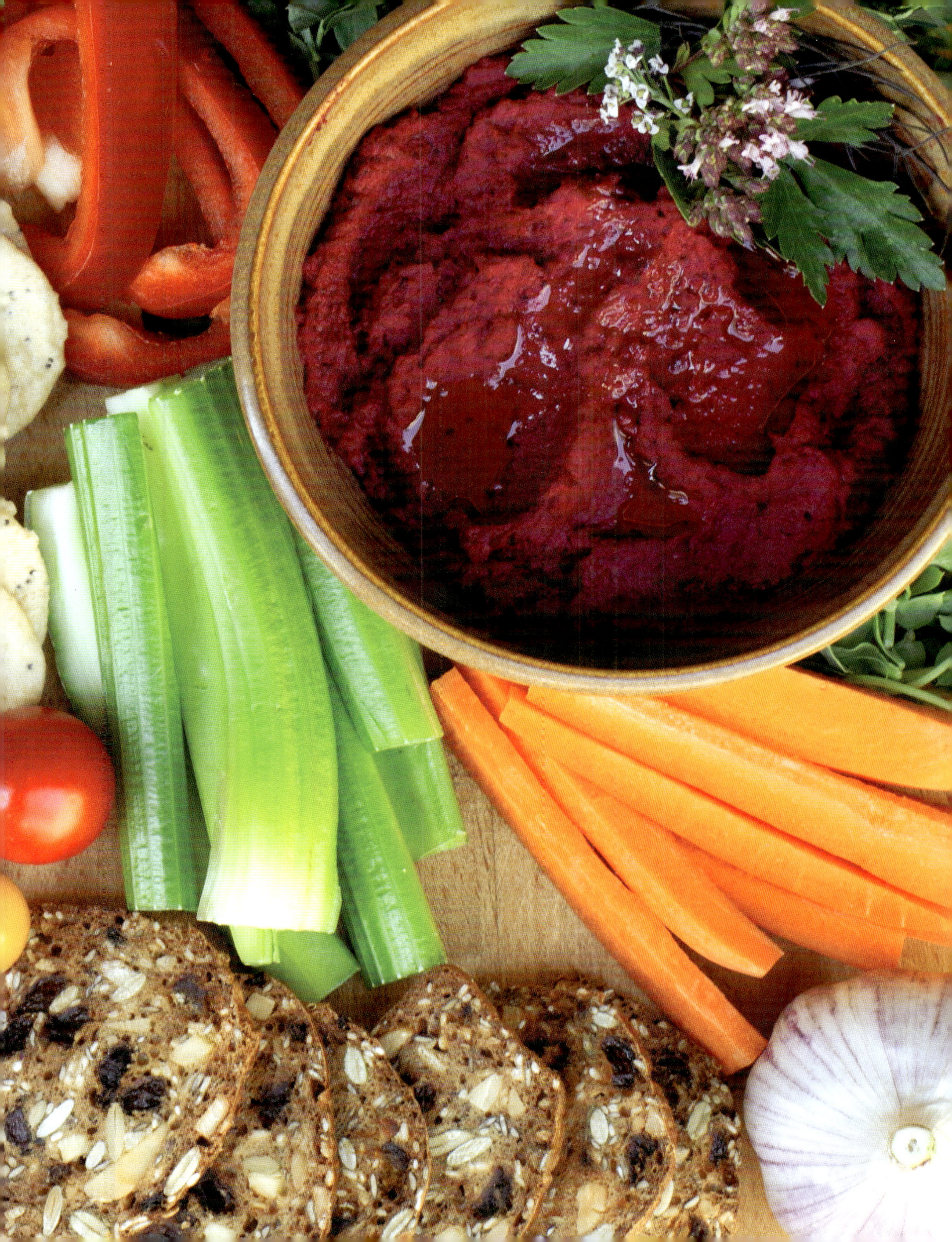

Balsamic Tomato Onion Conserve

This sauce is divine with all the notes of honey, balsamic and fresh herbs. When we have a teen garden harvest workday, this is a great way to use the bounty of tomatoes. During the harvest, teens go on a fresh herb treasure hunt, then spend time identifying and coming up with a description of what each herb smells like and how they would imagine using it in a recipe. When tomatoes aren't in season, make this using halved cherry tomatoes or even canned whole tomatoes with their juice.

— The Caring Kitchen Project Team

Serves 8
Prep time: 10 minutes
Cooking time: 80 minutes
Gluten-free
Dairy-free

Ingredients

2 Tbsp olive oil
2 medium sweet onions, quartered and thinly sliced lengthwise
1 tsp plus 6 Tbsp honey, divided
2 ½ cups quartered fresh tomatoes
¼ cup balsamic vinegar
½ tsp ground black pepper
salt to taste

Instructions

In a deep skillet, heat olive oil over a medium-low flame. Add onions and 1 tsp honey and cook, covered, for 10 to 15 minutes. Remove the lid and continue cooking, stirring often, until onions are brown but not burned, about 20 to 30 minutes more. You may need to lower the heat to keep onions from burning.

Add tomatoes and bring to a boil over medium heat. Cook until soft, about 5 minutes. Reduce heat and simmer until the liquid evaporates, about 30 minutes. Stir often, scraping the sides of the skillet.

Remove from heat and add the remaining honey, vinegar, pepper and salt. Stir well.

Optional: For a smoother texture, purée half of the finished conserve in a blender or food processor.

Nutrition info. *Serving size, ¼ cup: 137 calories, 2 g fat, 3 g protein, 32g carbohydrate, 162mg sodium*

Health and Healing Spice Blend

Using this blend is a simple way to add more vitamins, minerals, antioxidants, protein, fiber, and Omega 3s to every dish you make at home! It is a delicious and nutritious addition to vinaigrettes, marinades, eggs, grains, soups, stews, side dishes, stir fry, etc. Just add to your food to taste while seasoning with salt and pepper and other herbs, spices, and aromatics of your choice.

— The Meals 4 Health and Healing Team

Yields ½ cup

Ingredients

2 Tbsp ground flax seeds
2 Tbsp ground hemp seeds
1 Tbsp powdered turmeric
1 Tbsp dried oregano
1 Tbsp powdered garlic
1 Tbsp organic powdered onion
1 tsp fine Himalayan sea salt
½ tsp organic powdered ginger
½ tsp organic spirulina powder

Instructions

Mix ingredients and store refrigerated in an airtight container.

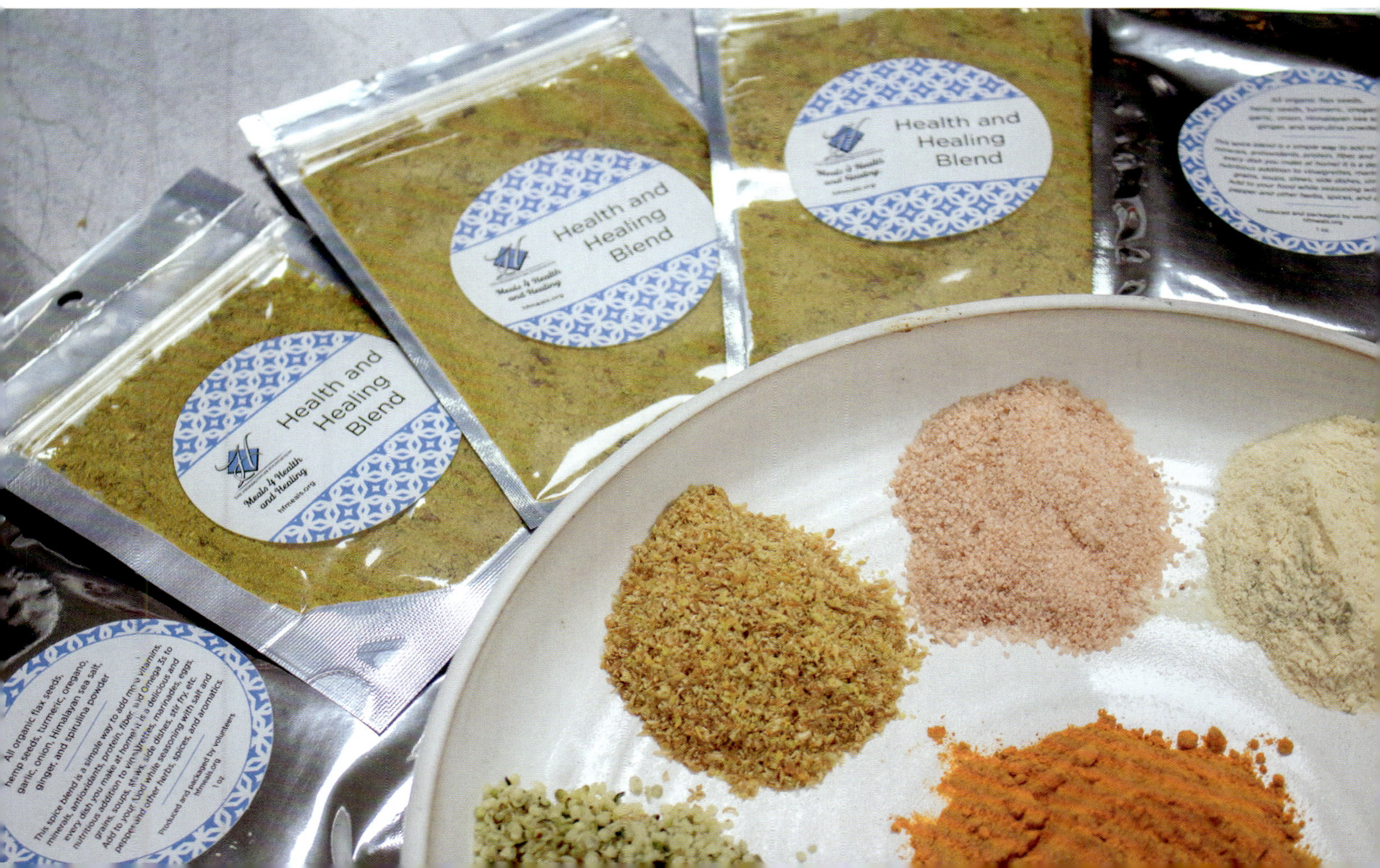

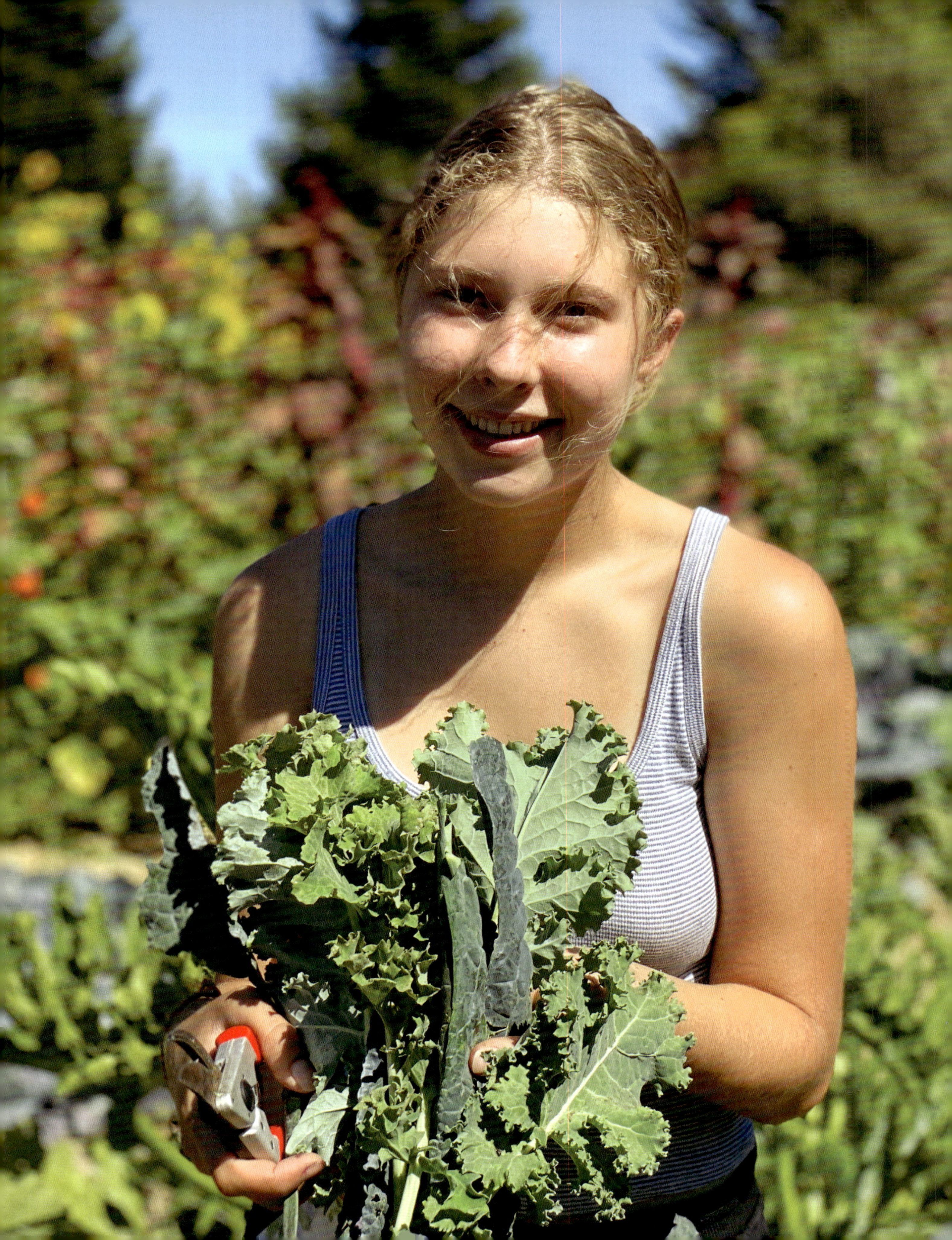

SALADS

Grilled Peach, Black Rice and Arugula Salad

Black rice, also known as forbidden rice or purple rice, provides more than a punch of color to your dish. This ingredient boasts fiber, iron, and protein as well as several antioxidants. This recipe was developed by Shanna Hutton, who leads Nourish: Food for Life cooking demos in our Eugene community. Shanna has served with Positive Community Kitchen since its early days and worn all the hats including head chef, board president, and more!

— The Positive Community Kitchen Team

Serves 6
Prep time: 15 minutes
Cooking time: 6 to 8 minutes
Vegan, if made without cheese
Gluten-free

Ingredients

1 ½ cup cooked black rice, prepared according to package directions and cooled

3 medium peaches, quartered
1 Tbsp olive oil
¼ tsp salt
¼ tsp ground black pepper

3 Tbsp apple cider vinegar
1 Tbsp Dijon mustard
2 Tbsp olive oil
2 Tbsp pure maple syrup
1 Tbsp finely chopped shallot
½ tsp salt
¼ tsp cayenne pepper (optional)

6 cups fresh arugula (about 4 ounces)
½ cup crumbled goat cheese (optional)

Instructions

Place peaches in a small bowl, drizzle with a little olive oil, sprinkle with salt and pepper.

Place peaches on an oiled grill rack over medium heat. Grill, covered, until lightly browned, 6 to 8 minutes, turning occasionally.

While peaches are grilling, make the dressing. In a mason jar container with a lid, pour in vinegar, mustard, olive oil, maple syrup, shallot, salt, and cayenne pepper (if using). Shake jar until the dressing is combined. Alternately, you can whisk together in a small bowl. Toss about ¼ of the dressing with the rice to coat evenly.

Line a platter with arugula; top with rice mixture and peaches. Drizzle with remaining dressing, top with cheese (if using) and serve.

Nutrition info. *1 serving: 291 calories, 11g fat, 7g protein, 52g carbohydrate, 335mg sodium*

Previous page: Ceres teen volunteer Sarah picking kale.

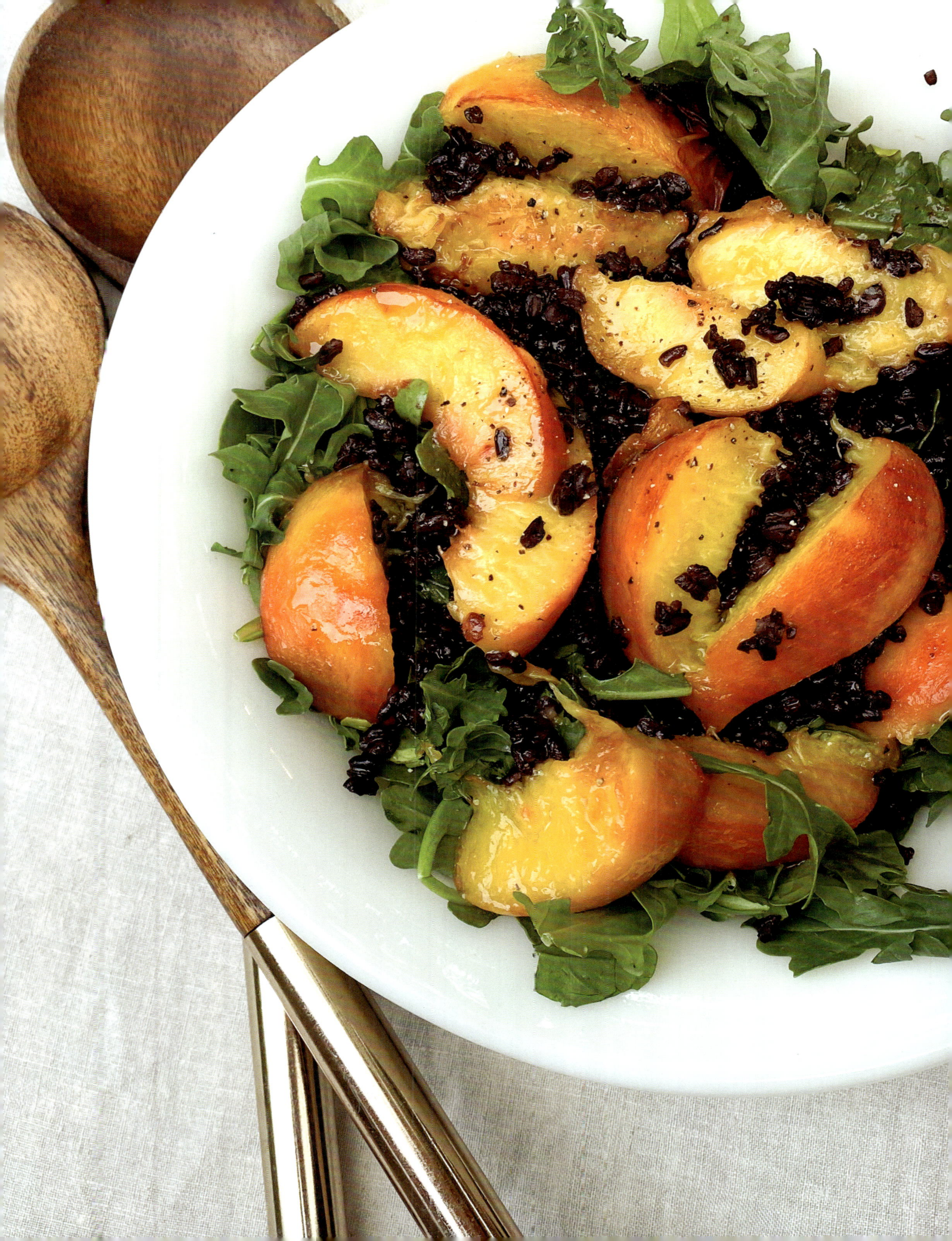

Watermelon Salad

The mint and feta cheese make this salad so refreshing and light. It's the perfect dish to bring to a summertime barbeque.

— The Revive & Thrive team

Serves 8
Prep time: 30 minutes
Vegan, if made without cheese
Gluten-free

Ingredients

1 large watermelon, peeled and cut in bite-size pieces
1 bunch fresh mint, chopped
6 limes, juiced
1 tsp salt
6 ounces feta cheese, crumbled (optional)

Instructions

In a large bowl, toss together the watermelon, mint, lime juice, and salt. Plate and garnish with feta cheese.

Nutrition info. *1 Serving: 241 calories, 5g fat, 7g protein, 49g carbohydrate, 429mg sodium*

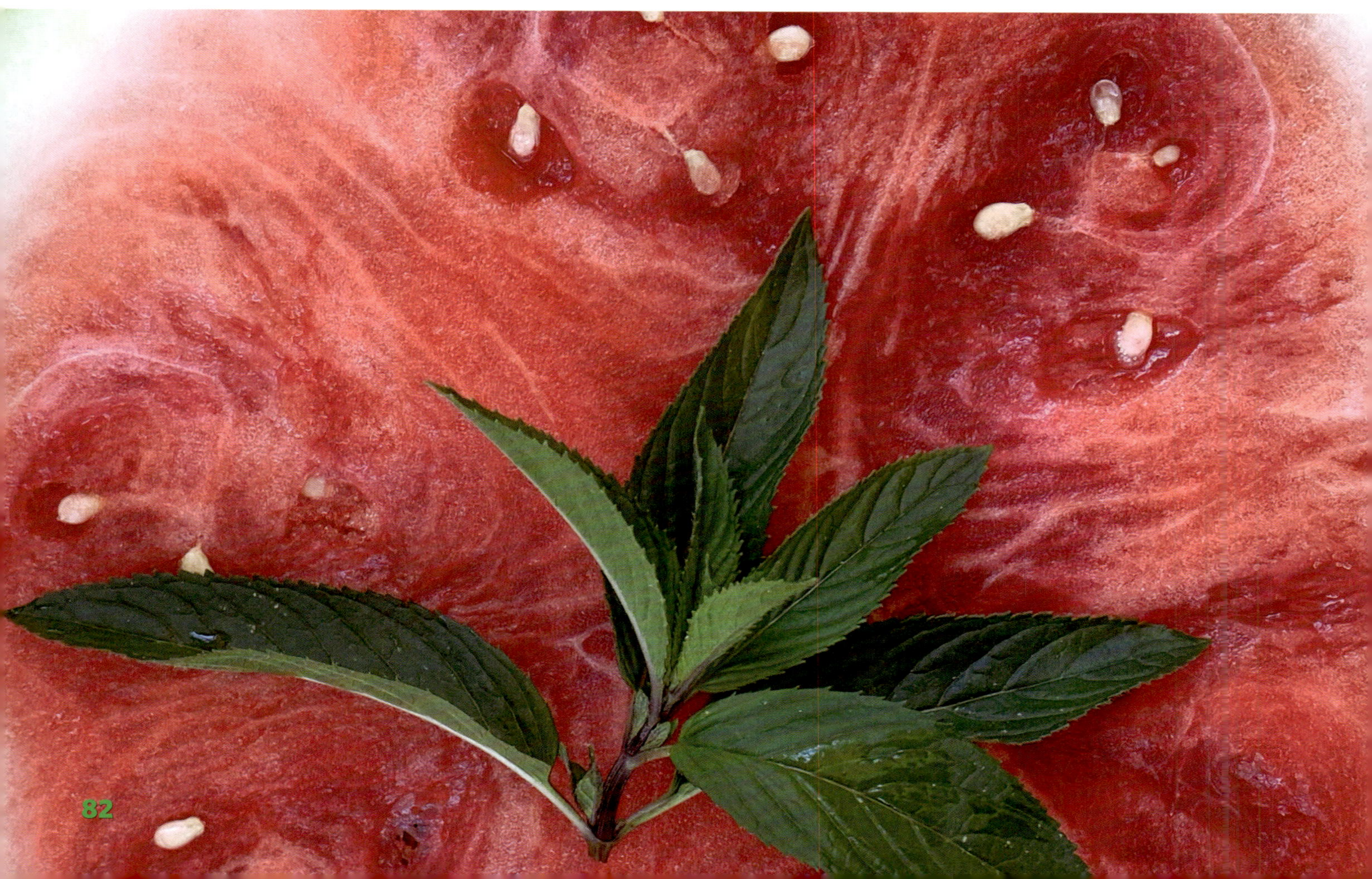

Cabbage, Beet and Blueberry Salad

This salad from Det Kærlige Måltid is beautiful and colorful. You become happy when both eating and looking at it.

— Det Kærlige Måltid Team

Serves 6
Prep time: 60 minutes
Vegan
Gluten-free

Ingredients

1 ¼ pounds beets (to yield about 2 cups cooked and chopped)
½ cup almonds
1 ¼ pounds red cabbage, shredded or thinly sliced (about 4 cups)
¼ cup olive oil
2 Tbsp lime juice
1 tsp honey
1 tsp Dijon mustard
½ tsp salt
ground black pepper to taste

1 ¾ cups fresh blueberries

Instructions

Preheat oven to 325°F.

Put the almonds on a baking tray and toast them in the oven until golden, about 8 minutes. Cool completely, then process in a food processor until finely chopped.

Scrub the beets well, then boil with skin on until easily pierced with a fork, approximately 25 to 35 minutes depending on size.

Rinse the beets with cold water and cool. Rub off the skins, then cut the beets in small cubes and mix with the red cabbage.

Whisk together olive oil, lime juice, honey, mustard, salt and pepper, and pour over the salad. Add the blueberries. Toss and serve.

Nutrition info. *1 serving: 304 calories, 21g fat, 8g protein, 27g carbohydrate, 309mg sodium*

Wedge Salad with Southwestern Dressing

The herbs and spices in this southwestern dressing meld seamlessly with the mayonnaise and create the perfect dressing atop the crisp lettuce wedge. Add your favorite organic vegetables for the ultimate wedge salad.

— The Meals 4 Health and Healing Team

Serves 4
Prep time: 30 minutes
Dairy-free
Gluten-free

Ingredients

½ cup avocado mayonnaise, or other good-quality mayonnaise
¼ cup lime juice
1 large clove garlic, minced into a paste
¼ tsp dried oregano or ½ to 1 tsp chopped fresh oregano
2 Tbsp finely finely chopped cilantro
½ tsp ground cumin
½ tsp ground coriander
½ tsp chili powder
Pinch ground cayenne pepper
2 Tbsp cold-pressed avocado or extra-virgin olive oil
½ tsp sea salt
Ground black pepper to taste
Water, if needed, to thin dressing

2 small heads Romaine lettuce, ends trimmed and sliced in half lengthwise to yield 4 portions

Optional: 1 cup chopped vegetables, such as radishes, cucumber, cherry tomatoes or zucchini

Instructions

Place first nine dressing ingredients in a bowl and whisk to combine.

Whisk in oil, then season to taste with salt and pepper. If needed, whisk in a small amount of water to reach your desired consistency.

Divide lettuce wedges on four salad plates and drizzle with dressing.

Top with chopped vegetables and serve.

Nutrition info. *1 serving size, 1 wedge: 290 calories, 26g fat, 5g protein,13g carbohydrate, 438mg sodium*

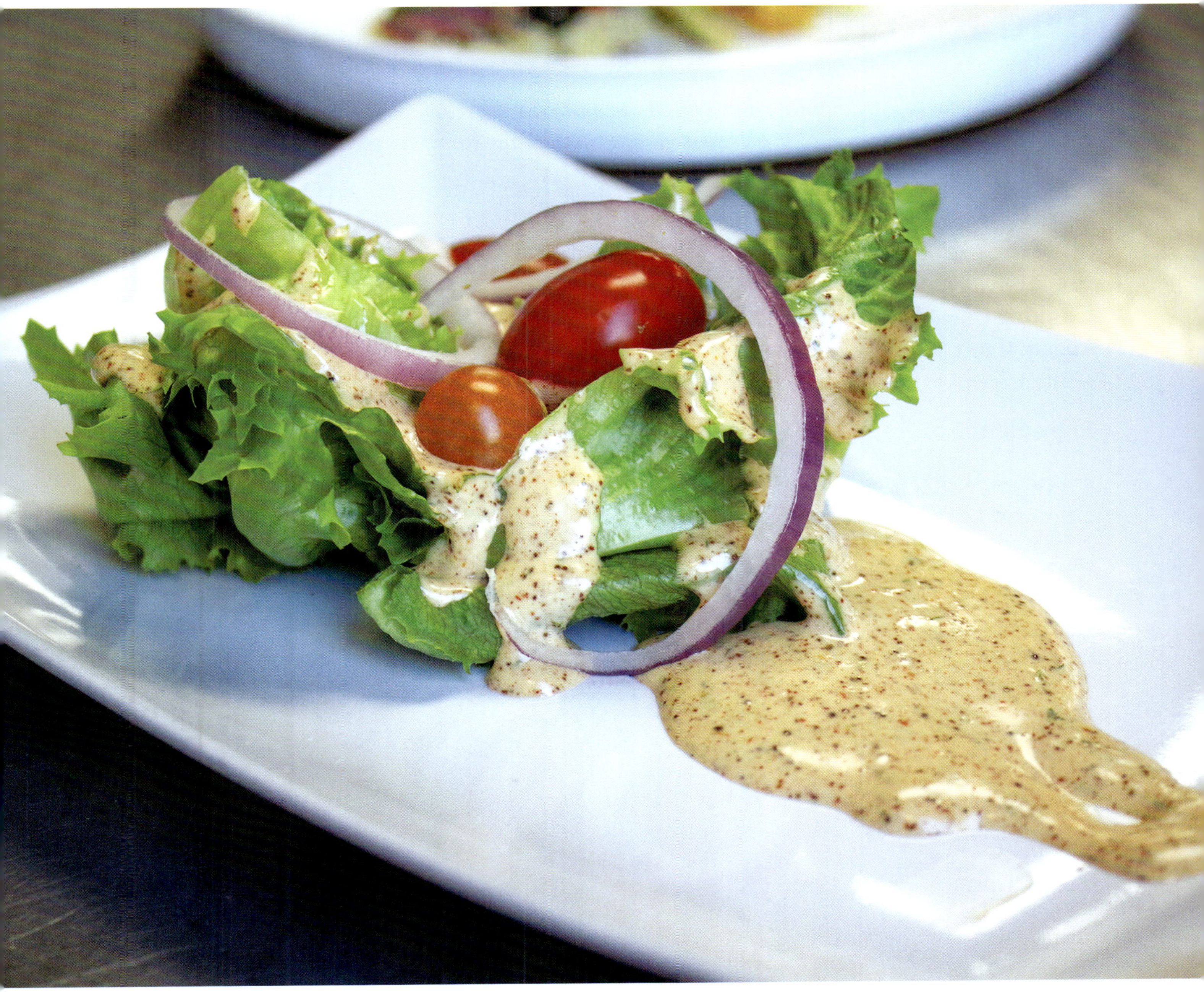

Cauliflower Salad with Cumin and Roasted Peppers

The cauliflower, roasted peppers, olive oil, and cumin are ingredients commonly used in Middle Eastern dishes. Maple syrup, apple cider vinegar, and pumpkin seeds: pure Ceres!

— Chef John Littlewood, Ceres Community Project

Serves 6
Prep time: 20 minutes
Cooking time: 30 minutes
Vegan, if not using Parmesan cheese
Gluten-free

Ingredients

8 cups small cauliflower florets
2 cups red bell peppers, diced in ½-inch pieces
2 Tbsp olive oil
10 Tbsp pumpkin seeds
1 ¼ tsp whole cumin seeds
½ cup olive oil
2 cups halved and thinly-sliced red onions
3 Tbsp apple cider vinegar
1 tsp pure maple syrup
1 tsp minced garlic
1 tsp salt
½ cup chopped parsley
¼ cup Parmesan cheese (optional)

Instructions

Preheat oven to 350°F. Line sheet pan with parchment paper or lightly oil.

Steam the cauliflower just until it is "tooth tender," 3 to 4 minutes, then plunge in a bath of ice water to stop the cooking. Drain well and set aside.

Toss the diced peppers with first measure of oil and roast in oven until softened and slightly blackened around edges, 20 to 30 minutes. At the same time, on another baking sheet, roast pumpkin seeds for 10 to 12 minutes. Cool completely.

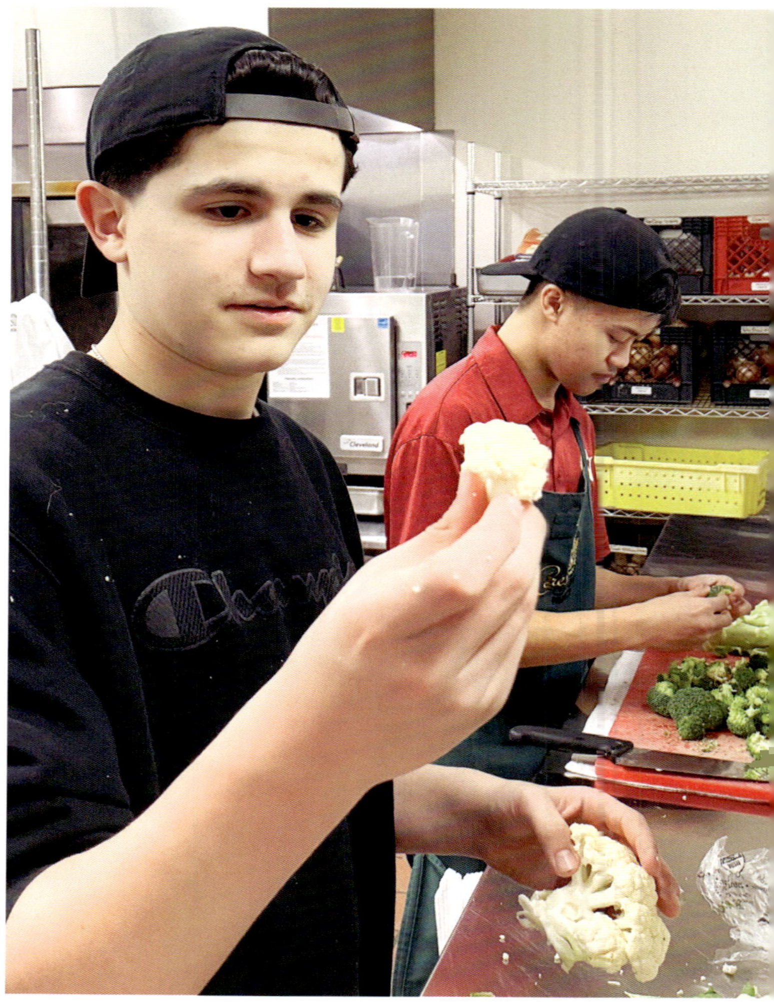

Pulse cumin seeds in spice grinder until broken up but not very fine.

Heat a skillet over medium heat. Add the second measure of olive oil, then add the red onion and pulsed cumin seeds. Cook until the onion is very soft, about 20 minutes. Onions may get slightly brown but try not to caramelize them. You may need to reduce the heat slightly or cover the pan. Scrape into a small bowl and cool completely, then mix in cider vinegar, garlic, maple syrup, and salt.

Combine cauliflower, peppers, onion mix, parsley, pumpkin seeds, and parmesan (if using) in a large bowl, tossing to mix everything evenly.

Nutrition info. *Serving size, 1½ cups: 349 calories, 27g fat, 7g carbohydrate, 429mg sodium*

Getting to know cauliflower in Ceres kitchen.

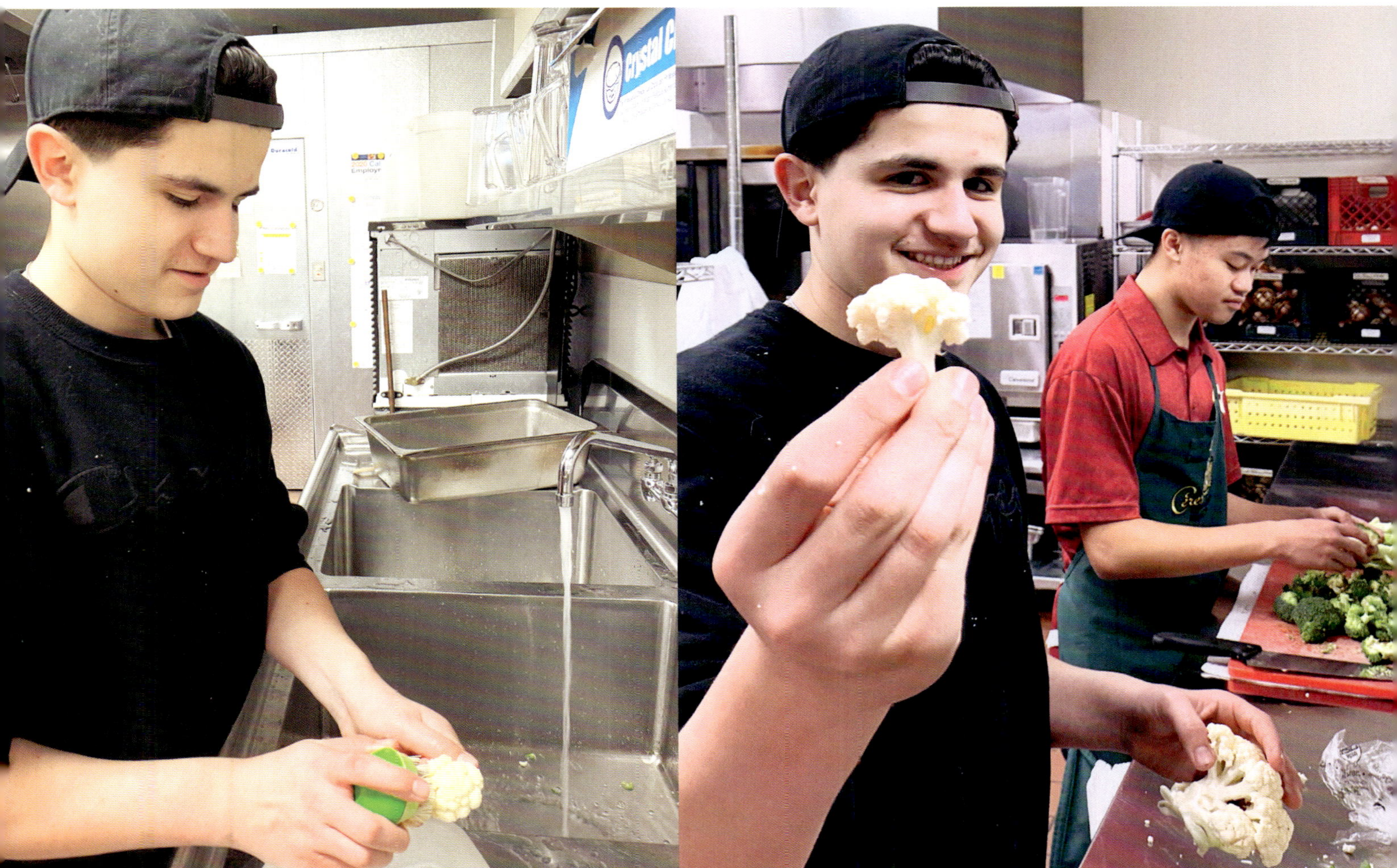

Broccoli Salad

Why not let one of the most nutritious vegetables be the key ingredient with a touch of sweetness from dried fruits? Best of both worlds.

— Det Kærlige Måltid Team

Serves 5
Prep time: 5 minutes
Cooking time: 5 minutes
Gluten-free
Dairy-free

Ingredients

Salad

4 cups small broccoli florets
1 medium red onion, diced
1 cup sunflower seeds
⅓ cup raisins
⅓ cup dried cranberries

Dressing

½ cup mayonnaise
2 Tbsp honey
2 Tbsp red wine vinegar
¾ tsp salt

Instructions

Place broccoli, onion, sunflower seeds, raisins, and cranberries in a large salad bowl.

In a small bowl, whisk together the mayonnaise, honey, red wine vinegar and salt.

Pour the dressing into the salad bowl and toss well to combine.

Nutrition info. *1 serving: 318 calories, 22g fat, 4g protein, 31g carbohydrate, 516mg sodium*

Kale Salad with Creamy Cashew Dressing

This hearty salad comes together quickly, and you'll have enough dressing left over for dipping and future salads.

— The Revive & Thrive Project Team

Serves 4
Prep time: 15 minutes, plus soaking nuts overnight
Vegan
Gluten-free

Ingredients

Salad

1 large bunch kale, stemmed and chopped
1 medium carrot, chopped
½ cucumber, peeled, seeded and chopped
¼ cup raisins

Dressing

1 cup cashews, soaked in 2 cups water overnight, then drained
1 clove garlic
1 ½ tsp ground onion powder
1 ½ tsp dried Italian seasoning
3 Tbsp water
2 tsp apple cider vinegar
2 tsp extra-virgin olive oil
¼ tsp salt
¼ tsp ground black pepper
Water as needed for consistency

Instructions

Combine salad ingredients in a large bowl and set aside.

For the dressing, combine all ingredients except water in a food processor or blender and blend until creamy. Add one tablespoon of water at a time to get the consistency you like.

To assemble, toss salad ingredients with enough dressing to lightly coat the greens and serve.

Nutrition info. *1 serving: 275 calories, 16g fat, 10g protein, 28g carbohydrate, 838mg sodium*

Citrus Burst Kale Salad with Spiced Chickpeas

"The food is so colorful it brightens my day."

— **Healing Meals Community Project Client**

Serves 8
Prep time: 20 minutes
Cooking time: 45 minutes
Vegan
Gluten-free

Ingredients

Spiced Chickpeas
2 cans low-sodium chickpeas, drained and rinsed
1 Tbsp salt
1 Tbsp smoked paprika
½ tsp chili powder
¼ tsp cayenne

Salad
2 pounds kale, stems removed and thinly sliced
1 head red cabbage, cored and shredded
2 cups shredded carrot

Dressing
1 Tbsp minced garlic
1 Tbsp fresh ginger, grated and squeezed for juice. Discard pulp.
1 Tbsp Dijon mustard
½ cup orange juice
1 cup olive oil
1 tsp salt
½ tsp fresh ground pepper

4 navel oranges, peeled and sectioned

Instructions

Spiced Chickpeas
Preheat oven to 400°F. Line a baking sheet with parchment paper or lightly oil.

Combine chickpeas with salt, paprika, chili powder and cayenne and toss to combine evenly. Spread chickpeas on the prepared sheet tray and bake for 45 minutes until they are lightly browned. Cool completely.

Salad
In a large bowl, toss the kale, red cabbage and carrots until evenly combined.

Dressing
Combine the garlic, ginger, mustard, and orange juice in a bowl. Slowly whisk in the olive oil. Add salt and pepper to taste.

To assemble, pour the dressing over the kale and toss well. Garnish the salad with orange sections and spiced chickpeas.

Nutrition info. *1 serving: 504 calories, 30g fat, 13g protein, 62g carbohydrate, 1mg sodium*

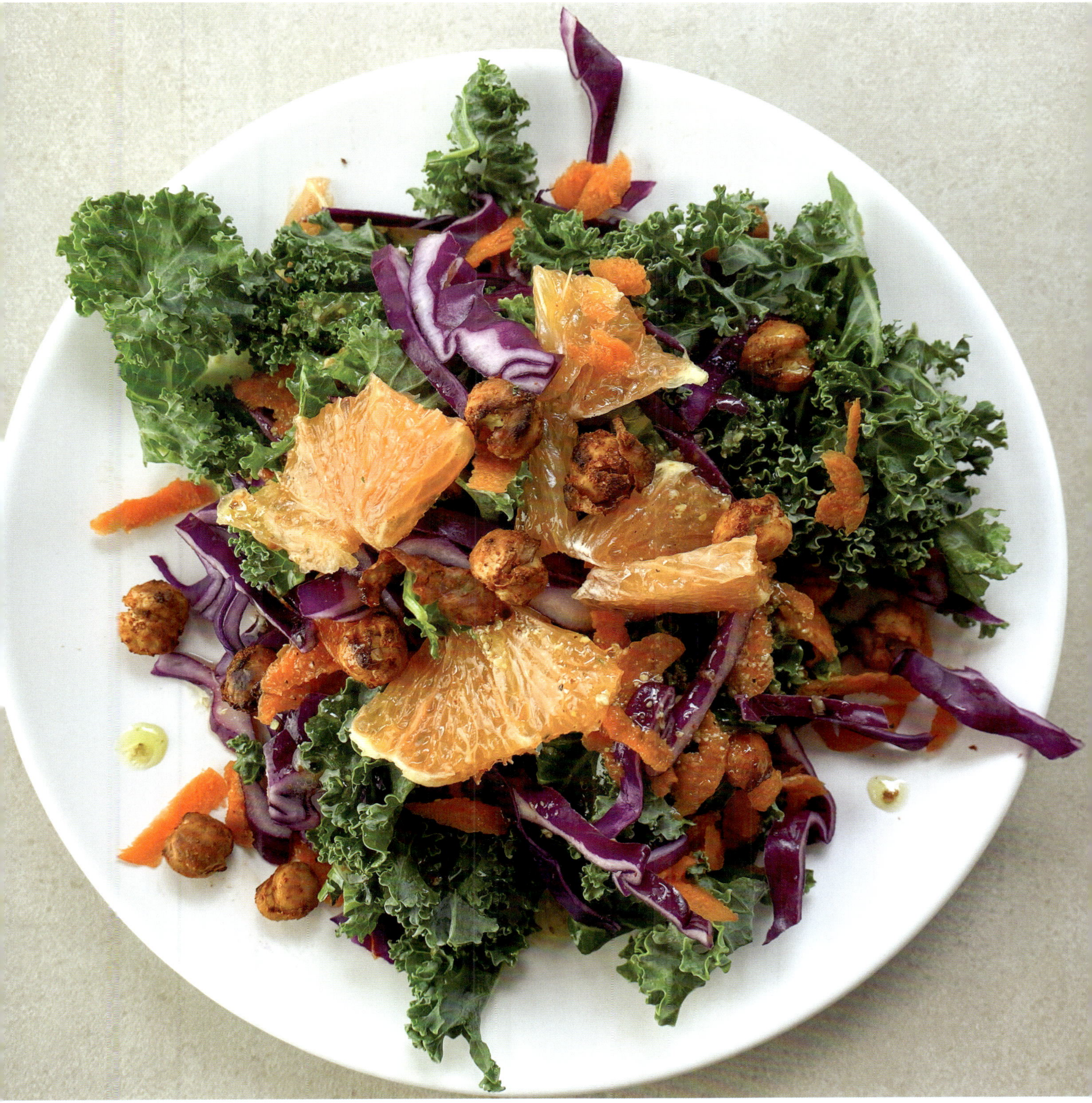

Harvest Kale Salad

Our farm and garden partners keep us covered in greens all growing season. We are amazed by their contributions to our meals and all the "healthy green" that is made possible because of their generosity. Everybody loves this salad rendition with a simple vinaigrette. For a heartier dish, serve it in a baked delicata squash half.

— The Meals 4 Health and Healing Team

Serves 4
Prep time: 10 minutes
Cooking time: 10 minutes
Vegan (if using agave syrup and almond cheese)
Gluten-free

Ingredients

2 Tbsp apple cider vinegar
¼ cup olive oil
½ Tbsp honey or agave syrup
¼ tsp salt
¼ tsp ground black pepper
3 cups baby kale, stemmed and chopped
1 golden beet, peeled, roasted and diced small; or raw and grated
¼ cup unsweetened dried cranberries
¼ cup raw shelled pumpkin seeds (pepitas)
¼ cup crumbled almond cheese or feta

Delicata squash, roasted and halved (optional)

Instructions

In a small bowl, make the dressing by whisking together vinegar, oil and honey. Taste, then add salt and ground black pepper to taste.

In a large salad bowl, mix together the kale, beets, dried cranberries, pepitas, and cheese. Toss with dressing. Refrigerate or serve immediately.

Nutrition info. *1 serving: 220 calories, 17g fat, 3 protein, 17g carbohydrate, 207mg sodium*

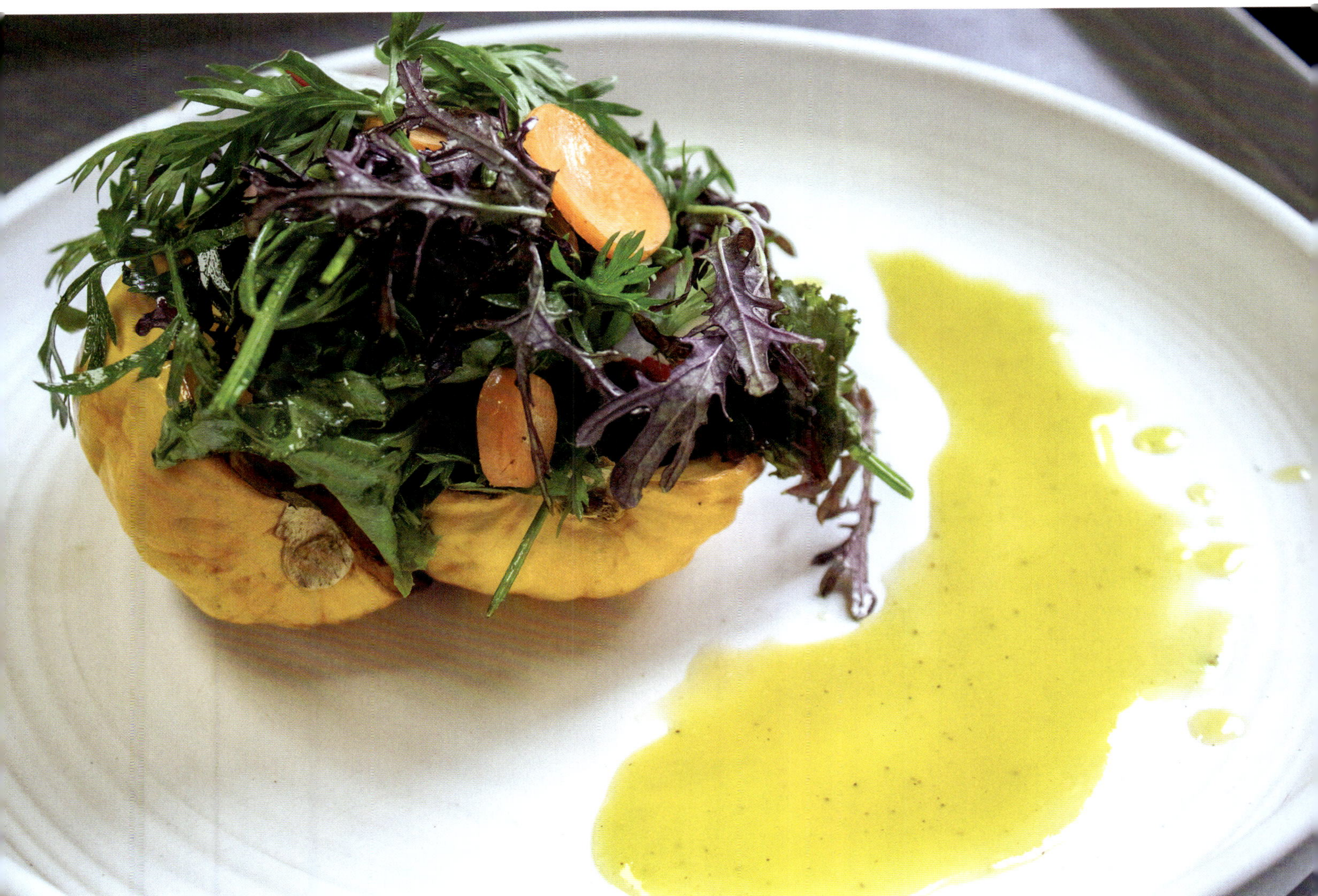

Spring Sweet Potato Thai Noodle Salad

This colorful salad features vegetable noodles. If you do not have a spiralizing tool, you can use a vegetable peeler to make long thin slices of the peeled sweet potato and the zucchini.

— Sarah Leathers, Healing Meals Community Project

Serves 4
Prep time: 15 minutes
Cooking time: 5 minutes
Vegan
Gluten-free

Ingredients

½ cup coconut milk
3 Tbsp almond butter
1 Tbsp curry paste

1 sweet potato, peeled and spiralized into thick noodles
1 cup spiralized zucchini
1 cup thinly sliced red pepper
1 cup thinly sliced green pepper
3 cups baby spinach
¼ cup fresh chopped cilantro
⅓ cup very thinly sliced scallions
¼ cup chopped cashews
4 lime wedges

Instructions

Heat coconut milk over medium heat, add almond butter and curry paste and stir until well combined. Cool completely.

Toss sweet potato, zucchini, peppers, spinach, cilantro and scallions together in a large bowl.

Pour sauce evenly over the vegetables and toss gently so that everything is evenly coated.

Serve with lime and cashews.

Nutrition info. *1 serving: 236 calories, 17g fat, 7g protein, 20g carbohydrate, 224mg sodium*

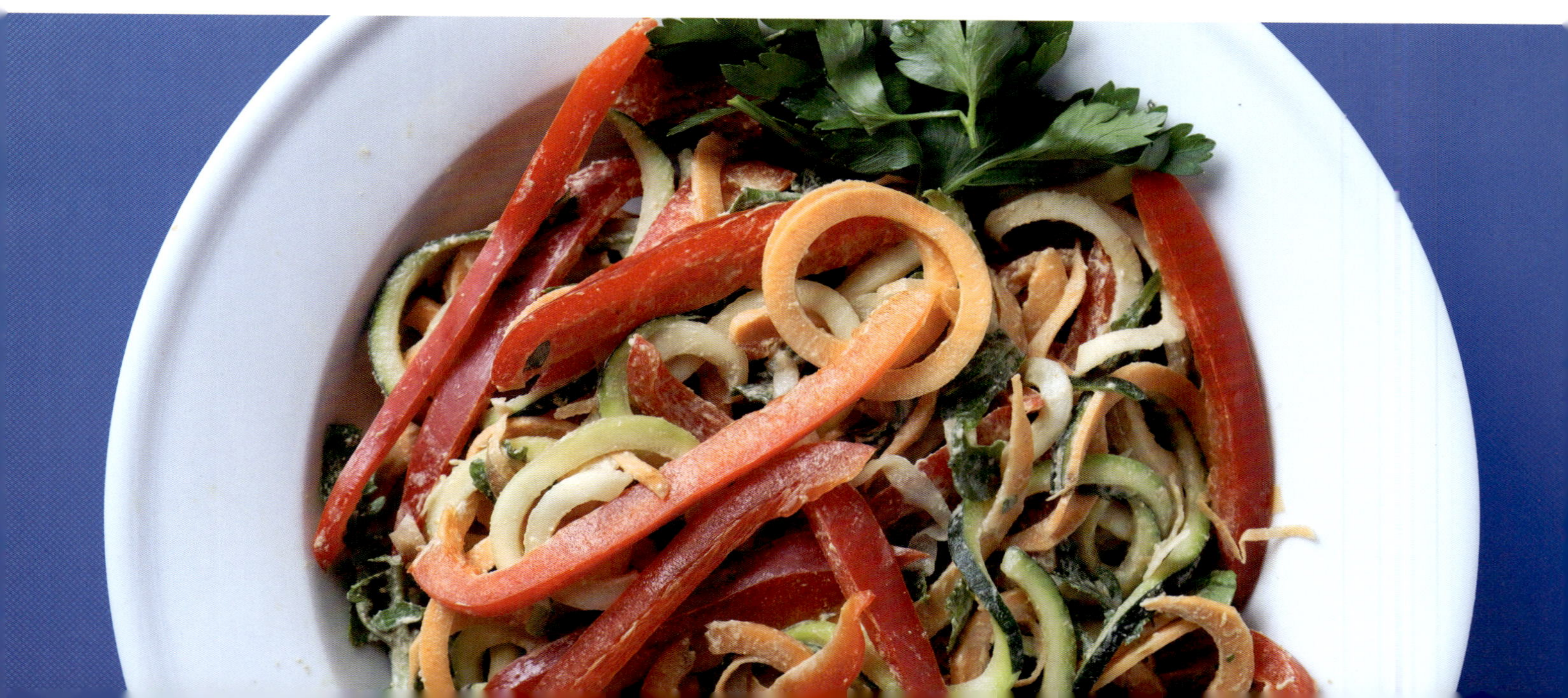

Farm Vegetable Chickpea Salad

With a solid, satisfying base like chickpeas, the sky is the limit for the variety of vegetables you can add to this dish – squashes, celery, carrots – your pick of what you can find at your farmer's market or in your own garden.

— The Meals 4 Health and Healing Team

Serves 6
Prep time: 45 minutes
Vegan
Gluten-free

Ingredients

1 Tbsp olive oil
½ orange bell pepper, diced
½ small red onion, thinly sliced in half-moons
2 cloves garlic, minced
½ tsp ground coriander
½ tsp ground cumin
2 cups assorted seasonal vegetables (sliced carrots, quarter slices of summer squash, small broccoli florets, small cauliflower florets)
1 cup cherry tomatoes, halved
3 Tbsp white wine vinegar
2 tsp chopped parsley
3 cups cooked chickpeas, or 2 cans chickpeas, drained and rinsed
Shaved fennel (optional)
Sliced celery (optional)
½ tsp salt
Ground black pepper to taste

Instructions

In a large skillet, heat olive oil over medium-high heat. Add the peppers, onion and garlic and sauté for 2 minutes until just starting to soften. Add the coriander, cumin, and seasonal vegetables. Sauté 3 to 5 minutes longer, just until vegetables are crisp tender. Let cool.

In a large bowl, combine the sautéed vegetables, tomatoes, vinegar, parsley, chickpeas, and fresh fennel and celery, if using. Gently toss to combine. Season to taste with salt and pepper.

Nutrition info. *1 serving: 189 calories, 5g fat, 8g protein, 28g carbohydrate, 235mg sodium*

Moroccan Lentil Salad with Cauliflower Rice

We love this salad because not only does it give you all the flavors you often crave (salty olives, sweet apricots, satisfying lentils) but it is also gluten- and dairy-free! While we make our own spice blend, you can also purchase a ready-made mix.

— Chef Molly Evans, Fox Valley Food for Health

Serves 7
Prep time: 1¼ hours
Cooking time: 30 minutes
Gluten-free
Vegan

Ingredients

Ras El Hanout (Moroccan spice blend)

½ tsp ground cumin
½ tsp ground ginger
½ tsp salt
Mounded ¼ tsp ground black pepper
¼ tsp ground coriander
¼ tsp cayenne pepper
¼ tsp ground allspice

1 cup dried green lentils, sorted and rinsed
4 cups water
½ tsp salt

5 cups purchased cauliflower rice, defrosted
2 Tbsp olive oil

4 cups loosely packed Tuscan kale, stems removed and chopped in 1″ pieces
2 tsp Ras El Hanout
1 ¼ cups shredded carrots
½ cup chopped pistachios or almonds, toasted in a 325°F oven for 8 minutes
¼ cup chopped dried Turkish apricots
¼ cup quartered or chopped Kalamata olives

Dressing

⅔ cup olive oil
½ cup apple cider vinegar
2 Tbsp Dijon mustard
4 tsp pure maple syrup
1 small shallot, minced
1 tsp salt
¼ tsp ground black pepper

Instructions

In a small bowl, whisk Ras El Hanout spice blend ingredients together. Set aside.

Place lentils in a saucepan with water and ½ teaspoon salt. Bring to boil, then reduce heat and cover. Simmer for about 30 minutes or until just tender. Do not overcook. Drain in a sieve and set aside to cool.

While the lentils are cooking, preheat oven to 400°F. In a large bowl, toss defrosted cauliflower rice with the olive oil. Transfer rice to two oiled 13″ x 18″ sheet pans, spreading it evenly across the pan. Roast for 10-15 minutes, stirring occasionally, until tender and beginning to brown. Set aside on a rack to cool. If you only have one pan, roast in two batches.

Meanwhile in a large bowl toss kale with Ras El Hanout spice mix. Add carrots, toasted nuts,

apricots, and olives. Add cooled cauliflower rice and lentils; toss until evenly combined.

For the dressing, in a small bowl, whisk together olive oil, vinegar, mustard, maple syrup, shallot, salt, and pepper. Add two-thirds of the vinaigrette to the lentil mixture; toss to coat. Taste and, if needed, add more dressing.

Cover salad and chill for at least 30 minutes or until ready to serve. You may add additional chopped toasted nuts, olives and apricots as garnishes.

***Nutrition info.** 1 serving: 395 calories, 27g fat, 10g protein, 40g carbohydrate, 640mg sodium*

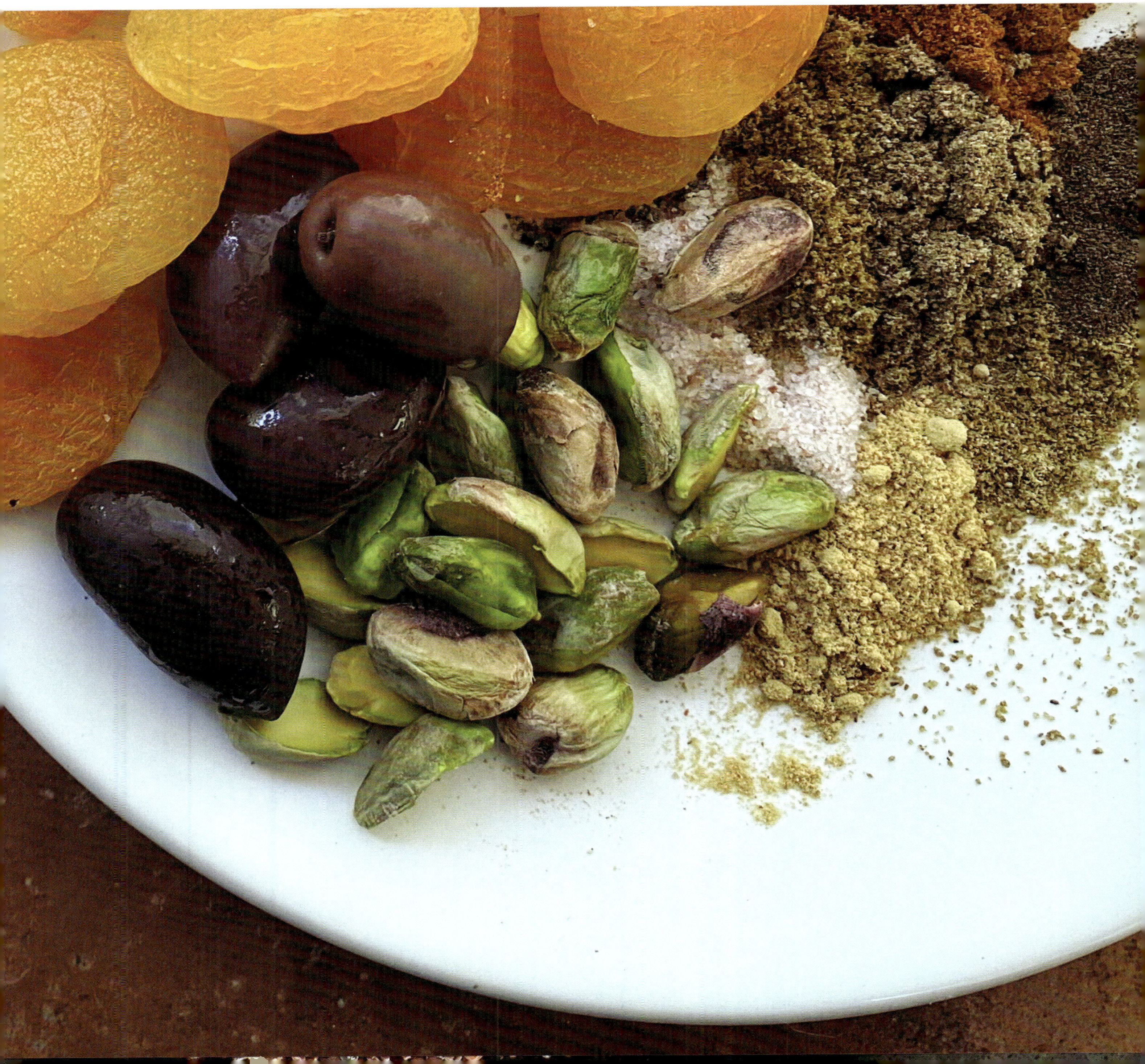

Orange Pistachio Quinoa Salad

"Thank you very much for your kindness, and your delicious food. I can tell you all put a lot of thought and love in your food."

— Healing Meals Community Project client

Serves 6
Prep time: 15 minutes
Cooking time: 15 minutes
Vegan
Gluten-free

Ingredients

½ cup raw pistachios
1 ½ cups quinoa
2 ½ cups Healing Vegetable Broth (see page 106) or water
2 tsp salt, divided
1 tsp ground cumin
½ tsp ground coriander
⅛ tsp freshly ground black pepper
½ cup chopped fresh mint
2 scallions, both green and white parts, finely chopped
2 Tbsp freshly squeezed orange juice
zest of 1 orange
1 ½ Tbsp olive oil
1 ½ Tbsp freshly squeezed lemon juice
½ cup raisins
1 cup cooked or canned chickpeas, drained and rinsed (optional)

Instructions

Preheat the oven to 325°F. Line a sheet pan with parchment paper or lightly oil.

Spread pistachios in an even layer on sheet pan and bake for 7 to 10 minutes, until aromatic and slightly browned. Let cool.

Place the quinoa in a fine-mesh strainer and rinse well under cold running water to remove all the resin.

In a pot, bring the broth or water and 1 tsp salt to a boil. Add the quinoa and cover. Decrease the heat to low and simmer for 15 minutes. Transfer from the heat and fluff with a fork. Spread mixture out on a sheet pan and "rake" with a fork occasionally until cooled.

Transfer the quinoa from the sheet pan to a large bowl. Stir in the cumin, coriander, 1 tsp salt, and pepper. Add the mint, scallions, orange juice, orange zest, olive oil, lemon juice, toasted pistachios, and raisins. Mix well and taste; you may need a pinch of salt, a squeeze of lemon, or a dash of olive oil. If desired, mix chickpeas into salad. Serve chilled.

Nutrition info. *1 serving: 329 calories, 10g fat, 11g protein, 50g carbohydrate, 649mg sodium*

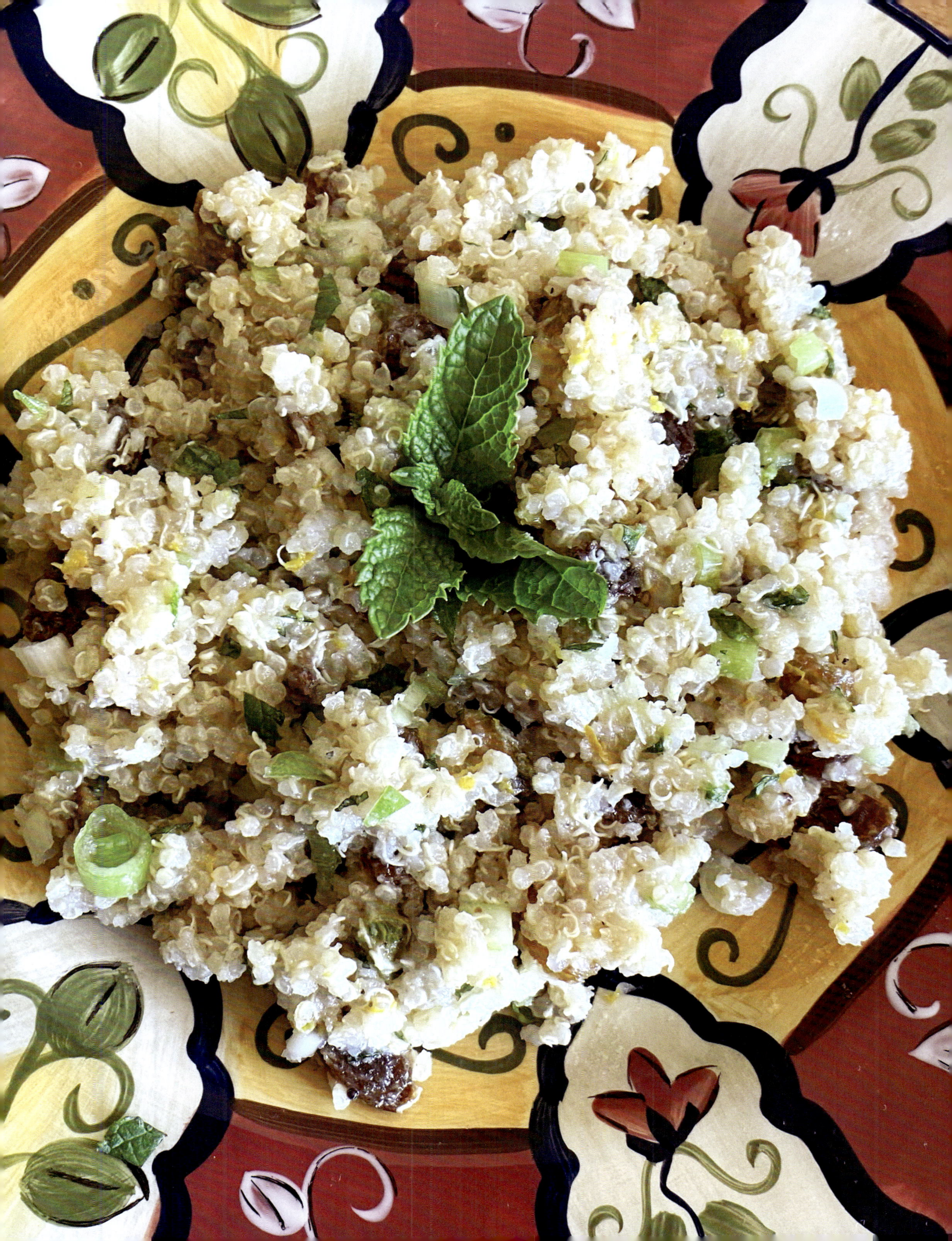

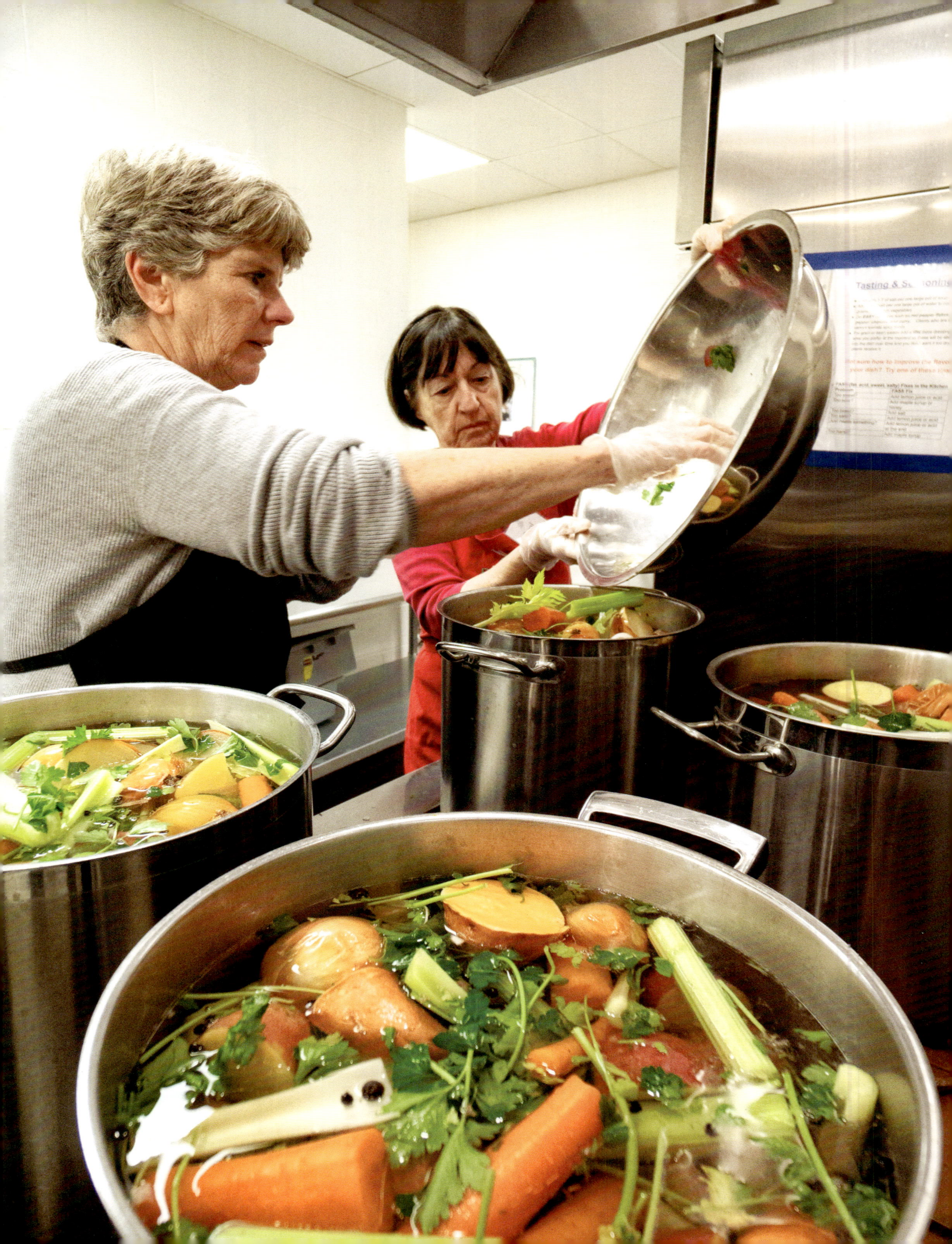

SOUPS & STEWS

Healing Vegetable Broth

Thanks to Rebecca Katz, long-time Ceres supporter and author of Cancer Fighting Kitchen, for her Magic Mineral Broth which we adapted for this recipe. This broth can be sipped on its own if you aren't feeling well, but it's also a great base for soup or for cooking grains.

— The Ceres Community Project Team

Serves 6 (about 12 cups)
Prep time: 10 minutes
Cooking time: 2 to 4 hours
Gluten-free
Vegan

Ingredients

3 carrots
1 medium yellow onion
4 stalks celery, chopped
2 cloves garlic, not peeled
1 cup chopped parsley
2 red potatoes, quartered
1 sweet potato, chopped in 1-inch cubes
1 bay leaf
1 6-inch strip dried kombu seaweed
¼ tsp whole peppercorns
¼ tsp whole allspice
16 cups water

Instructions

Wash all vegetables well, but don't peel.

Place all the ingredients in a large soup pot. Add water and bring to a boil.

Reduce the heat to low, partially cover, and simmer for at least 2 hours and up to 4, adding more water if needed.

Let the broth cool, then strain the stock with a fine mesh strainer, pressing out as much liquid as possible.

Package the broth in containers and store in the refrigerator or freezer.

NOTE: For Immune Broth, add these items to base recipe: ½ ounce (15 grams) dried sliced reishi mushrooms (a small handful), 1 ounce (30 grams) dried codonopsis root (about ¼ cup), and 1 ounce (30 grams) astragalus root slices (a handful).

Nutrition info. *Serving size, 2 cups: 157 calories, 6g fat, 4g protein, 35g carbohydrate, 291mg sodium*

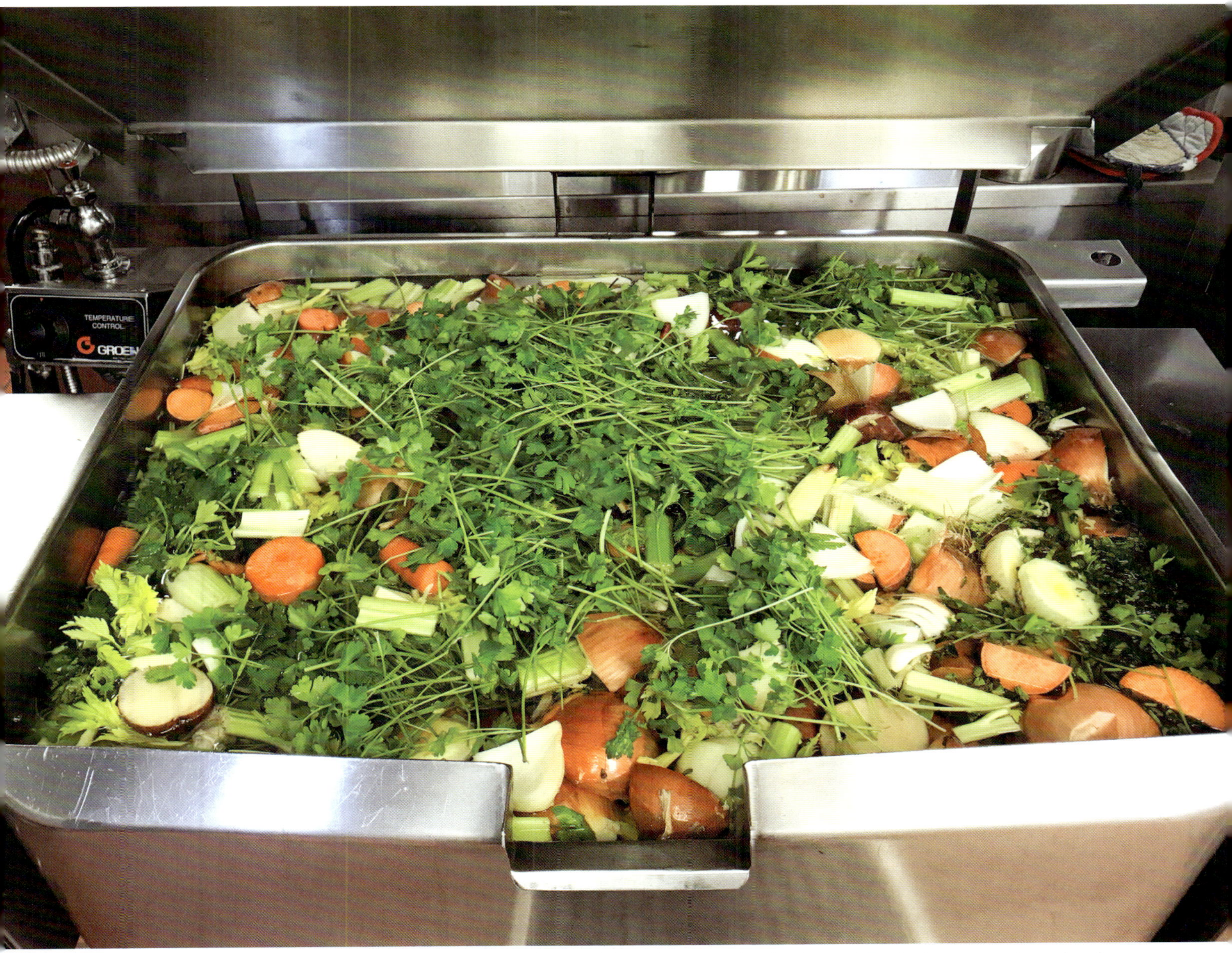

Healing Vegetable Broth brewing in the Ceres kitchen and (previous page) volunteers at Fox Valley preparing a broth.

Healing Chicken Broth

A terrific way to use leftover chicken or beef bones, this can cook unattended in a crock pot or even in a stock pot on your stove. Start it early in the morning and let it cook all day. You'll be rewarded with rich broth full of nutrients.

— The Ceres Community Project Team

Serves 6 (about 12 cups)
Prep time: 30 minutes
Cooking time: 12 to 24 hours
Gluten-free
Dairy-free

Ingredients

1 whole chicken, or 2 to 3 pounds bony chicken parts such as wings, necks, and backs
20 cups water
2 Tbsp apple cider vinegar
1 6-inch strip dried kombu seaweed
1 medium yellow onion, chopped
3 carrots, chopped
4 stalks of celery, chopped
1 bay leaf
¼ tsp peppercorns
¼ tsp whole allspice
2 garlic cloves, not peeled
1 cup chopped parsley

Instructions

Place the chicken and water in a large soup pot. Bring to a boil, cover and simmer until the meat is tender and will easily fall off of the bones, about 1 hour.

Strain the broth into a second large pot. Place the chicken in a bowl to cool. Remove all of the meat from the bones and store in the refrigerator for another use.

Put the bones back in the soup pot with the broth. Add the vinegar, kombu, onion, carrots, celery, bay leaf, peppercorns, allspice, garlic and parsley. Cover and bring the broth to a low boil.

Reduce the heat to very low. Simmer for 12 to 24 hours, covered, adding more water if needed to keep the ingredients all covered.

Let the broth cool. Strain the stock with a fine mesh strainer. When the broth is cool, the fat will solidify on the top and can be removed with a spoon.

Package the broth in containers and store in the refrigerator or freezer.

Nutrition info. *Serving size, 2 cups: 200 calories, 8g fat, 18g protein, 13g carbohydrate, 310mg sodium*

Zucchini and Eggplant Summer Soup

"What do you do with all that zucchini?" asks every first-time gardener. Here's the answer from Positive Community Kitchen. To chiffonade the basil, stack the leaves atop one another, then roll them into a cigar shape and cut into thin ribbons using a very sharp knife.

— The Positive Community Kitchen Team

Serves 4
Prep time: 20 minutes
Cooking time: 40 minutes
Vegan
Gluten-free

Ingredients

1 Tbsp olive oil
2 cups peeled ½-inch cubes eggplant
½ cup small diced onion
2 cups ½-inch cubes zucchini
½ cup carrot half moons
¾ cup diced tomatoes, with juice (fresh or canned)
2 Tbsp small diced red bell pepper
1 tsp dried thyme, or 2 tsp chopped fresh thyme
½ tsp dried oregano, or 1 tsp chopped fresh oregano
1 Tbsp tomato paste
3 cups vegetable broth
¾ tsp salt
½ tsp ground white pepper
½ cup uncooked gluten-free pasta, preferably rotini or bowtie
2 Tbsp fresh basil chiffonade

Instructions

In a large soup pot, heat oil over medium-low heat. Add eggplant and cook, stirring often, until it starts to brown, about 5 to 7 minutes. Eggplant soaks up a lot of oil, so you may need to add more as you go.

Add onion and cook an additional 5 minutes. Add zucchini, carrot, tomatoes, peppers, thyme, oregano, tomato paste, broth, salt, and pepper. Bring to a simmer, partially cover, and cook until vegetables are just tender. Partially purée using an immersion blender. Return to the stove and add the pasta. Cook until pasta is al dente, about 15 minutes.

Taste for seasoning and add more salt and pepper, as necessary. Stir in basil just before serving.

Nutrition info. *1 serving: 192 calories, 4g fat, 5g protein, 36g carbohydrate, 438mg sodium*

Mexican Cabbage Soup

Farm partners frequently supply our Meals 4 Health and Healing program with cabbage. We love cabbage as a comforting cruciferous vegetable rich in nutrients that boost digestion and keep inflammation in check.

— The Meals 4 Health and Healing Team

Serves 4
Prep time: 10 minutes
Cooking time: 45 minutes
Vegan
Gluten-free

Ingredients

1 Tbsp avocado or olive oil
1 small onion, diced
1 small red bell pepper, diced
4 cups chopped green cabbage
4 cloves garlic, minced
1 tsp ground cumin
½ tsp ground coriander
½ tsp dried oregano
1 (6-ounce) can tomato paste
1 (14-ounce) can diced or crushed tomatoes
3 cups vegetable broth
2 cups cooked black beans, or 1 (14-ounce can), rinsed and drained
2 Tbsp chopped fresh cilantro
1 lime, zested and juiced
Salt and ground black pepper

Instructions

Warm a large stockpot over medium high heat. Coat the bottom of the pan with oil and sauté onions, peppers, and cabbage with a pinch of salt for 3 to 5 minutes until softened.

Add garlic, cumin, coriander, and oregano and sauté for 30 to 60 seconds, until aromatic. Add tomato paste, tomatoes, broth and black beans and bring to a boil.

Turn down to a simmer and cook, slightly covered, until flavors combine, about 35 to 40 minutes. Stir in cilantro and lime juice and zest (to taste). Season to taste with salt and pepper and serve hot.

Nutrition info *1 serving: 136 calories, 3g fat, 5g protein, 26g carbohydrate, 97mg sodium*

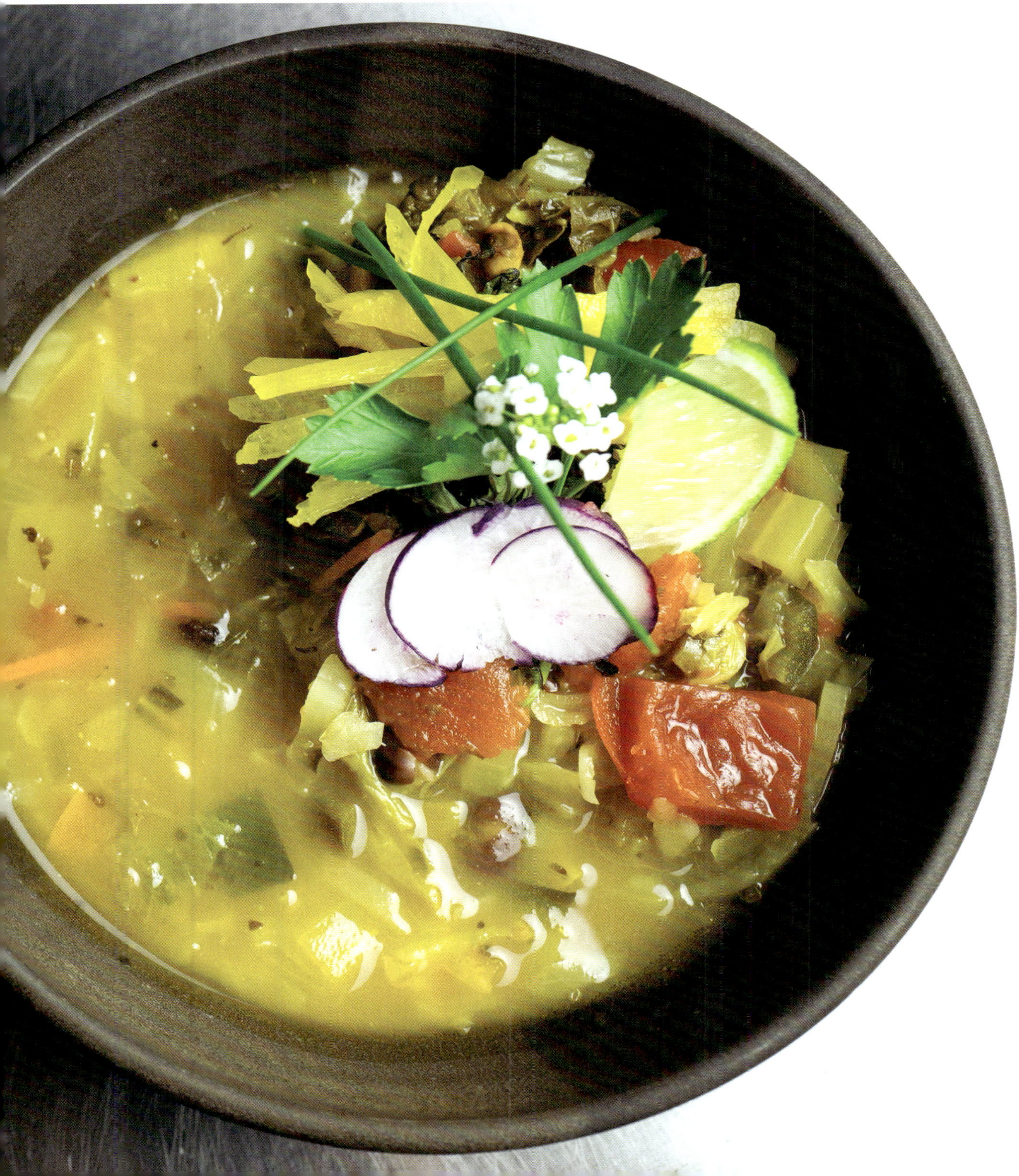

Tomato and Roasted Red Pepper Soup

We have many varieties of sweet red peppers pouring into our kitchen during the summer thanks to our local farmers and the Mendocino College Agriculture Department who grow produce for us! We take the time to roast them and purée into a concentrated paste that adds a flavorful punch to our recipes in the winter.

— The Caring Kitchen Project Team

Serves 6
Prep time: 20 minutes
Cooking time: 60 minutes
Vegan, if made with vegetable broth
Gluten-free, if made with rice or gluten-free pasta

Ingredients

2 medium red peppers
3 Tbsp olive oil, divided
1 cup diced onion
1 Tbsp minced garlic
½ cup grated carrots
4 ½ cups vegetable or chicken broth
5 cups tomato juice
1 ½ cups diced potatoes
1 Tbsp lemon juice
1 tsp salt
¼ tsp ground black pepper
⅛ tsp ground cumin
⅛ tsp ground coriander
1 cup diced carrots
1 ½ cup cooked short grain brown rice or cooked orzo pasta

***Nutrition info.** Serving size, 2 cup: 217 calories, 8g fat, 5g protein, 35g carbohydrate, 963mg sodium*

Instructions

Preheat the oven to 375°F. Line a sheet pan with parchment paper or lightly oil.

Cut peppers in half lengthwise and remove seeds. Toss the peppers in 1 tablespoon olive oil to coat and place cut side down on your prepared sheet pan. Cook in oven for 20 minutes. Reduce oven to 325°F and cook for 45 minutes more, or until very soft. Let cool, then peel and set aside.

While cooking the peppers, heat remaining olive oil in a large pot over medium heat. Add onions and cook for 10 minutes stirring often. Reduce heat if onions start to brown. Add garlic and grated carrots and cook for 2 more minutes.

Add broth, tomato juice, roasted peppers and potatoes and bring to boil. Simmer about 10 minutes or until potatoes are soft. Add lemon juice, salt, pepper, cumin, and coriander. Purée until smooth.

While the soup is cooking, cook the diced carrots in simmering water until tender.

After the soup is puréed, add the diced carrots and cooked rice or orzo.

NOTE: You can prepare extra red bell peppers by puréeing with oil and water as needed and freezing in 1 cup containers to enjoy this soup year-round, or to use in any soup or sauce.

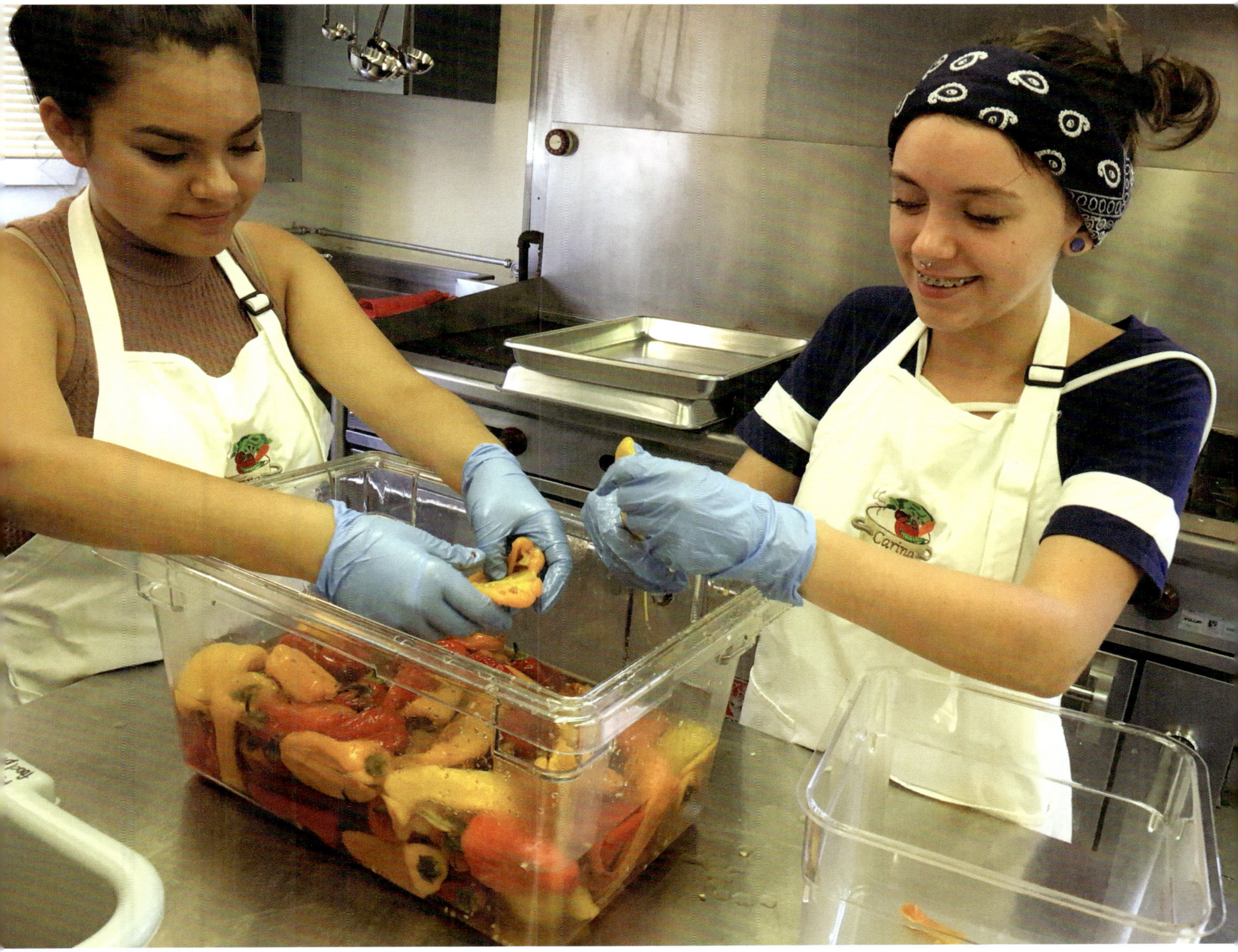

Teens from the Caring Kitchen Project preparing peppers.

Potato Soup

We love potatoes in Denmark and when winter's chill sets in, this is our go-to warm-you-up-from-the-inside dish.

— Det Kærlige Måltid Team

Serves 4
Prep time: 10 minutes
Cooking time: 30 minutes
Gluten-free

Ingredients

2 Tbsp olive oil
2 pounds potatoes, peeled and cubed
3 cups roughly chopped leeks
1 to 2 cloves garlic
5-½ cups vegetable broth
½ tsp salt
½ tsp ground black pepper
¾ cup heavy whipping cream
1 Tbsp apple cider vinegar

Instructions

In a large pot, heat olive oil over medium heat. Sauté potatoes, leeks and garlic until garlic is aromatic, 2 to 3 minutes.

Add vegetable broth, salt and pepper. Put the lid on, bring to a boil and then lower heat and simmer, covered, for 20 minutes or until the potatoes have softened.

Blend the soup with an immersion blender until smooth and creamy. Add the cream and season with apple cider vinegar and additional salt and pepper to taste.

Nutrition info: *1 serving. 427 calories, 23g fat, 7g protein, 51g carbohydrate, 404g sodium*

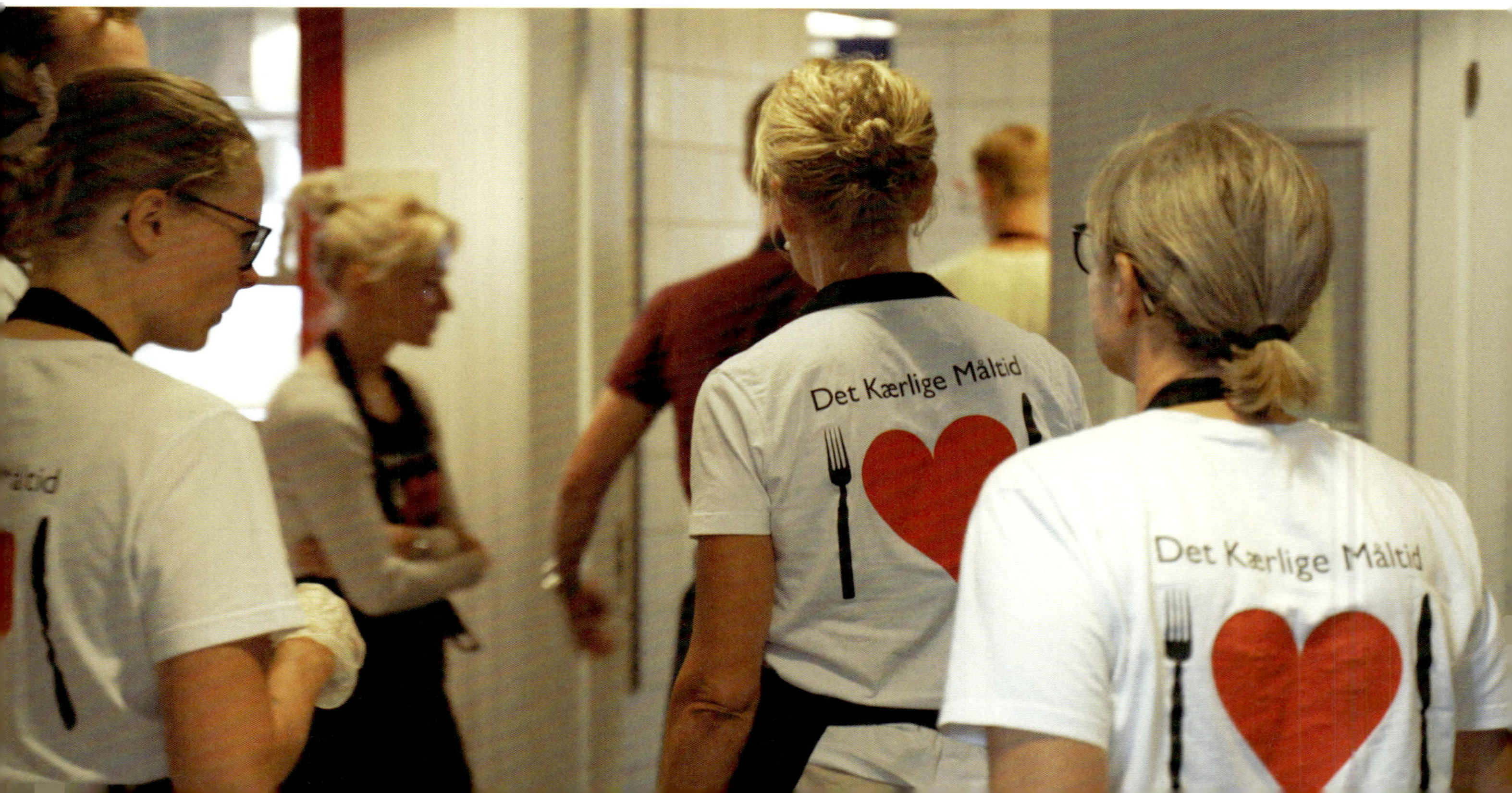

Butternut Squash Bisque

We love this rich, hearty bisque so much. Nothing says comfort like butternut squash. We enhanced its presentation once by pouring it into hollowed out miniature pumpkin bowls. So fun!

— The Meals 4 Health and Healing Team

Serves: 4
Prep time: 20 minutes
Cooking time: 55 minutes
Vegan
Gluten-free

Ingredients

2 tsp coconut oil
1 leek, sliced
1 turnip, diced
4 cups peeled 2-inch cubes butternut squash
3 cloves garlic, smashed
½ tsp Health and Healing Spice Blend (see page 77)
4 cups vegetable broth
1 sprig of thyme
8 sprigs of sage, divided
Salt and ground black pepper to taste

Instructions

Warm a soup pot over medium high heat and melt coconut oil. Sauté leeks and turnips until softened, about 5 minutes, adding a pinch of salt and pepper. Add squash, spice blend, broth, thyme, and half of the sage with another pinch of salt and pepper. Bring to a boil.

Reduce heat and simmer until squash is fork tender, about 45 minutes. Remove thyme sprig and purée with an immersion blender until smooth.

Garnish with remaining sage leaves and serve hot.

Nutrition info. *1 serving: 143 calories, 3g fat, 3g protein, 30g carbohydrate, 149g sodium*

Creamy Delicata Soup

One of our volunteers provided this recipe when we had an abundance of delicata squash from our garden. It makes for easy prep since the squash does not have to be peeled.

— Chef Molly Evans, Fox Valley Food for Health

Serves: 10
Prep time: 15 minutes
Cooking time: 45 minutes
Gluten-free

Ingredients

5 pounds delicata squash
¼ cup olive oil
2 ½ cups chopped onions
6 to 8 cloves garlic, peeled and minced
10 cups vegetable or chicken broth
1 tsp salt
1 tsp hot sauce
1 ½ cups whole milk
½ cup heavy cream

Instructions

Preheat oven to 375°F. Line a baking sheet with parchment paper or lightly oil.

Trim ends off squash, cut lengthwise and scoop out seeds (leave skin on). Place cut side down on prepared sheet pan, cover squash with foil and bake for 30 minutes or until tender. A fork should pierce the squash easily.

While the squash is baking, heat the olive oil in a large stockpot over medium heat. Add onions and cook for about 5 minutes or until tender and translucent. Add the garlic and cook for 2 to 3 more minutes, stirring to prevent browning.

When squash is tender, cut into half moons (leave the skin on—it is edible) and add to the pot along with stock.

Using an immersion blender, purée the soup until it is very smooth. Add salt and hot sauce to taste. Add the milk and cream as needed until you reach desired consistency. Taste and adjust the seasonings, if necessary.

Nutrition info. *Serving size, 1 ½ cups: 271 calories, 14g fat, 6g protein, 36g carbohydrate, 311mg sodium*

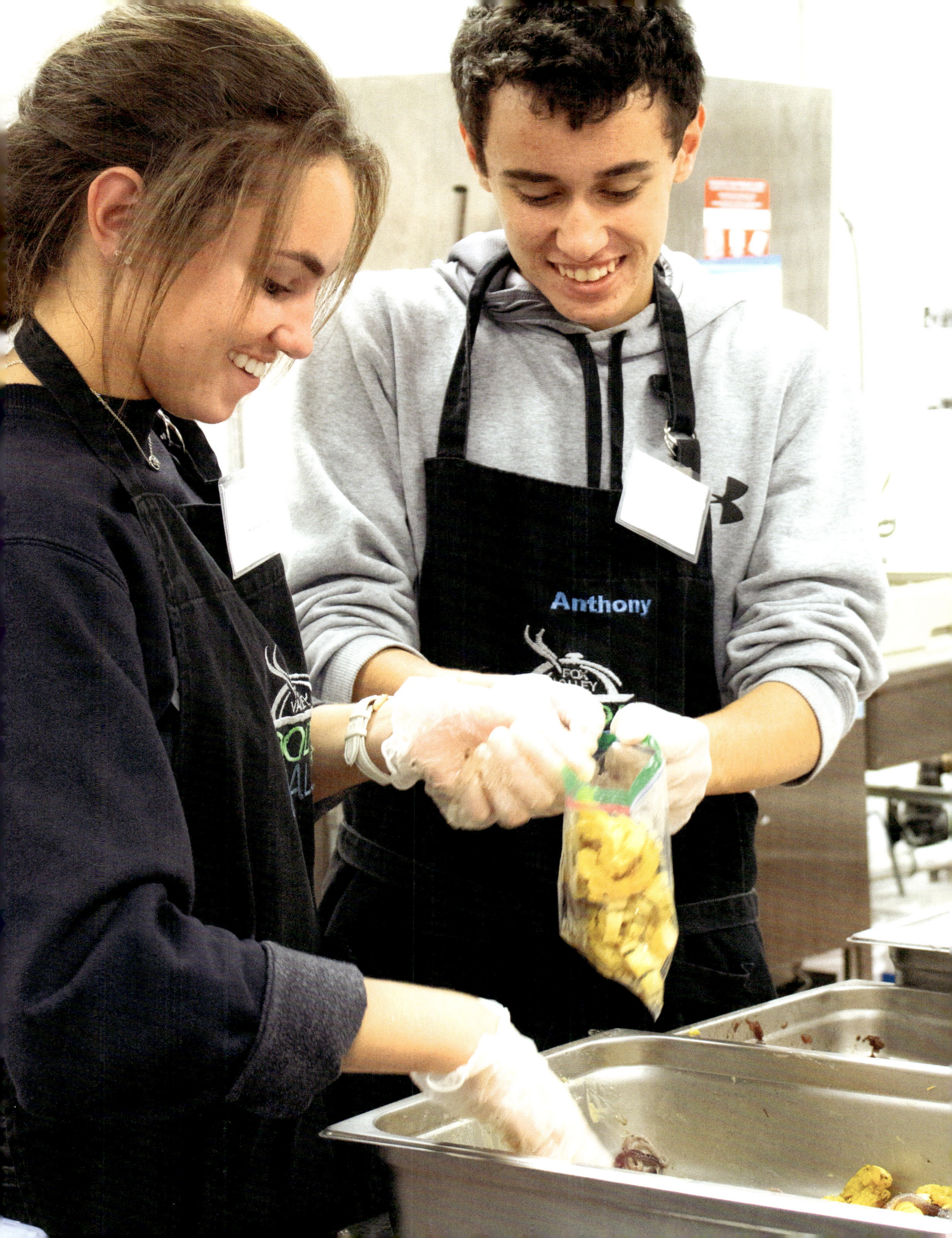
Anthony

Chickpea Miso Soup

The softened cabbage and bok choy, along with the chickpea pasta, add the bulk in this creamy, sweet soup. But it's the ginger, a distinct spice with anti-inflammatory properties, that definitely adds the exotic punch of flavor!

— The Meals 4 Health and Healing Team

Serves: 4
Prep time: 20 to 25 minutes
Cooking time: 15 minutes
Vegan
Gluten-free

Ingredients

2 Tbsp olive oil
1 small onion, thinly sliced into half moons
1 Tbsp ginger juice, grate, squeeze and discard pulp
3 to 4 cloves garlic, minced
1 cup shredded cabbage
1 cup sliced baby bok choy
¼ tsp toasted sesame oil
3 cups low-sodium vegetable broth
2 Tbsp coconut aminos or 1 Tbsp low-sodium tamari
½ cup chickpea miso paste or white miso paste
1 cup cooked chickpea pasta, any small shape
2 Tbsp bias-sliced scallions

Instructions

Heat oil in a soup pot over medium heat.

Add onions and sauté until softened, about 3 minutes. Add ginger juice and garlic. Cook until onions are starting to turn golden, about 5 minutes.

Add 2 tablespoons water, cabbage, bok choy and sesame oil. Cook for another 2 minutes.

Add broth and bring to a boil. Cover and simmer for another 3 to 5 minutes.

Stir in coconut aminos (or tamari) and miso paste. Taste for flavor. Add pre-cooked chickpea pasta and heat just until simmering. Do not allow to boil.

Serve, garnished with scallions.

Nutrition info. *1 Serving: 213 calories, 7g fat, 2g protein, 35g carbohydrate, 1400mg sodium*

Mulligatawny Soup

Our go-to for a heartwarming, comforting meal. This is one of Chef Nicole's family favorites which she graciously shared with Positive Community Kitchen.

— The Positive Community Kitchen Team

Serves: 4
Prep time: 20 minutes, plus soaking time
Cooking time: 1 hour
Vegan
Gluten-free

Ingredients

⅔ cup lentils, soaked 4 to 6 hours, drained, and rinsed
1 Tbsp coconut oil
¾ cup small diced onion
¾ tsp salt, divided
1 Tbsp minced garlic
1 Tbsp minced fresh ginger
1 tsp ground cumin
1 tsp ground coriander
½ tsp ground cinnamon
1 tsp curry powder
¾ cup cooked chickpeas
¾ cup thinly sliced celery
⅓ cup thinly sliced carrot half moons
¾ cup peeled and ½-inch cubes apple
3 cups vegetable broth
⅓ cup coconut milk
1 Tbsp lemon juice
1 Tbsp chopped fresh cilantro

Instructions

Heat oil in a soup pot over low heat. Add the onion, a sprinkle of salt and cook until translucent, about 5 minutes. Add the garlic and ginger and let cook for several more minutes. Add cumin, coriander, cinnamon and curry powder and stir to release their flavor.

Add the chickpeas, celery, carrot, and apple and stir to coat with the spices. Add lentils, broth, salt, and coconut milk. Bring to a boil, then reduce to a simmer and cook, partially covered, until lentils and vegetables are tender, about 1 hour.

Finish with lemon juice. Garnish with cilantro when serving.

Nutrition info. *1 serving: 268 calories, 9g fat, 12g protein, 39g carbohydrate, 467mg sodium*

Curried Red Lentil Soup

The blend of spices and ginger make this soup deliciously fragrant. The red lentils cook down quickly and make a thick, smooth soup, even better when puréed in the blender. Clients who thought they didn't like lentil soup, found a new favorite in this one.

— The Caring Kitchen Project Team

Serves 8
Prep time: 30 minutes
Cooking time: 30 minutes
Vegan
Gluten-free

Ingredients

Spice mix

½ tsp ground coriander
½ tsp paprika
½ tsp ground turmeric
½ tsp ground cumin

Soup

3 Tbsp avocado or olive oil
⅓ cup diced onion
2 tsp minced fresh garlic
2 tsp fresh ginger, grated and squeezed for juice. Discard pulp. Or use peeled and finely chopped ginger
½ tsp salt, or to taste
9 cups vegetable broth
2 Tbsp roasted tomato purée or tomato paste
1 large garnet sweet potato, peeled and cut into ¼-inch cubes
¾ cup diced carrots
1 ¼ cups dried red lentils, rinsed and drained
1 Tbsp lemon juice

Garnish

Vegan or regular yogurt, pomegranate seeds (optional)

Instructions

Combine spice mix ingredients in small bowl. Set aside.

Heat oil in a soup pot over medium heat. Add onion. Cook, stirring often until tender and beginning to brown, about 6 minutes. Add garlic and ginger and cook 2 more minutes.

Add spice mix and salt. Cook, stirring constantly until fragrant, 1 to 2 minutes.

Add broth, tomato, sweet potatoes, carrots, and lentils. Bring to a boil, reduce heat, and simmer until lentils are tender, about 20 minutes.

Working in batches, transfer mixture to a blender (or use an immersion blender). Carefully process until smooth. Stir in lemon juice and salt to taste.

Garnish with yogurt and pomegranate seeds if desired.

NOTE: Some broths may be salty, so wait to add salt until after you taste the finished soup.

Nutrition info. *Serving size, 1 ¾ cups: 194 calories, 4g fat, 9g protein, 32g carbohydrate, 220mg sodium*

"The soups are my favorite!" says Ceres client, Mary Lou

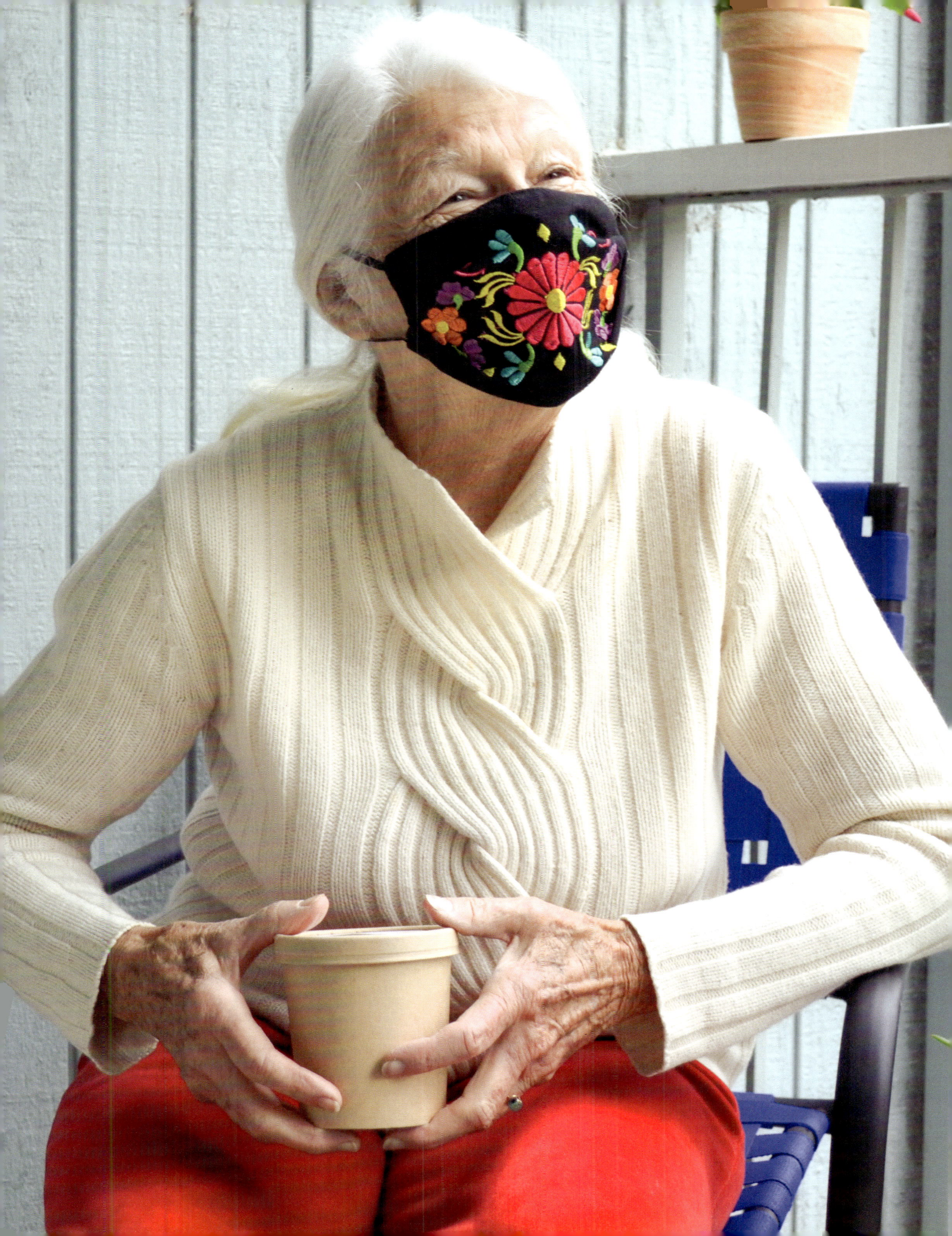

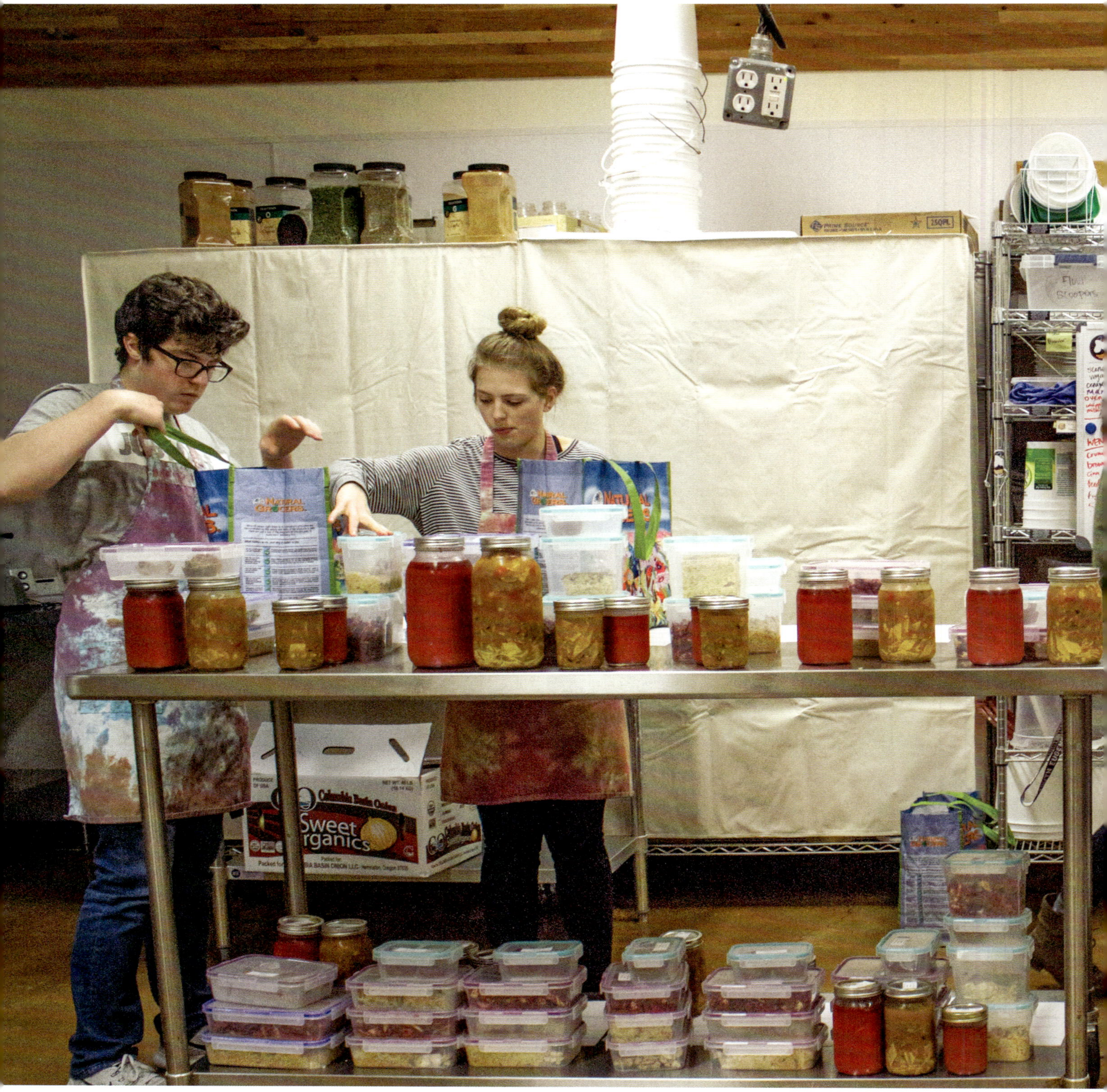
NATURAL GROCERS
Sweet Organics

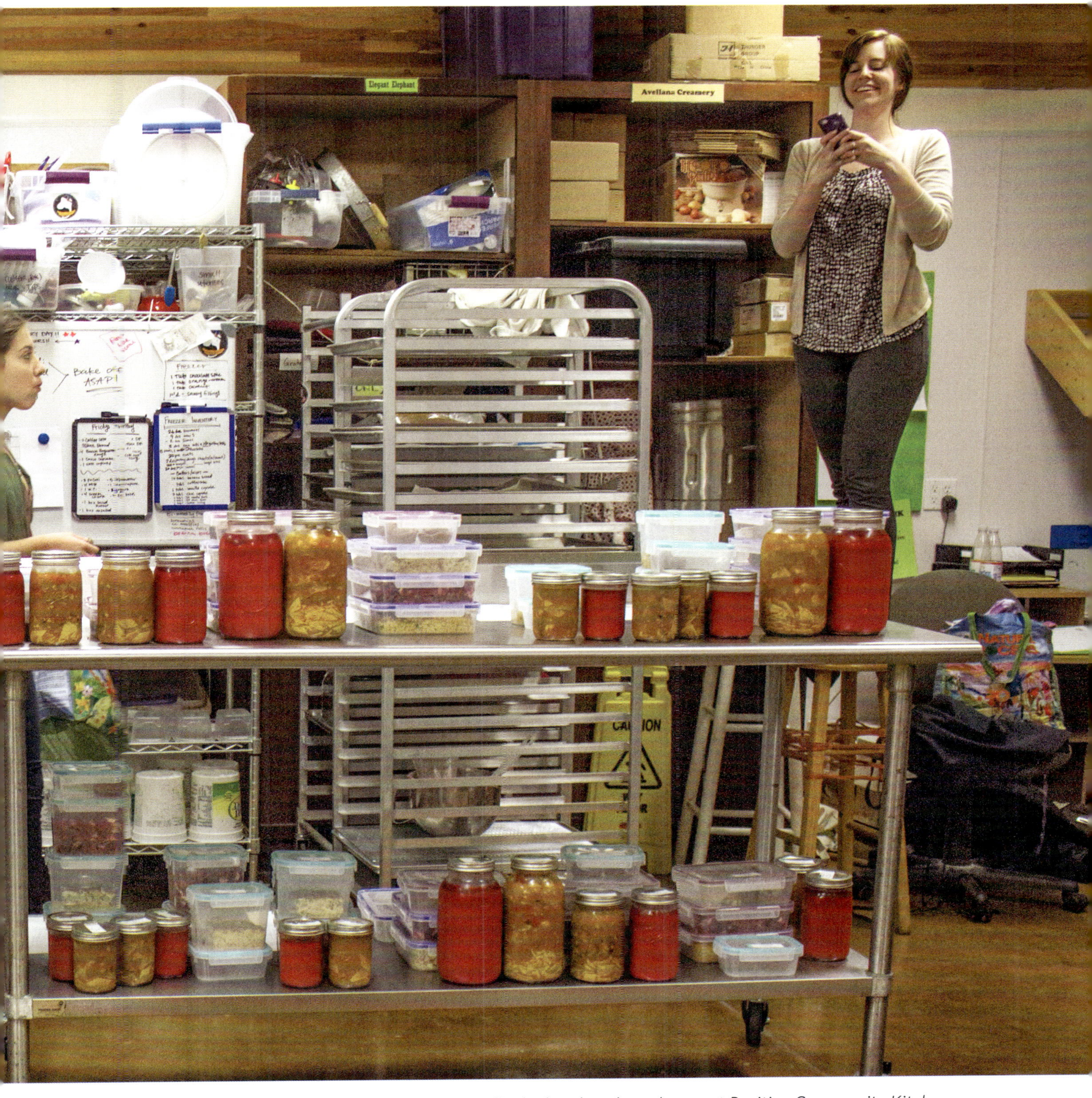

Cooked and packaged soup at Positive Community Kitchen

Hearty Tomato Lentil Soup

This soup makes a hearty one-dish lunch or a delicious dinner paired with a green salad and some warm bread (gluten-free or otherwise!). This is a flexible recipe. You can use any dark leafy greens for this recipe. If you are using kale or chard, add the greens when you add the quinoa instead of when you add the lentils. You can also increase the greens to 2 packed cups. In place of the tomato puree, you can use 1 cup canned tomato sauce, 1 cup diced tomatoes with 1 Tbsp. tomato paste, or ¼ cup tomato paste whisked with ¾ to 1 cup of water or extra broth.

— A Positive Community Kitchen Mentor

Serves 4
Prep time: 20 minutes
Cooking time: 45 minutes
Vegan
Gluten-free

Ingredients

½ cup lentils, rinsed and soaked
½ cup quinoa, soaked for at least 6 hours and drained

1 Tbsp olive oil
½ cup small diced onion
½ cup small diced carrot
½ cup small diced celery
1 Tbsp minced garlic
¾ tsp smoked paprika
¾ tsp ground cumin
½ tsp chili powder
4 cups vegetable broth
1 cup tomato purée
1 cup stemmed and rough chopped collard greens
¾ tsp salt
½ tsp ground black pepper
2 tsp lemon juice

Instructions

In a 3-quart soup pot, heat the oil over medium heat. Add the onions, carrots and celery and let them sweat, stirring often, until softened, about 5 to 7 minutes.

Add the garlic, paprika, cumin and chile powder. Stir to coat evenly and cook for several more minutes.

Add the broth, tomato purée, drained lentils, collard greens, salt, and pepper. Bring to a boil and then lower heat. Cover and simmer for 30 minutes.

Stir in the soaked quinoa and cook for an additional 12 minutes. Remove from heat and stir in the lemon juice. Adjust seasonings as necessary.

Nutrition info. *1 Serving: 274 calories, 5g fat, 13g protein, 46g carbohydrate, 567mg sodium*

Adding some spice! A volunteer at Positive Community Kitchen

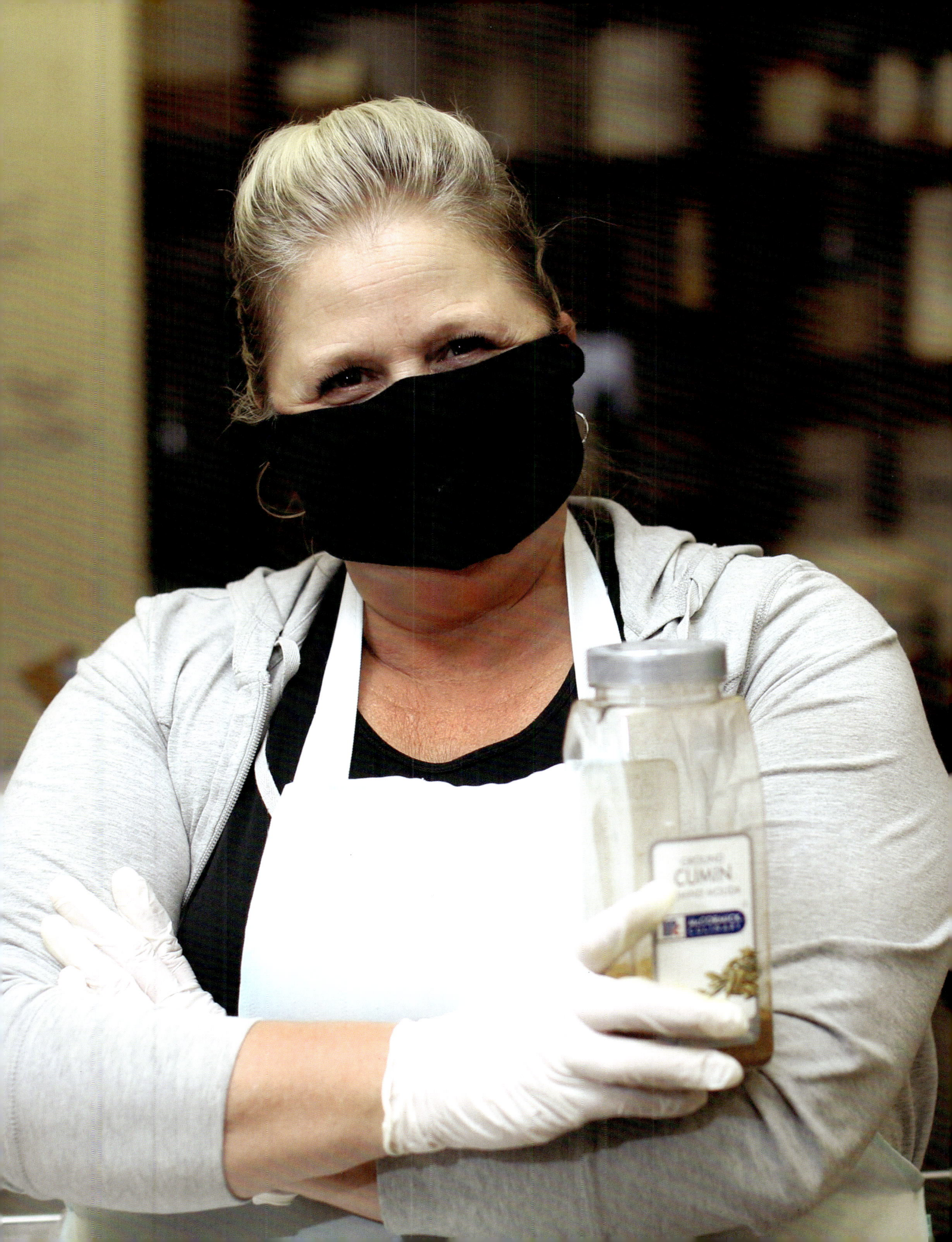
CUMIN

Minestrone Barley Soup

This is a great soup for using up the bounty of summer produce. We harvest from our garden on campus and make substitutions to the recipe depending on what's growing that week. The barley adds fiber and helps make this a very satisfying soup.

— The Caring Kitchen Project Team

Serves 8
Prep time: 20 minutes
Cooking time: 2 hours
Vegan (without Parmesan cheese)

Ingredients

¾ cup dry kidney beans, covered with 4 cups of water and soaked overnight, or 1 (15-ounce) can kidney beans, drained and rinsed
¾ cup hulled barley
3 Tbsp olive oil
2 ½ cups diced onions
1 ½ Tbsp minced garlic
1 cup diced celery
3 cups sliced carrots
6 cups diced tomatoes with juice
2 Tbsp chopped fresh oregano (or 1 Tbsp dried)
3 Tbsp fresh chopped basil (or 1 Tbsp dried)
14 cups vegetable broth or water
1 ½ pounds small red potatoes, quartered
2 tsp salt
¼ tsp ground black pepper
2 bay leaves
½ pound green cabbage, shredded
1 ½ cups shredded kale or chard, or sliced zucchini
Garnishes (optional): chopped parsley, a drizzle of extra-virgin olive oil, julienned basil, croutons or Parmesan cheese

Instructions

If using dry beans, drain and rinse soaked beans, then cover with 4 cups of fresh water. Bring to a boil, reduce to a simmer and partially cover. Cook until the beans are tender all the way through, 40 to 60 minutes depending on freshness.

Rinse barley well and put in saucepan with 3 cups water or stock. Bring to boil and simmer for about 35 minutes or until tender. Drain any excess liquid.

Heat the olive oil in a large soup pot. Add the onion and cook on medium heat for about 5 minutes or until the onion is translucent.

Add the garlic, celery, and carrots and cook for another 2 minutes.

Add tomatoes, oregano, and basil; cook for 2 more minutes.

Add remaining 11 cups broth or water, potatoes, salt, pepper, and bay leaves. Bring to a low boil. Reduce heat to simmer and cook for 30 minutes.

Add cabbage, cooked beans, kale, chard or zucchini and simmer for 5 minutes.

Remove 2 to 3 cups of soup and purée in a blender until smooth. Return to the pot. Bring to simmer. Add barley to pot.

To serve, garnish with chopped parsley, drizzled extra virgin olive oil, julienned basil, croutons or Parmesan cheese.

Nutrition info. *Serving size, 2 cups: 278 calories, 5g fat, 9g protein, 531g carbohydrate, 421g sodium*

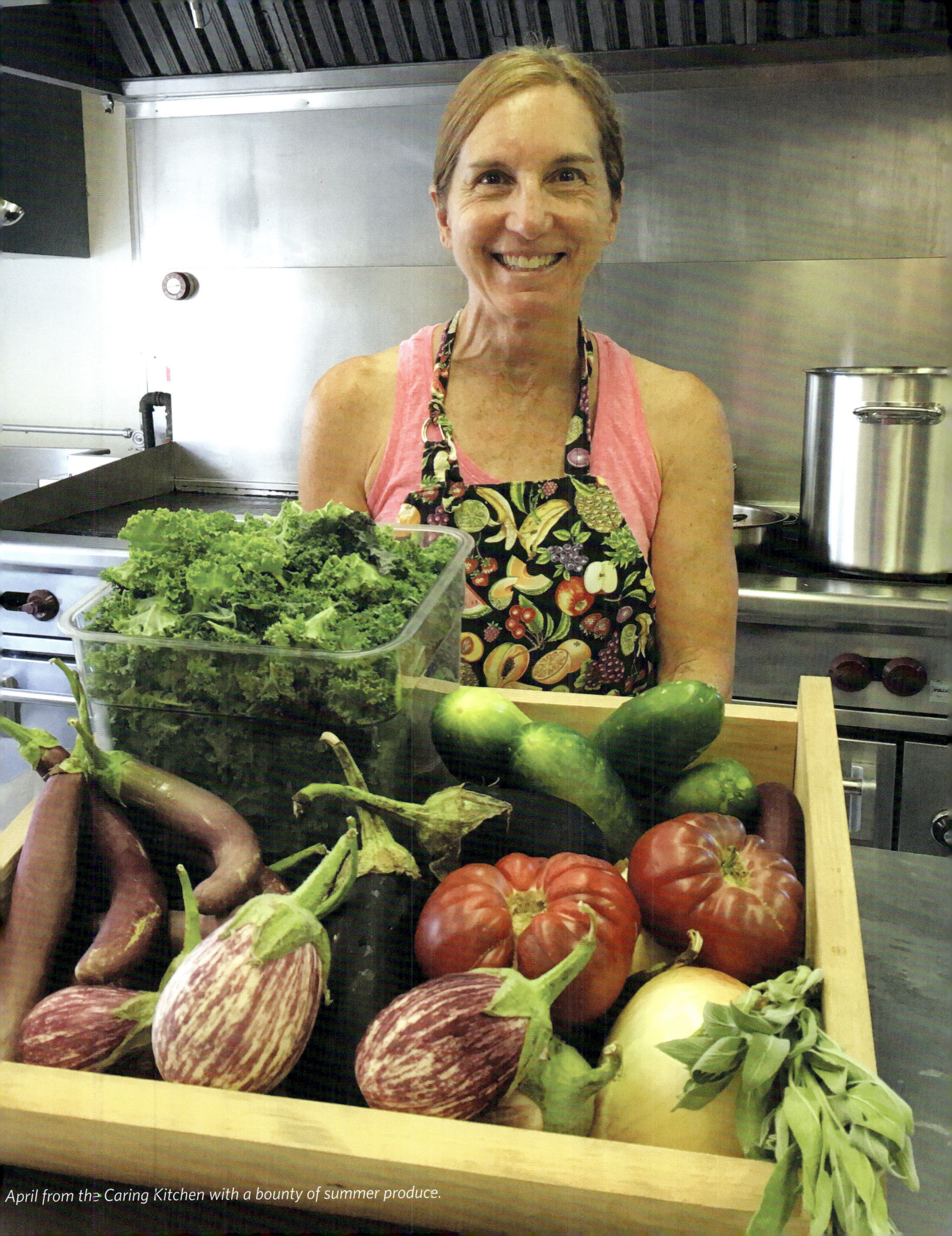

April from the Caring Kitchen with a bounty of summer produce.

Black Bean Pumpkin Chili

This is a mild but flavorful chili. The recipe makes a generous quantity and leftovers make for a quick, nutritious lunch. The chili will keep for three to four days in the fridge and will also freeze well for up to 3 months.

— The Healing Meals Community Project Team

Serves 8
Prep time: 15 minutes
Cooking time: 45 minutes
Vegan
Gluten-free

Ingredients

2 Tbsp olive oil
1 medium yellow onion, diced
2 stalks celery, diced
1 green or red bell pepper, seeded and diced
1 medium carrot, peeled and diced
2 large cloves garlic, minced
1 tsp chili powder
1 tsp ground cumin
1 tsp oregano
¼ tsp ground cinnamon
3 (15-ounce) cans low-sodium diced tomatoes
1 (15-ounce) can pumpkin purée
3 (15-ounce) cans low-sodium black beans, drained and rinsed
1 tsp salt
1 tsp ground black pepper
1 cup water or broth, as needed

Instructions

Heat oil in a large pot over medium heat. Add the onion, celery, bell pepper, and carrot. Sauté until the onion is translucent, about 5 minutes.

Add garlic, chile powder, cumin, oregano, and cinnamon, and cook until spices are fragrant, 1 to 2 minutes.

Add tomatoes with their juices and pumpkin purée. Stir until thoroughly combined. Add black beans, salt, and pepper. Add water or broth if needed to produce the desired consistency. Bring to a low simmer, slightly cover, and let simmer for at least 30 minutes, stirring often.

Nutrition info. *Serving size, 1 ¾ cups: 237 calories, 5g fat, 12g protein, 40g carbohydrate, 618mg sodium*

Hearty Fish Stew

"The meals you provided and the TLC saved our lives in a difficult time"

— Client, Healing Meals Community Project

Serves 8
Prep time: 15 minutes
Cooking time: 55 minutes
Dairy-free
Gluten-free

Ingredients

1 Tbsp coconut oil
1 medium onion, thinly sliced
3 cloves garlic, smashed
¼ cup fresh lemon juice
1 tsp ground turmeric
1 tsp ground cumin
1 tsp paprika
1 (13.5-ounce) can coconut milk
1 tsp salt
3 pounds firm white fish, such as Alaskan true cod, Ling cod, or rock cod
2 red bell peppers, seeded and cut into strips
1 (18-ounce) jar low-sodium diced tomatoes
½ cup coarsely chopped cilantro leaves and thin stems
2 cups cooked brown rice
3 scallions, trimmed and thinly sliced
salt and black pepper, to taste

Instructions

Preheat oven to 400°F.

In a large, high-sided skillet, heat the coconut oil over medium heat, add the onion and cook, stirring, until the onion just begins to soften, about 2 minutes.

Add the garlic, lemon juice, turmeric, cumin, paprika, coconut milk, and salt; raise the heat to bring the liquid to a low boil, then lower the heat to achieve a gentle simmer. Let simmer until sauce thickens a bit, about 20 minutes.

While the stew is simmering, place the fish on an oiled baking dish and bake in preheated oven until just cooked through, about 8 minutes. Fish will easily flake with fork when cooked. Let cool and then gently cube the fish.

Add the peppers and tomatoes to the stew, cover, and cook until the peppers are softened slightly, about 5 minutes more. Add cooked fish. Stir gently so as not to break up the fish.

Turn off the heat. Serve over brown rice, garnish with scallions and cilantro and season with salt and pepper to taste.

Nutrition info. *1 Serving: 262 calories, 13g fat (11g saturated fat), 29g protein, 9g carbohydrate, 760mg sodium*

Salmon and Fennel Chowder

This delicate and flavorful stew makes a wonderful lunch, or you can add a half cup of grains and a green salad for dinner. We love to make this in the spring when fennel is showing up at the farmers' markets. Use a spice grinder to process the whole spices before measuring them. Cashew milk is quick and easy to make. Soak 1 cup of raw cashews overnight, then drain and rinse. Place the cashews and 4 cups water in a high-powered blender and blend on high for one minute.

— Chef John Littlewood, Ceres Community Project

Serves 6
Prep time: 20 minutes
Cooking time: 30 minutes
Dairy-free
Gluten-free

Ingredients

1 ½ tsp salt
¼ tsp ground black pepper
¼ tsp ground celery seed
1 tsp dill weed
½ tsp thyme
¼ tsp ground bay leaf
1 tsp paprika
¼ tsp ground fennel seed
1 Tbsp brown rice flour
1 Tbsp olive oil
1 ½ cup small diced yellow onion
1 cup peeled and small diced carrots
1 cup small diced celery
1 ½ cup finely diced fennel bulb
¾ cup white wine
2 ½ cups Healing Vegetable Broth, page 106 (or vegetable broth of your choice)
2 ½ cups cashew milk
1 ½ cup unpeeled 1-inch cubes red potato
1 pound salmon fillet, cubed
3 Tbsp chopped parsley

Instructions

Combine the first 9 ingredients and set aside.

In a large soup pot, heat oil, then immediately add onions, carrots, celery, and fennel bulb. Sauté about 3 minutes, stirring, until onion is translucent. Add spice/rice flour mix and continue cooking, stirring constantly, about 2 to 3 minutes, until spices are very fragrant (the rice flour will make it very thick).

Add wine and broth, bring to a boil, stirring constantly. Reduce heat and simmer 5 minutes, uncovered.

Add cashew milk and potatoes, bring back to a simmer, cover and cook for 5 to 7 minutes until potatoes are very tender.

Add salmon and cook another 3 to 5 minutes until salmon is just cooked through. Stir in parsley and serve.

Nutrition info. *Serving size, 1-⅔ cup: 273 calories, 10g fat, 21g protein, 25g carbohydrate, 587g sodium*

Sancocho Columbian Chicken Stew

The technique of "blitzing" some of the main flavoring ingredients in a blender early on in this recipe makes it unique. You may want to try it with other brothy soups.

— Chef John Littlewood, Ceres Community Project

Serves 6
Prep time: 20 minutes
Cooking time: 2 hours and 15 minutes

Ingredients

3 pounds bone-in chicken thighs
1 Tbsp minced garlic
1 cup peeled, medium-diced carrots
1 cup diced red peppers
¾ cup diced yellow onion
¾ cup chopped fresh cilantro (divided)
6 cups Ceres Healing Vegetable Broth, page 106 (or vegetable broth of your choice)
1 tsp salt
½ tsp ground black pepper
1 ½ tsp ground cumin
½ tsp oregano
3 cups unpeeled 1-inch cubes red potato
1 ½ cups 1-inch cubes zucchini
1 ½ cups corn kernels

Instructions

Place thighs in stockpot and add cold water (not listed in ingredients) until you have about 3 inches of water above the thighs. Bring to a boil, reduce heat, and simmer until meat is very tender and cooked all the way through (this will take about 30 to 45 minutes). When done, remove chicken from water and let cool. Pull meat from bones and place in two piles: one pure meat, one all bones and skin. Check meat for bones. Dice meat into 1-inch chunks.

Place bones and skin back into stockpot and simmer on very low heat for at least an hour, and up to 4 hours. Strain broth and chill (discard bones and skin).

Use a blender to purée the garlic, carrots, peppers, onion and half of the cilantro. Use just enough broth to make the mixture liquid enough to blend, not totally smooth, a little texture is good.

In a large stockpot, combine the purée with the broth, salt, pepper, cumin and oregano. Bring to a boil, lower heat and simmer for 10 minutes.

Add potatoes and simmer for another 10 minutes, or until potatoes are just starting to get tender. Add zucchini and corn, then simmer another 5 minutes. Do not overcook; zucchini should be just barely cooked.

Stir in chicken meat and remaining cilantro and heat through before serving.

Nutrition info. *Serving size, 2 cups: 535 calories, 19g fat, 60g protein, 29g carbohydrate, 616mg sodium*

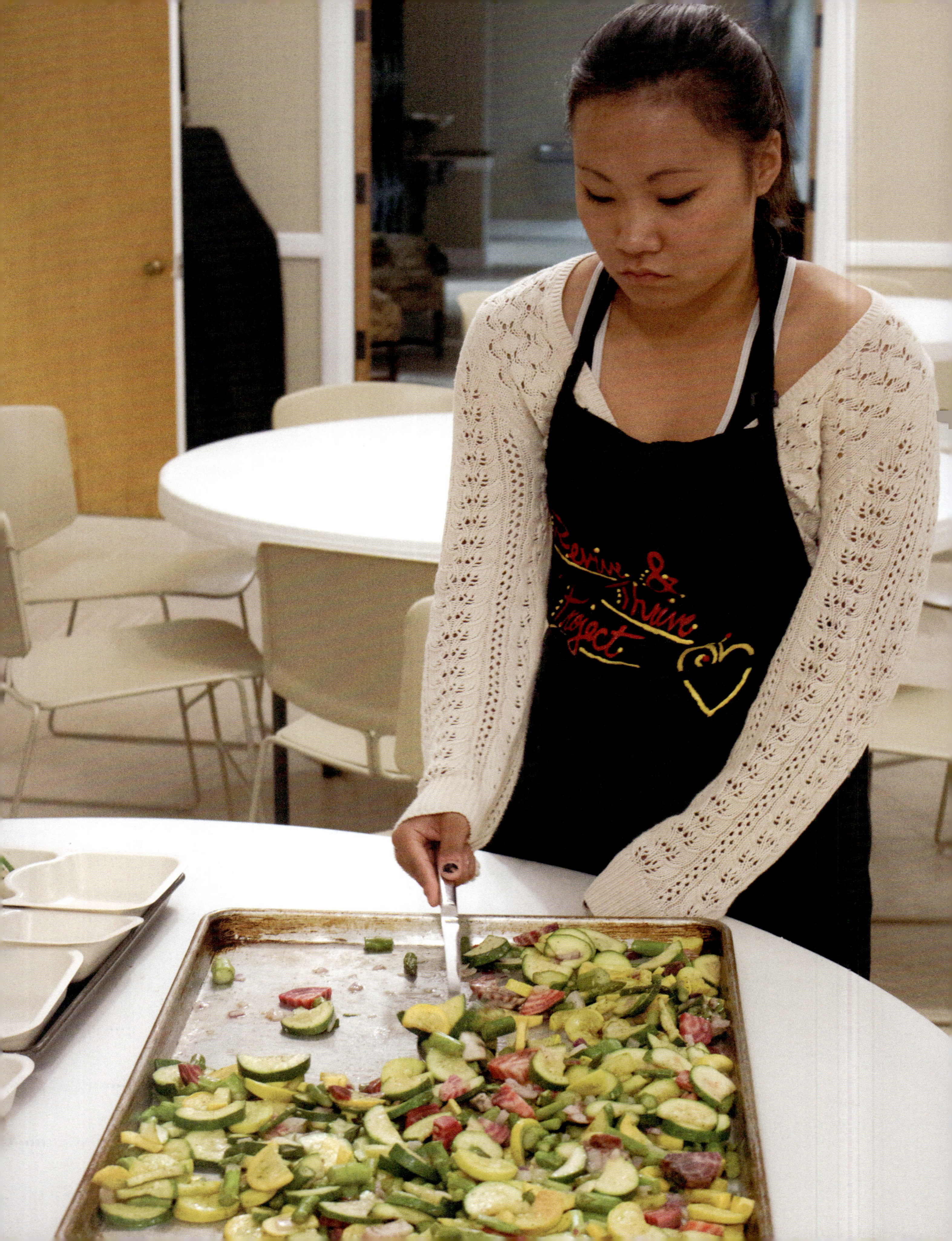
Revive & Thrive Project

SMALL PLATES & SIDES

Creole Pan-Fried Cabbage

We love using this pan-fried cabbage as a complementary side dish full of comfort and flavor. It works with various proteins, and the blended creole flavor is reminiscent of the blended cultures of its origin. Fresh ginger and oregano are a plus for flavor, but dried substitutes are fine.

— The Meals 4 Health and Healing Team

Serves 4
Prep time: 15 minutes
Cooking time: 30 minutes
Gluten free
Dairy-free

Ingredients

2 Tbsp avocado oil
1 large onion, diced (about 2 cups)
Pinch of salt
Ground black pepper, to taste
2 large cloves garlic, minced
1 Tbsp peeled and minced fresh ginger, or ¼ tsp ground ginger
1 tsp minced fresh oregano, or ¼ tsp dried oregano, crumbled
Scant ½ tsp ground allspice
2 tsp paprika or smoked paprika
1 small head cabbage (about 1½ pounds), cored and diced
2 Tbsp honey
2 tsp lemon juice
2 tsp apple cider vinegar
2 Tbsp finely chopped fresh parsley, plus extra for garnish

Instructions

Warm a large skillet or wok over medium-low heat.

Coat the bottom of the pan with the avocado oil and sauté onion with a pinch of salt and pepper, stirring frequently until lightly browned, about 12 minutes. Lower heat if needed to prevent burning.

Stir in garlic, ginger, oregano, allspice and paprika and cook until aromatic, about 30 seconds.

Add cabbage and remaining ingredients.

Cook, stirring frequently, until cabbage is tender and flavors combine.

Taste, adjust salt and pepper, garnish and serve.

Nutrition info. *1 cup serving: 165 calories, 5g fat, 4g protein, 30g carbohydrate, 182mg sodium*

Previous page: Roasting vegetables at Revive and Thrive.
Right: Martha with Meals 4 Health and Healing and teen volunteers package meals

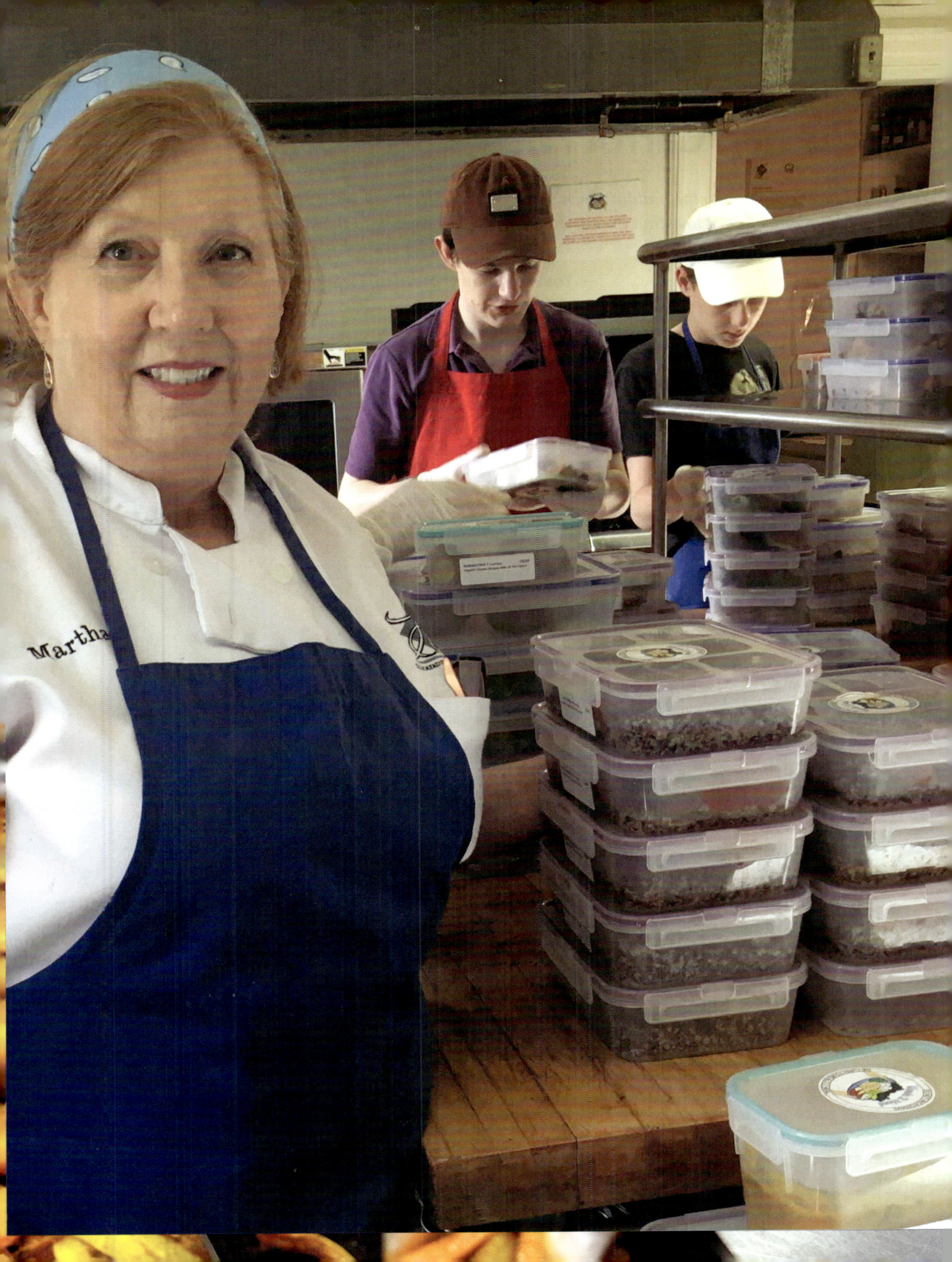
Martha

Turmeric Roasted Cauliflower

This vibrant yellow side dish is even better made ahead, so the turmeric and fennel flavors permeate the vegetables. Reheat in an oven-proof casserole dish and serve. Do-ahead perfection!

— Chef John Littlewood, Ceres Community Project

Serves 8
Prep time: 15 minutes
Cooking time: 30 to 40 minutes
Gluten-free
Vegan

Ingredients

½ cup plus 2 Tbsp olive oil
1 ½ cups halved and thinly sliced yellow onions
1 Tbsp apple cider vinegar
1 ½ tsp turmeric
½ tsp salt
1 tsp ground fennel
1 tsp granulated garlic
¼ tsp ground black pepper
12 cups cauliflower florets

Instructions

Preheat oven to 350°F. Line two sheet pans with parchment paper or lightly oil.

In a small skillet, heat 2 tablespoons olive oil and sauté the onion over low to medium heat until very soft, about 20 minutes. Don't hurry this process or you will burn the onion rather than melt it. Let cool.

In a large bowl, whisk together remaining ½ cup olive oil, vinegar, turmeric, salt, fennel, garlic, and pepper.

Toss the cauliflower with this dressing and spread out on sheet pans. Roast in oven until browned and soft. Check cauliflower after 10 minutes, then every 5 minutes after that, stirring with spatula as needed to create evenly browned cauliflower. Cauliflower should be tender, not crunchy.

Mix onion and cauliflower well. Serve warm.

Nutrition info. *1 serving, ¾ cup: 199 calories, 17g fat, 3g protein, 10g carbohydrate, 106mg sodium*

Teen volunteer in Ceres kitchen cooking turmeric cauliflower.

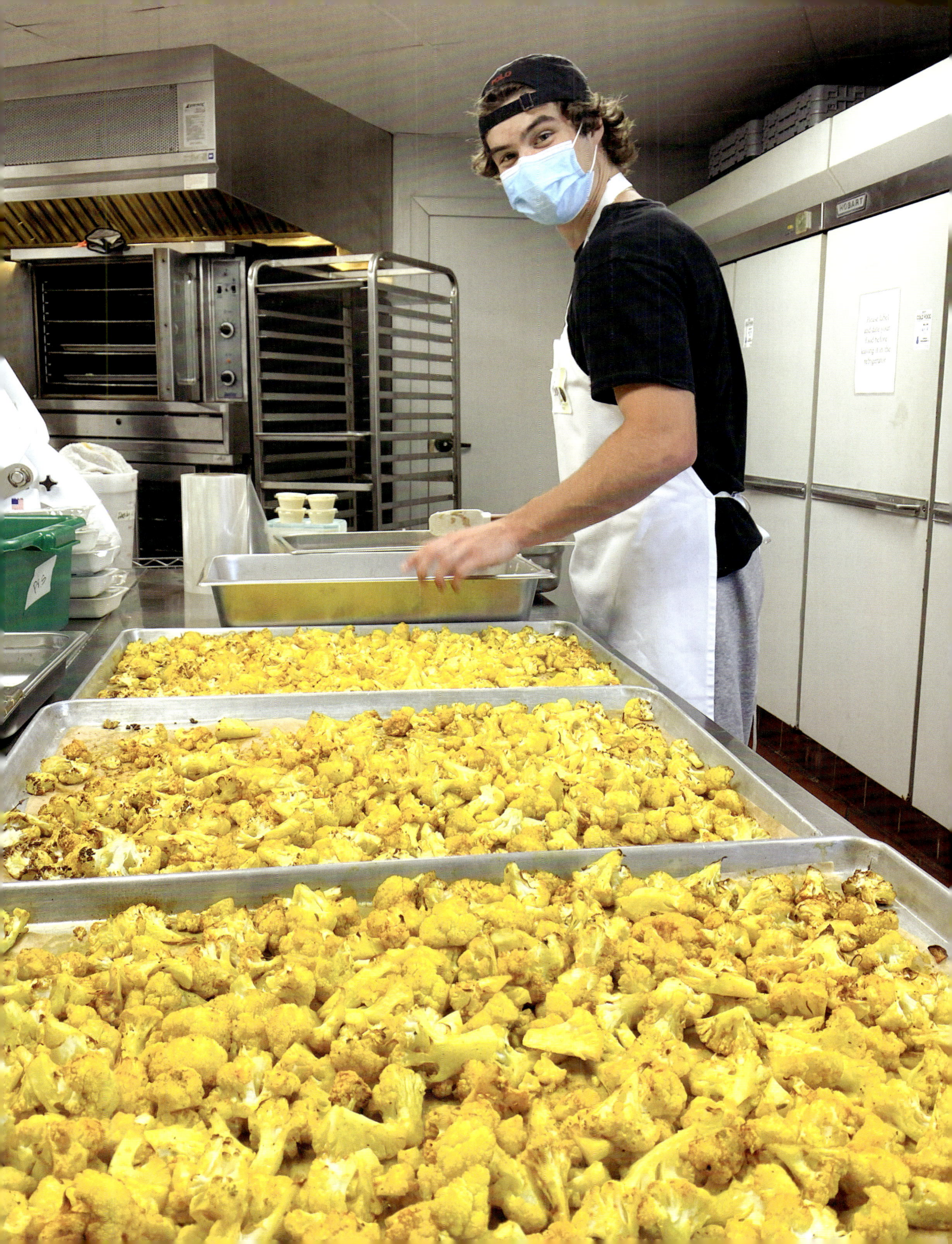

Roasted Squash with Fennel and Green Beans

Fennel richly complements the other vegetables in this unforgettable fall dish. Roasting partially caramelizes the fennel, bringing out a natural sweetness and mellow flavor. Entirely edible, this vegetable with a bulbous base and feathery fronds supplies vitamins A and C, dietary fiber and potassium.

— **Assistant Chef Marcie Carlson, Fox Valley Food for Health**

Serves 6
Prep time: 1 hour
Cooking time: 40 minutes
Vegan
Gluten-free

Ingredients

1 pound haricots verts (or thin green beans), cut on diagonal into 2-inch pieces
Bowl of ice water for blanching process
1 large butternut squash (around 2 pounds) peeled, seeded and cut into ½ inch pieces
1 large fennel bulb, halved, cored and thickly sliced
5 medium shallots, quartered (about 2 cups)
5 cloves garlic, peeled
3 Tbsp olive oil
2 tsp balsamic vinegar
½ tsp salt
2 pinches red pepper flakes
Chopped fresh parsley, for garnish

Instructions

Bring a medium pot of water to boil. Add beans, cover and bring back to boil. Cook 2 to 3 minutes, just until tender-crisp. Drain and chill beans immediately in ice water bath to stop cooking and preserve color. Drain well when cool. Dry thoroughly in a clean dish towel and set aside.

Preheat oven to 400°F. Line a sheet pan with parchment paper or lightly oil.

In large bowl, combine squash, fennel, shallots, garlic, olive oil, vinegar, salt, and red pepper flakes; toss to coat. Spread evenly on sheet pan.

Roast for about 40 minutes, or until vegetables are tender. Turn off oven. Lightly salt green beans and add to tray. Return sheet to oven for 2 to 3 minutes, letting beans warm in the oven's residual heat. Garnish with parsley and serve.

Nutrition info. *1 serving: 581 calories, 25g fat, 53g protein, 40g carbohydrate, 713mg sodium*

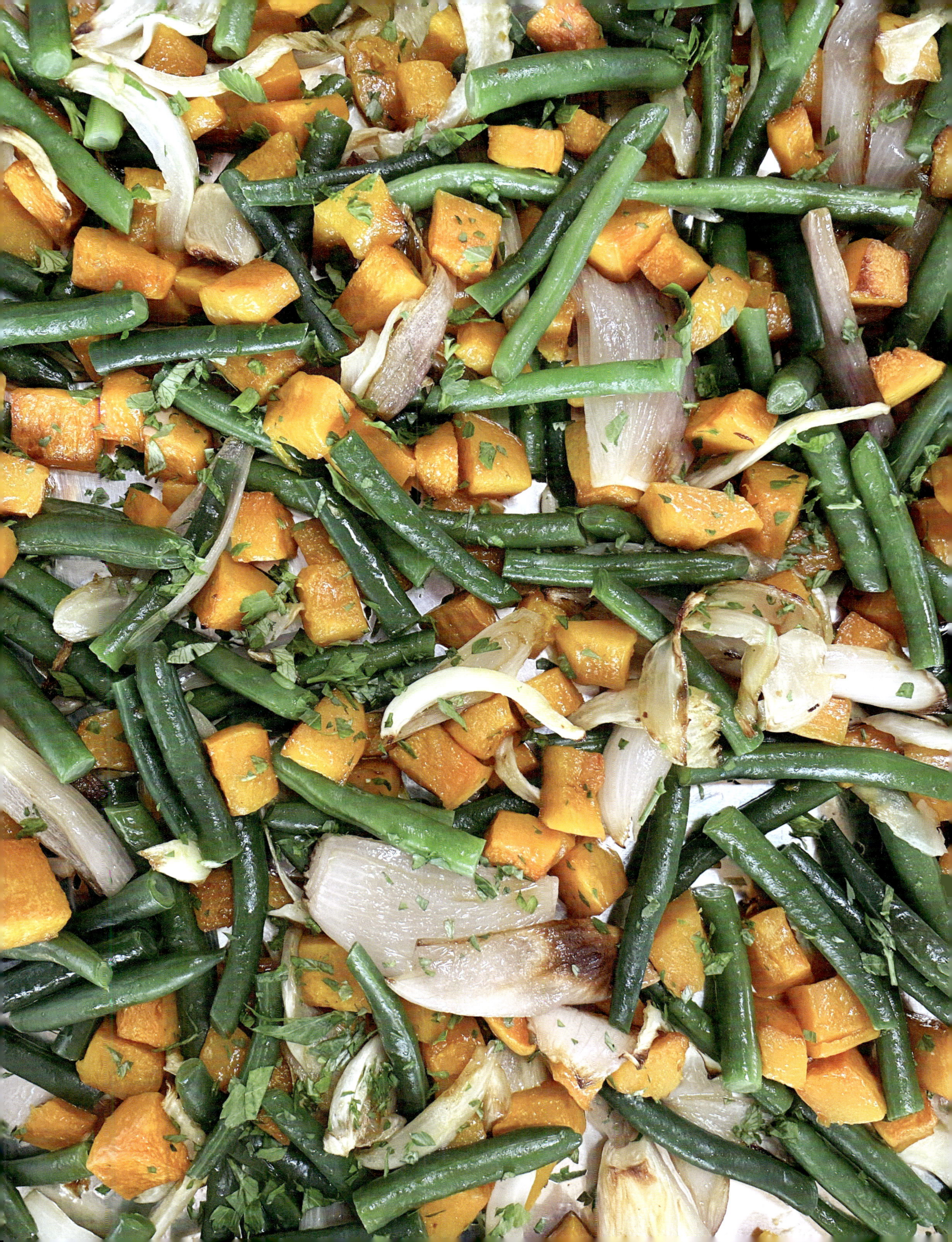

Delicata Squash & Kale with Cranberries

Delicata squash is considered a winter squash but is actually planted in the spring and grown in the summer. It grows on long vines producing about 4 to 6 squash per plant. The skin is edible, which adds to the high fiber content. Roasted and mixed with kale and cranberries, it makes a colorful and nutritious side dish.

— The Caring Kitchen Project Team

Serves 4
Prep time: 45 minutes
Cooking time: 20 minutes
Vegan
Gluten-free

Ingredients

1 small bunch Lacinato kale
2 large or 3 medium Delicata squash, about 3 pounds
3 Tbsp olive oil, divided
½ tsp ground allspice
½ tsp paprika
¾ tsp salt, divided
Pinch red pepper flakes
½ cup dried cranberries
1 Tbsp white balsamic vinegar or lemon juice

¼ cup shelled and lightly toasted pistachios, for garnish

Instructions

Preheat oven to 425°F. Line a baking sheet with parchment paper or lightly oil.

Cut squash in half lengthwise. Scoop out the seeds, and slice crosswise into half moons, about ¼ inch thick.

Mix allspice, paprika, and ½ teaspoon salt together in a small bowl.

In a large bowl, toss the squash with 2 tablespoons olive oil and the spice mix, coating each piece. Spread the squash in a single layer on the prepared baking sheet.

Roast for 20 to 25 minutes, or until tender and lightly browned.

While the squash is roasting, remove ribs and stems from kale and tear into 1-inch pieces. Sprinkle with remaining ¼ teaspoon salt.

Heat skillet over medium low heat. Add remaining tablespoon of oil, pepper flakes and cranberries. Stir for 20 seconds.

Add the kale. Sauté until tender, about 3 to 5 minutes. Add a tablespoon of water, if needed, to finish cooking.

Add kale mixture to the roasted squash in a serving bowl. Stir in balsamic vinegar.

Garnish with toasted pistachios.

Nutrition info. *1 serving: 358 calories, 15g fat, 7g protein, 60g carbohydrate, 421mg sodium*

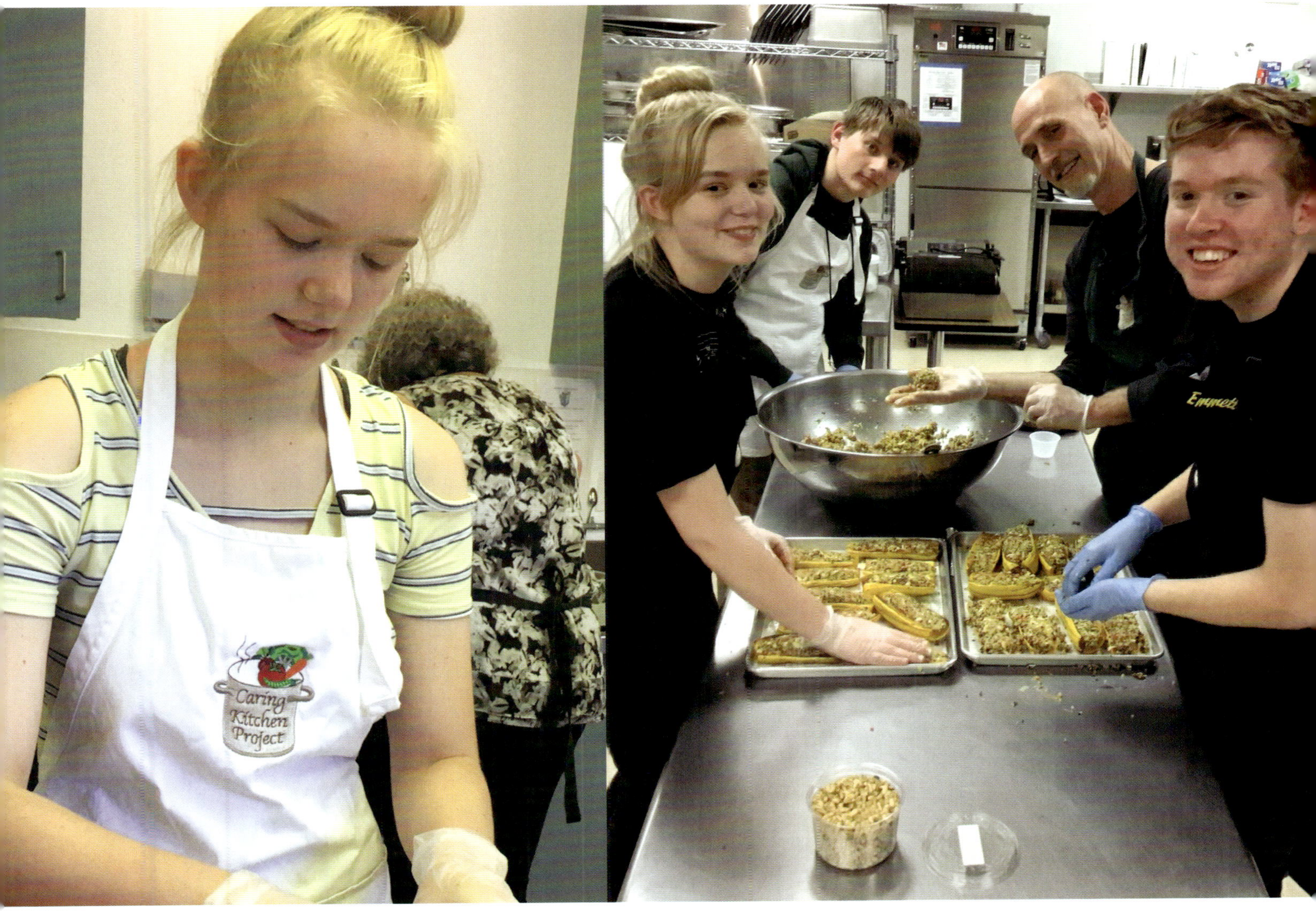

Cooking delicata squash at the Caring Kitchen.

Maple-Roasted Butternut Squash

When our gardens are overflowing with butternut squash, we love this simple side dish alongside almost any of our entrées, or even as a topping for a fresh green salad.

— Chef Molly Evans, Fox Valley Food for Health

Serves: 6
Prep time: 20 minutes
Cooking time: 35 to 60 minutes
Vegan
Gluten-free

Ingredients

1 large butternut squash (2 to 3 pounds), peeled, seeded, and cut into ¾ to 1 inch cubes
4 cloves garlic, peeled
2 Tbsp olive oil
2 Tbsp pure maple syrup
½ tsp kosher salt
¼ tsp ground black pepper
16 whole fresh sage leaves, tossed with 1 tsp olive oil

Nutrition info. *1 serving: 189 calories, 7g fat, 2g protein, 33g carbohydrate, 386mg sodium*

Instructions

Preheat oven to 400°F. Line a sheet pan with parchment paper or lightly oil.

In a large bowl, combine squash cubes and whole peeled garlic cloves. Add olive oil, maple syrup, salt, and pepper; toss to coat. Spread squash mixture evenly on prepared sheet pan.

Bake for 20 to 30 minutes, or until squash begins to brown, turning once during baking.

Sprinkle sage leaves over squash and continue to bake for another 20 to 30 minutes, or until squash and garlic are tender and caramelized.

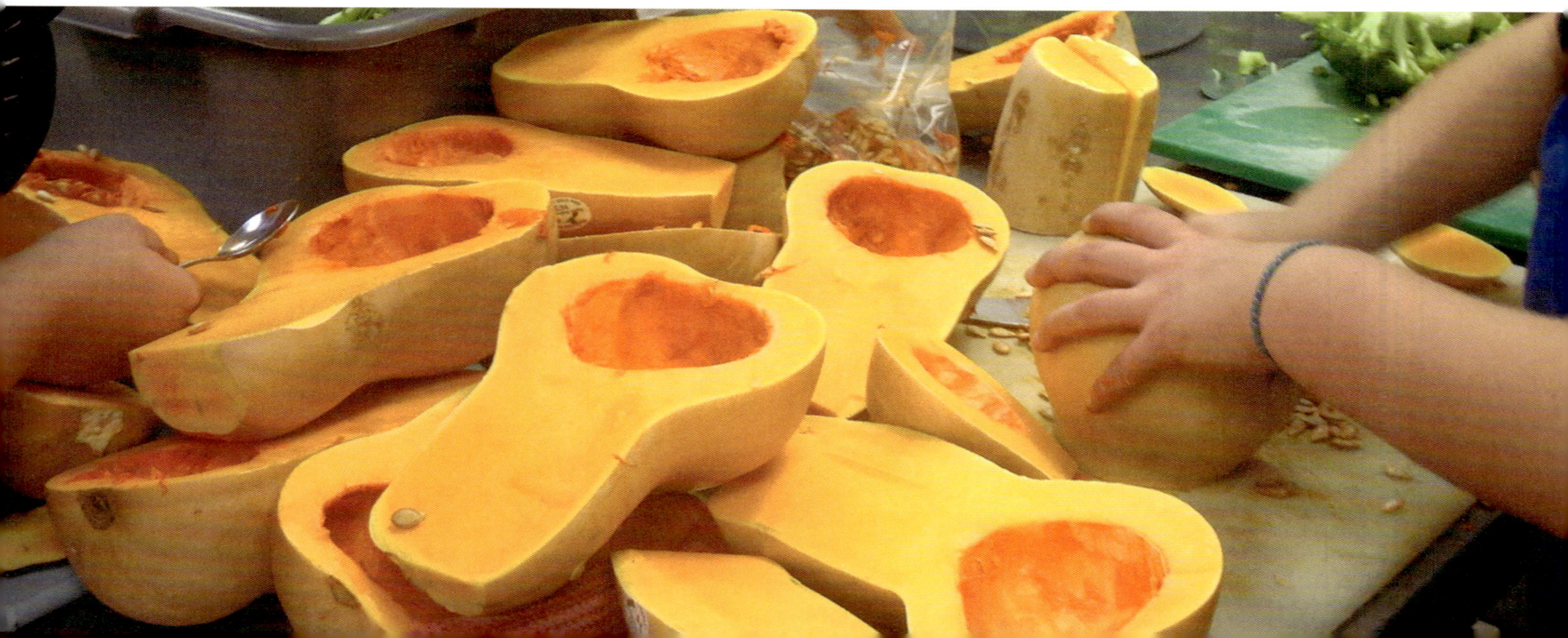

Lemon-Scented Saffron Rice

The rich golden hue and earthy flavor of this rice dish comes from saffron, a spice produced from the flower of the autumn-blooming crocus plant. Saffron contains carotenoids, which are thought to help reduce the risk of disease. Additionally, a recent study demonstrated that two saffron carotenoids may have anti-inflammatory and pain-relieving properties. Although saffron is expensive, a small amount goes a long way.

— Assistant Chef Marcie Carlson, Fox Valley Food for Health

Serves 6
Prep time: 10 minutes
Cooking time: 35 to 40 minutes
Gluten-free
Dairy-free

Ingredients

3 Tbsp olive oil
3 large shallots, thinly sliced
¼ tsp crumbled saffron threads
1 ½ cups short grain brown rice
3 cups low-sodium chicken or vegetable broth
3 Tbsp fresh lemon juice
2 Tbsp lemon zest
1 large bunch chives, chopped (about ½ cup), plus additional for garnish
¼ tsp salt
¼ tsp ground black pepper

Instructions

Heat the olive oil in a large skillet over medium heat. Add the shallots and saffron and sauté for 3 minutes, stirring occasionally. Add rice and stir for 2 to 3 minutes or until all grains are coated and translucent around the edges. Stir in broth and lemon juice; bring to a boil. Reduce heat to low, stir and cover.

Simmer until rice is creamy and tender, stirring vigorously every 10 minutes, for about 25 to 30 minutes. Remove from heat. Keep covered and let rest undisturbed for 10 minutes.

Add lemon zest and chives. Season with salt and pepper; mix well. Garnish with additional snipped chives before serving.

Nutrition info. *1 serving: 258 calories, 8g fat, 5g protein, 42g carbohydrate, 100mg sodium*

Asian-Style Rice Pilaf

This pilaf is a Positive Community Kitchen staple. It's a simple way to level up the love, to share techniques with our Teen Chefs and to incorporate hearty, nutrient-dense ingredients.

— The Positive Community Kitchen Team

Serves 4
Prep time: 15 minutes
Cooking time: 30 to 40 minutes
Vegan
Gluten-free

Ingredients

1 cup brown rice, soaked overnight in 2 cups water and 1 Tbsp apple cider vinegar
2 tsp coconut oil
2 tsp minced garlic
1 cup vegetable broth or water
4 Tbsp coconut aminos or 3 Tbsp low-sodium tamari
1 ½ tsp sesame oil
¼ cup chopped fresh cilantro

Instructions

Drain rice and rinse well.

In a medium saucepan, melt coconut oil over medium-low heat. Add garlic and sauté, stirring constantly, until fragrant, about 2 minutes.

Stir in rice and sauté over medium heat for 2 more minutes. Stir in broth or water, coconut aminos or tamari, and sesame oil.

Bring mixture to a boil, stirring frequently. Reduce heat to low simmer, cover and cook for 30 to 40 minutes, until liquid has been absorbed and rice is tender.

Fluff with a fork and stir in cilantro right before serving.

Nutrition info. *1 serving: 190 calories, 5g fat, 3g protein, 43g carbohydrate, 424mg sodium*

Vegetarian Spring Rolls

"Thank you so much for the healthy food. It nourished my body as well as my spirit. It is so nice to know there are good people who care. Keep shining your light and know that you make such a difference during a difficult time."

— A Positive Community Kitchen Client

Serves 3
Prep time: 30 minutes
Cooking time: 5 to 10 minutes
Vegan
Gluten-free

Ingredients

1 ounce vermicelli rice noodles
¾ tsp toasted sesame oil, or to taste
4 large leaves butter lettuce, ribs removed, creating 8 pieces
½ cup very thinly sliced red cabbage
1 small carrot, sliced into matchsticks or shredded
½ red bell pepper, seeded and membrane removed, sliced into matchsticks
½ cucumber, seeded and sliced into matchsticks
1 green onion, thinly sliced on diagonal
16 cilantro leaves
8 mint leaves
6 rice paper spring roll wrappers (depending on much you put in each roll, you may have extra ingredients to make more)

Instructions

Cook the noodles until al dente. Drain and rinse with cold water. Toss the noodles with sesame oil.

In a pie plate filled with warm water, soak the rice papers one at a time until just soft.

Lay a sheet of softened rice paper on a cutting board. Layer the ingredients, starting with 1 piece butter lettuce, then some rice noodles, cabbage, carrots, red bell pepper, cucumber, green onions, cilantro, and mint. Make sure they aren't too full. You should be able to roll them up comfortably. Roll them up tightly, like a small burr to.

Continue assembling and rolling until you've used up all your ingredients.

To serve, cut each roll in half.

NOTE: These rolls are excellent with "Peanut" Sauce (page 72) for dipping. Using a plastic cutting board rather than a wooden one will help reduce sticking when assembling and rolling the spring rolls.

Nutrition info. *1 spring roll: 70 calories, 1g fat, 2g protein, 14g carbohydrate, 52mg sodium*

Vegetarian Pad Thai with Millet

This recipe is super versatile. Make it a meal by using other seasonal vegetables. Change it up by using snap peas, broccoli or other seasonal vegetables in place of those listed. We love adding whatever plentiful herbs from our Giving Garden strike our fancy to this dish to keep the tastebuds guessing.

— The Meals 4 Health and Healing Team

Serves 4
Prep time: 30 minutes
Cooking time: 10 to 15 minutes
Gluten-free, if using coconut aminos
Dairy-free

Ingredients

1 Tbsp toasted sesame oil
3 Tbsp coconut aminos or soy sauce
3 Tbsp vegetable broth
1 Tbsp honey
2 Tbsp apple cider vinegar
2 Tbsp avocado oil
1 small red onion, diced
1 zucchini, julienned
1 red bell pepper, julienned
2 carrots, julienned
2 cups millet, cooked
salt to taste

¼ cup chopped fresh herbs (basil, cilantro, chives), for garnish
¼ cup chopped almonds, for garnish

Instructions

Make a sauce by whisking together the sesame oil, coconut aminos, broth, honey, and vinegar in a small bow; set aside, then warm a large wok or skillet over medium-high heat. Add avocado oil and sauté vegetables until tender crisp, just 3 to 4 minutes. Add sauce and cook until flavors combine. Season to taste with salt, if needed, and serve over millet. Garnish with fresh herbs and chopped almonds.

Nutrition info. *1 Serving: 281 calories, 13g fat, 6g protein, 42g carbohydrate, 343mg sodium*

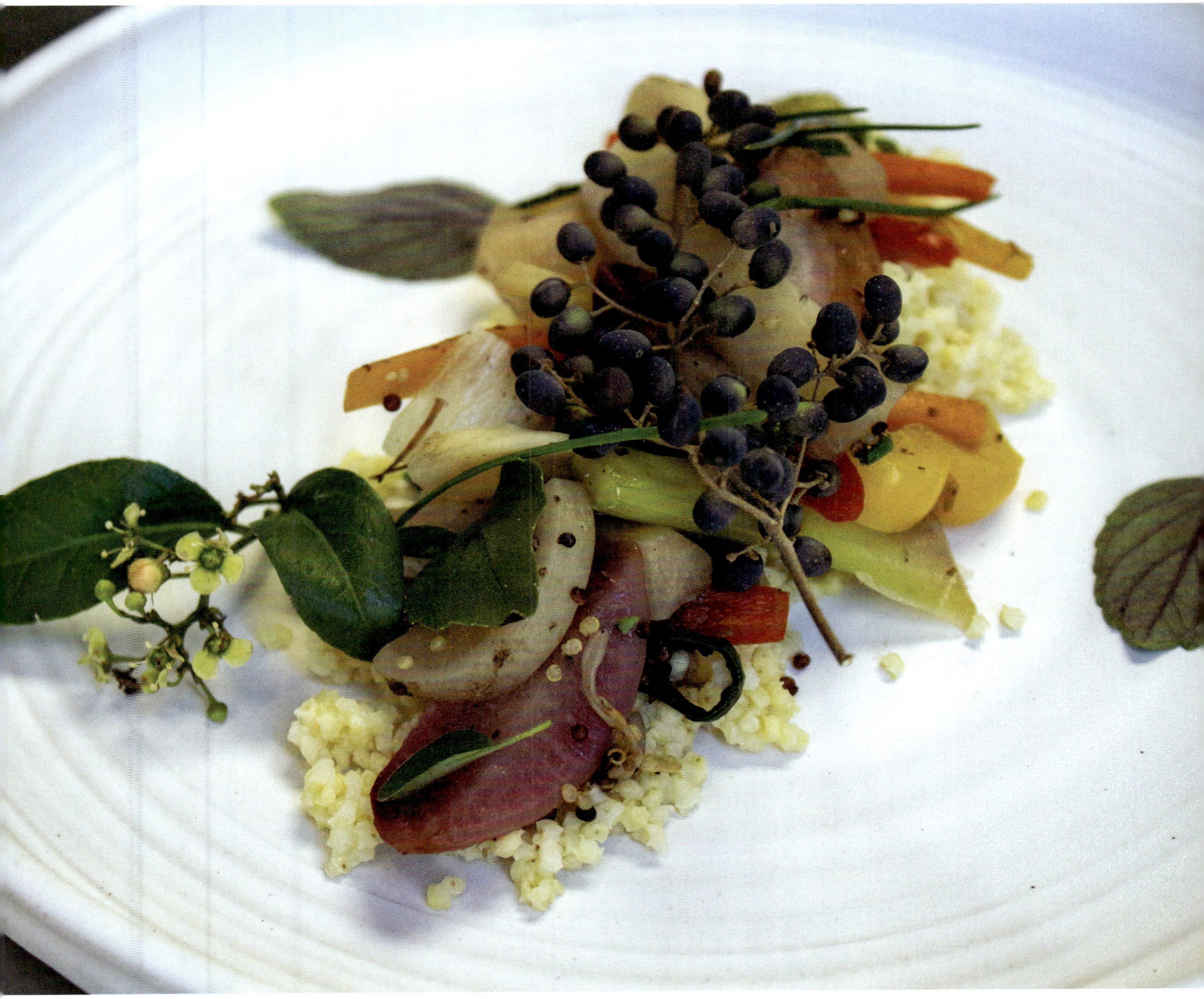

A beautifully garnished Pad Thai millet dish by Meals 4 Health and Healing

Millet Cakes with Herb Aioli

The creamy, tangy herb aioli is the perfect companion to the veggie and millet patties. Dressed up, these cakes are so special and nutritious!

— The Meals 4 Health and Healing Team

Serves 4
Prep time: 10 minutes
Cooking time: 1 ½ hours
Dairy-free

Ingredients

Aioli

½ cup good quality avocado or olive oil mayonnaise
1 Tbsp chopped fresh herbs (parsley, chives, basil, rosemary, oregano, etc.)
1 to 2 tsp lemon juice

Millet cakes

3 Tbsp extra-virgin olive oil
½ small red onion, diced
2 ½ cups vegetables, grated (carrot, potato, zucchini, greens, etc.)
2 cloves garlic, minced
2 cups cooked millet
1 egg, beaten
1 tsp Health and Healing Spice Blend (page 77)
Olive oil cooking spray for baking cakes
Salt and ground black pepper, to taste

Instructions

Preheat the oven to 375°F. Line a small baking sheet with parchment paper or lightly oil.

For the aioli, mix mayonnaise, minced herbs and lemon juice in a small bowl and season to taste with salt and pepper. Set aside.

For the millet cakes, warm a large skillet over medium-high heat. Coat the bottom of the pan with olive oil then sauté the onion and vegetables in a pinch of salt and pepper until tender, 3 to 5 minutes. Add garlic and sauté 30 more seconds, or until aromatic. Let cool, then add to millet with egg and spice blend. Mix to combine thoroughly.

Form into eight equal-sized patties and arrange evenly on baking sheet.

Season well with salt and pepper then spray generously with olive oil and bake for 30 to 35 minutes, until firm to the touch and lightly browned around the edges.

Serve hot with herb aioli.

Nutrition info. *2 patties: 601 calories, 39g fat, 12g protein, 53g carbohydrate, 734mg sodium*

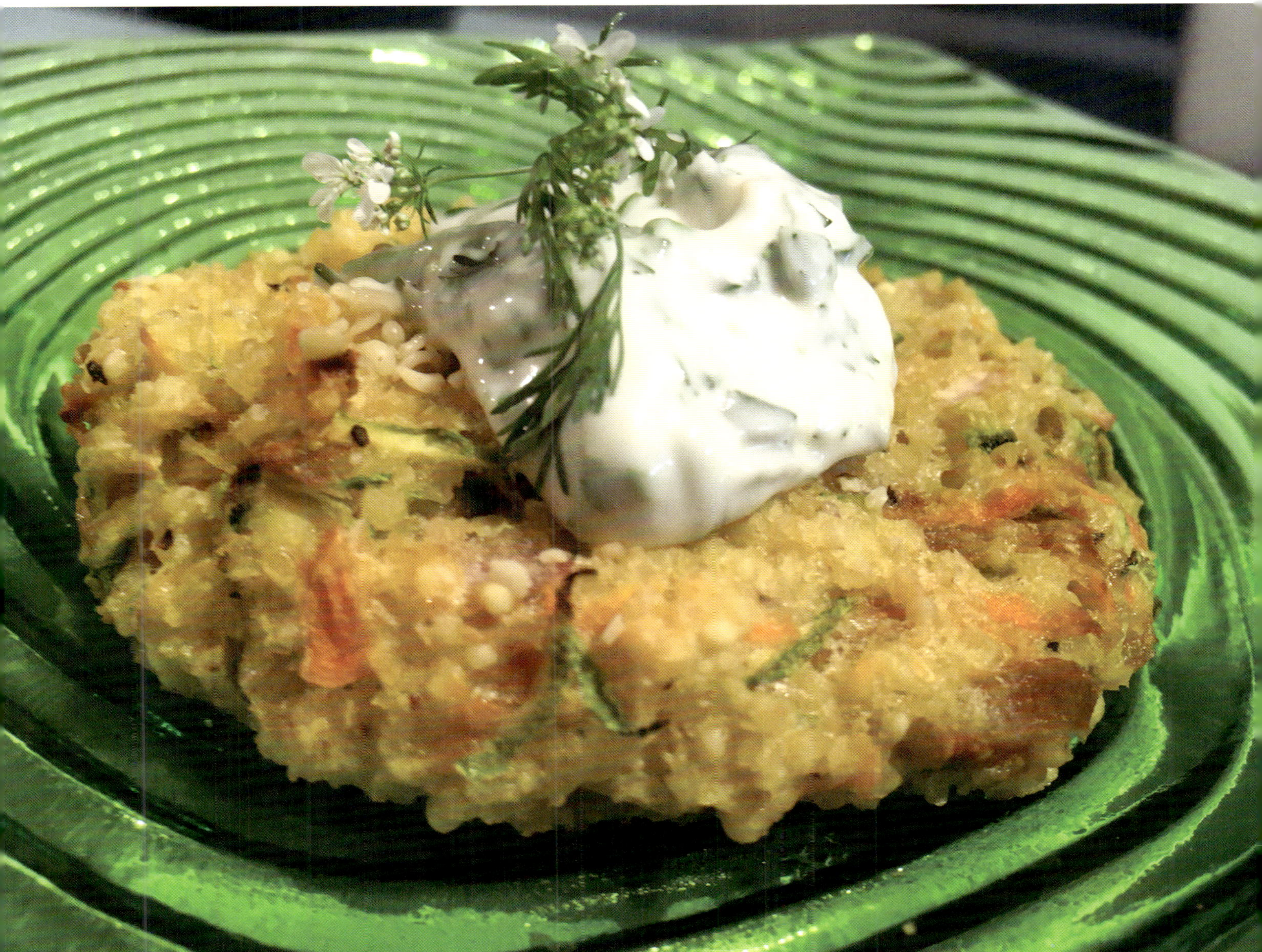

Stewed Chickpeas with Tomatoes and Rosemary

Hearty, simple and satisfying. Top with protein of choice and serve with a green salad for a tasty, nutritious dinner.

— Chef John Littlewood, Ceres Community Project

Serves 6
Prep time: Overnight for soaking plus 10 minutes
Cooking time: 2 hours
Gluten-free
Vegan

Ingredients

1 ½ cups dried chickpeas
1 ½ tsp apple cider vinegar
⅓ cup olive oil, divided
1 ½ Tbsp minced garlic cloves
½ cup small diced yellow onions
¾ cup canned chopped tomatoes, including the liquid
½ tsp salt
1 ½ tsp minced fresh rosemary

Instructions

The night before, place chickpeas into a large pot with 4-½ cups water and vinegar. Soak, unrefrigerated, overnight.

The next day, drain and rinse the chickpeas. Place chickpeas in a heavy-bottomed stock pot, add water to cover by several inches and bring to a boil over high heat. Reduce heat and cover, keeping lid slightly ajar. Simmer until chickpeas are soft, 1 to 2 hours depending on the freshness of your chickpeas. Drain and cool.

Heat large skillet over medium heat until hot. Add half the olive oil, plus the garlic and onions. Cook, stirring, for about 8 minutes, until lightly browned and tender.

Add tomatoes and their liquid, salt, and chick-peas. Simmer on low for 30 minutes. Add rosemary and remaining olive oil. Stir well to combine. Remove from heat and serve.

Nutrition info. *1 serving, ¾ cup serving: 308 calories, 15g fat, 11g protein, 35g carbohydrate, 252mg sodium*

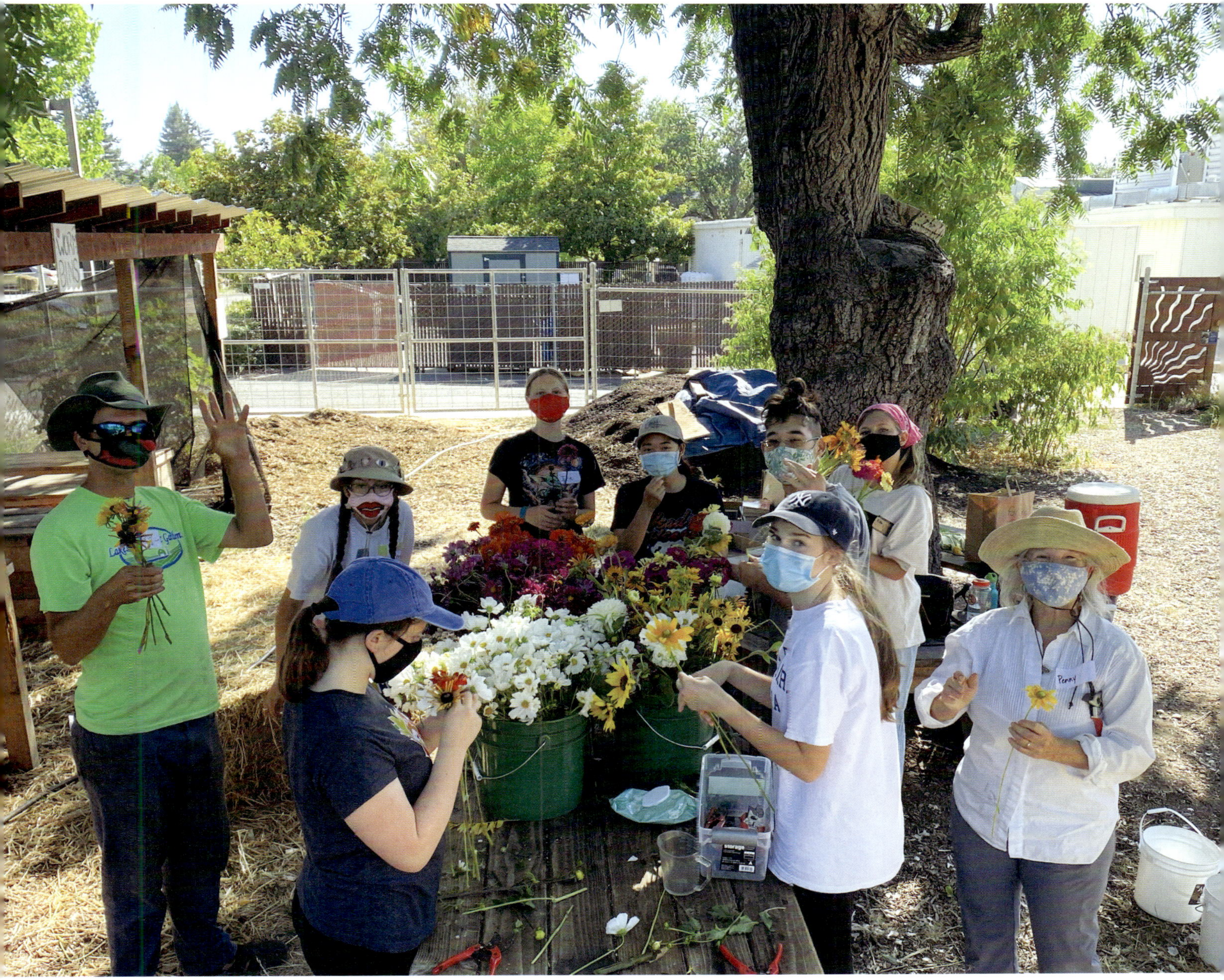

Preparing bouquets to be delivered with meals for clients in a Ceres garden.

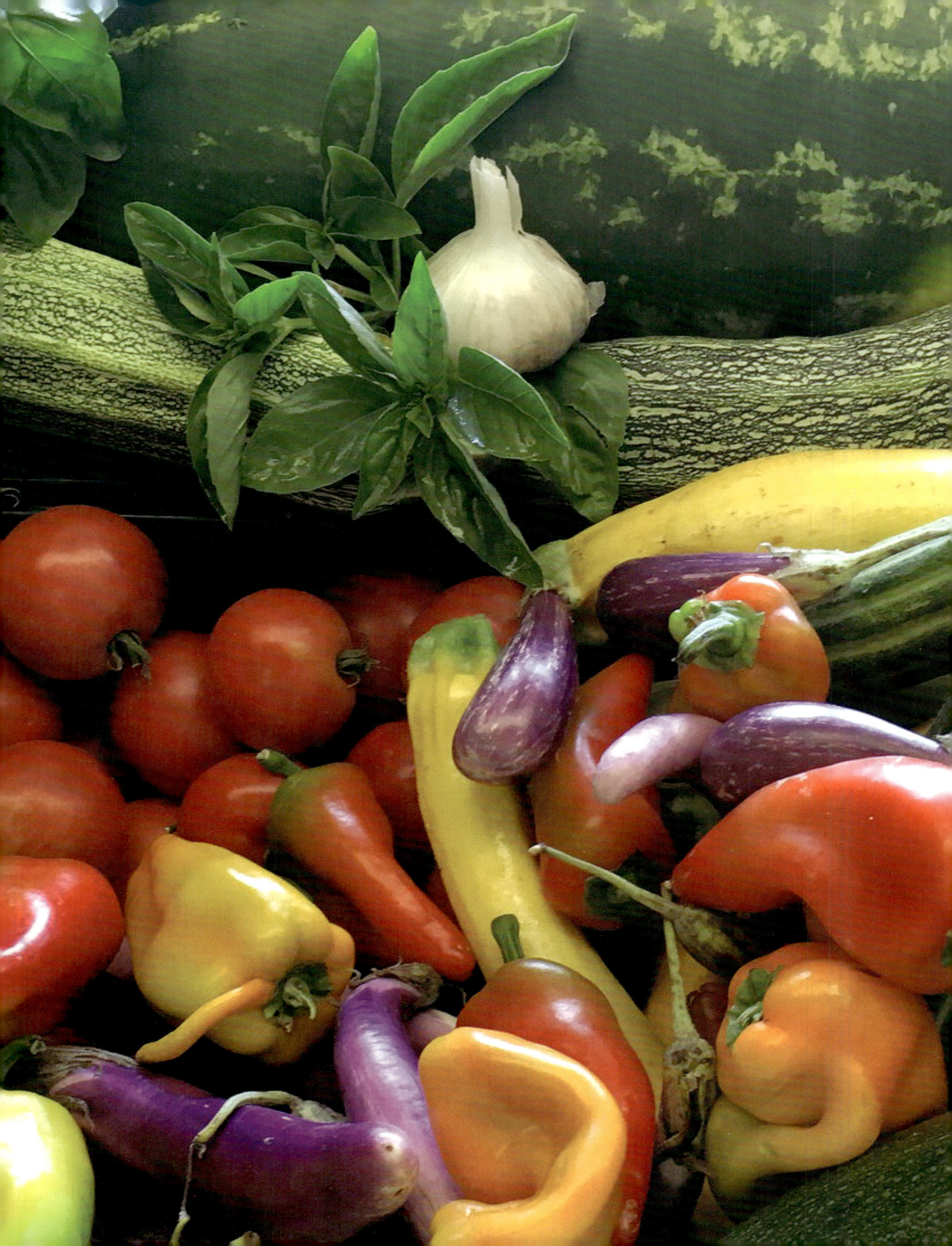

VEGETARIAN ENTREES

Zucchini Confetti Patties

The first time we were invited to showcase Caring Kitchen Project at a local event, we served this as an appetizer, and it was quite the hit. We spent weeks perfecting the recipe — pan after pan was cooked ahead, then cut into heart shapes, dusted with fresh parsley, and topped with our Balsamic Tomato Onion Conserve (page 76). You can either make this as a loaf, or individual patties. To serve as an entrée, add a cooked grain and a salad for a hearty, nourishing meal.

— The Caring Kitchen Project Team

Serves 4
Prep time: 40 minutes
Cooking time: 18 minutes

Ingredients

3 cups grated zucchini (from 3 medium zucchinis)
½ tsp salt
⅔ cup grated carrots
⅓ cup sliced green onion
⅔ cup finely diced red bell pepper
3 Tbsp chopped fresh parsley
¼ cup flour
½ tsp baking powder
1 cup Panko bread crumbs
3 eggs
1 cup grated Parmesan cheese (optional)
1 ½ tsp Old Bay seasoning
1 ½ tsp Dijon mustard
1 ½ Tbsp Greek yogurt
⅛ tsp cayenne pepper

Instructions

Put the grated zucchini in a colander and stir in the salt. Let the zucchini drain for 15 minutes. Squeeze out excess moisture with a towel or by hand.

Pre-heat oven to 400°F. Line a sheet pan with lightly oiled parchment paper for patties or lightly oil a loaf pan or 8′ square baking dish for a loaf.

Put the drained zucchini in a large bowl and mix in carrots, green onions, peppers, and parsley.

In a separate bowl, mix the flour, baking powder and breadcrumbs together. Stir this mixture into the vegetables.

In a small bowl, whisk eggs with Parmesan cheese, Old Bay seasoning, mustard, yogurt, and cayenne. Fold into vegetables until thoroughly combined.

Nutrition info. *2 patties: 283 calories, 11g fat, 17g protein, 33 g carbohydrate, 1g sodium*

Let the mixture sit for 10 minutes.

Shape the mixture into 8 patties or fill the prepared pan with the mixture.

Bake patties for 10 minutes, turn over, and bake for 8 minutes more. If making a loaf, bake for 30 minutes.

NOTE: To crisp patties more, reheat in an oiled frying pan.

Open house amongst the redwoods with the Caring Kitchen.

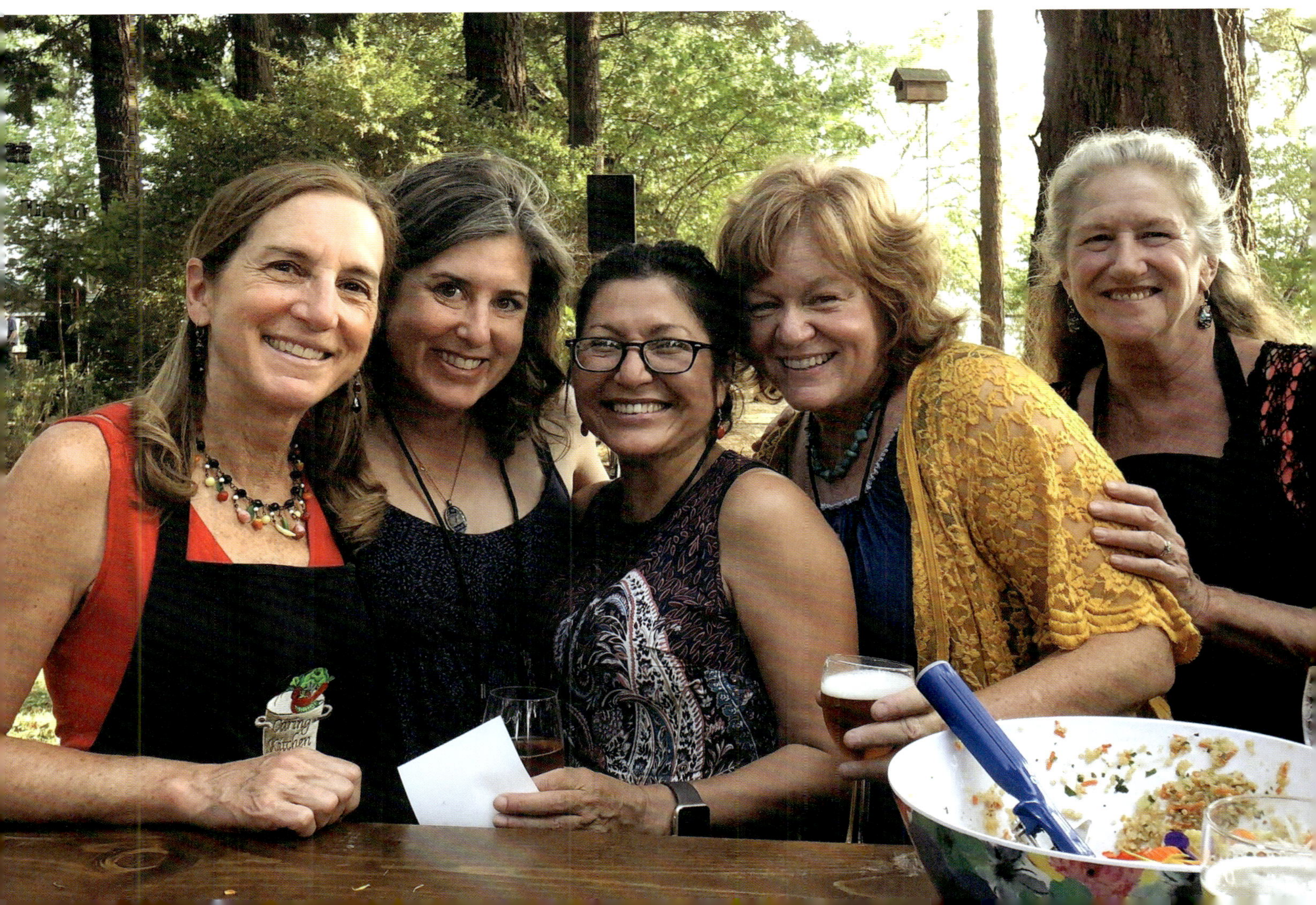

Broccoli Patties or Broccoli Hash

These broccoli patties are a great option when you are looking for a vegetable-focused dish. Eat them as a veggie burger, as an on-the-go snack, or with your favorite salad. We serve them with our Cabbage, Beet and Blueberry Salad (page 83).

— Det Kærlige Måltid Team

Serves 6
Prep time: 1 hour
Cooking time: 15 to 20 minutes
Gluten-free

Ingredients

1 ⅓ pounds broccoli (around 8 cups) finely chopped
1 cup finely chopped red onion
2 garlic cloves, minced
Zest of ½ lemon, minced
½ red chile, minced or ½ to 1 tsp hot sauce
½ cup almonds, ground finely in blender
¾ cup grated Parmesan cheese
⅓ cup finely chopped fresh parsley
1 tsp paprika
1 tsp salt
2 Tbsp water
3 Tbsp corn flour (blend cornmeal in a blender to make your own)
⅓ cup regular rolled oats
Salt and pepper to taste
¼ cup olive oil
3 eggs
For hash only: olive oil for frying

Nutrition info. *2 patties: 313 calories, 20g fat, 14g protein, 23g carbohydrate, 609mg sodium*

Instructions

Combine the first 8 ingredients (broccoli through parsley) in a large bowl and mix thoroughly.

Mix in paprika, salt, water, corn flour and oats. Add pepper and more salt if needed.

Beat eggs with olive oil and add to mixture, stirring well.

Refrigerate for at least 30 minutes, so the corn flour and oats can soak up the liquid and the mixture sets. This step is important for the patties to hold together.

If making patties, preheat oven to 375°F. Line a baking sheet with parchment paper or lightly oil.

Form patties using a ½ cup measure. Press down firmly on each patty in the measuring cup before reversing out onto the parchment. Then press down lightly to form slightly flattened patties.

Bake at 375°F for 20 minutes.

If making hash, heat 2 tablespoons olive oil in a large skillet over medium heat and swirl to coat pan. Add hash mixture to pan and press down firmly. Cook until bottom begins to brown and then turn hash over, breaking it up. Cook an additional 5 minutes or until broccoli is tender and nicely browned.

Mushroom Pâté with Cranberries and Quinoa Green Bean Salad

We recommend serving this with a homemade Greek yogurt and herb dressing, and crusty pumpernickel or rye bread. Sourdough-based, traditional rye bread is considered a national Danish food.

— Det Kærlige Måltid Team

Serves 8
Prep time: 30 minutes
Cooking time: 1 hour

Ingredients

Pâté

6 ounces large-grain couscous
1 cup boiling water
4 Tbsp olive oil, divided
7 cups finely chopped mushrooms
1 yellow onion, finely diced
1 cup almonds, chopped roughly
¾ cup dried cranberries
1 ¼ cups plain Greek yogurt
4 eggs, whisked
¼ tsp salt
¼ tsp ground black pepper

Salad

1 ¾ cups black quinoa (or other type)
10 to 12 ounces green beans
1 cup packed kale, stems removed and roughly chopped
½ cup pomegranate balsamic vinegar (or regular balsamic)
1 Tbsp olive oil
3 persimmons, chopped into bite-size pieces
½ cup pomegranate seeds
7 ounces feta cheese, cubed
⅔ cup toasted pumpkin seeds (pepitas)

Nutrition info. *1 serving: 573 calories, 25g fat, 24g protein, 68g carbohydrate, 752mg sodium*

Instructions

Preheat oven to 325°F. Lightly grease an 8 x 8-inch baking dish. For the pâté, put the couscous in a bowl and cover with boiling water. Let sit for 5 to 10 minutes.

In a large pan, heat 2 tablespoons of the oil over medium-high heat. Add the mushrooms and sauté for 5 minutes, until they are tender and all the liquid has evaporated. Put the mushrooms in a large bowl.

In the same pan, heat the remaining oil over medium heat and cook the onions for several minutes until just tender. Remove from heat. Add the onions to the mushrooms along with the remaining pâté ingredients. Mix until well combined.

Transfer to the baking dish and pat down to make an even layer. Bake until the internal temperature reaches 165°F, about 45 minutes. While the pâté, is baking, prepare the salad. Rinse quinoa well and cook according to the package. Let cool.

Cook beans in salted water for 5 to 7 minutes, until cooked through but still al dente. Rinse in cold water. If using frozen green beans, just cover them with boiling water to heat them up.

In a salad bowl, combine the quinoa, beans, kale, vinegar and oil. Add salt and pepper to taste. Carefully mix in persimmon, pomegranate seeds, and feta. Sprinkle pepitas over salad.

Swiss Chard and Goat Cheese Frittata

We make this frittata as an appetizer for events, cut into little triangles and topped with our Balsamic Tomato Onion Conserve (page 76). It's also great topped with Chimichurri sauce or pesto. For a nice color accent, choose red chard. The frittata combines sweet notes from the onion and a bit of tanginess from the goat cheese. Enjoy it warm or cold!

— The Caring Kitchen Project Team

Serves 6
Prep time: 40 minutes
Cooking time: 15 to 18 minutes
Gluten-free

Ingredients

1 small bunch (about ½ pound) Swiss chard with stems
3 Tbs olive oil
1½ cups diced onion
½ tsp salt, divided
1½ Tbsp minced garlic
8 eggs
½ pound goat cheese, at room temperature
3 Tbsp finely chopped fresh herbs (such as basil, thyme, oregano)
¼ tsp ground black pepper
¼ cup grated Parmesan cheese

Instructions

Preheat oven to 350°F. Grease an 8-inch casserole dish or baking round.

Wash chard thoroughly, drain well and remove stems and tough ribs. Dice stems and ribs and set aside. Roughly chop the leaves.

Heat olive oil in a large skillet over medium heat. Add the onion and chard stems and ribs. Sprinkle with ¼ tsp salt and sauté for 7 minutes, or until the onions are translucent and slightly browned.

Add the garlic and cook 1 more minute, stirring often to keep garlic from browning. Stir in the chard leaves and cook for another 2 minutes, until the leaves have wilted. Set aside to cool.

Whisk the eggs in a medium bowl. Add the cheese, herbs, remaining salt and pepper and whisk until combined. Add to the chard mixture and stir just to mix.

Pour into prepared dish and top with Parmesan cheese.

Bake, uncovered, for 15 to 18 minutes, or until cooked through. To test, insert knife in center. If it comes out clean, frittata is done.

Let cool slightly before cutting.

Nutrition info. *1 serving: 427 calories, 31g fat, 23g protein, 10g carbohydrate, 800mg sodium*

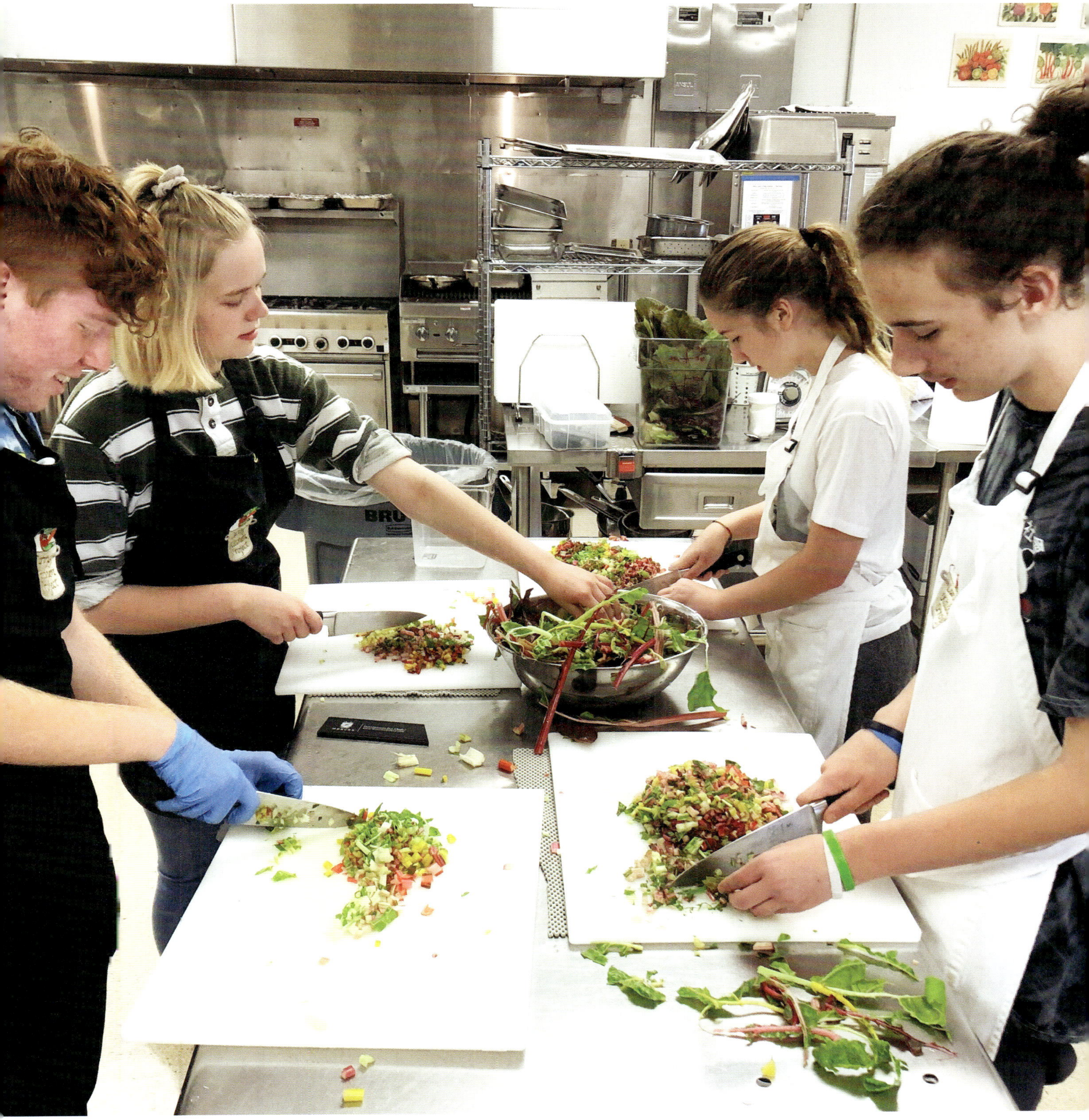

Teens volunteers chopping chard at the Caring Kitchen.

Broccoli and Kale Frittata

As members of the cruciferous family of vegetables, broccoli and kale power this frittata with vitamins, minerals, fiber, and phytochemicals such as as glucosinolates. Glucosinolates break down into several biologically active compounds that are being studied for possible cancer-protective effects.

— Assistant Chef Marcie Carlson, Fox Valley Food for Health

Serves 8
Prep time: 20 minutes
Cooking time: 45 minutes
Gluten-free

Ingredients

1 (10-ounce) package prepped kale, or 2 bunches, stems removed
5 cups broccoli florets and peeled stems, cut into ½ inch pieces
1 Tbsp olive oil
1 medium onion, chopped
2 cups grated cheddar cheese
12 eggs
1 ½ cups whole milk
½ tsp sea salt
½ tsp ground black pepper
3 Tbsp chopped fresh dill
1 cup crumbled feta cheese

Instructions

Preheat oven to 375°F. Grease a 9 x 13-inch baking dish.

In a large pot of boiling water, blanch kale for 2 to 3 minutes or until just tender. With a slotted spoon or spider, transfer kale to ice water to cool. Remove from ice water and drain well. Squeeze out any excess water and chop finely. Transfer kale to a large bowl.

In the same pot of boiling water, blanch broccoli for 2 to 3 minutes or until bright green, crisp and tender. With a slotted spoon or spider, transfer broccoli to ice water to cool. Remove from ice water and drain well. Transfer to bowl with kale.

In a large skillet, heat the oil over medium heat and cook onion for about 5 minutes or until tender and beginning to turn golden. Transfer onion to bowl with kale and broccoli. Toss the vegetables to combine. Spread the vegetable mixture evenly in prepared baking dish. Sprinkle with cheddar cheese.

In a large bowl, whisk together eggs, milk, salt, pepper and dill. Pour egg mixture over vegetable mixture. Sprinkle with feta cheese. Bake for 40 to 45 minutes, or until a knife inserted near the center comes out clean. Serve warm or at room temperature.

Nutrition info. *1 serving: 465 calories, 33g fat, 29g protein, 13g carbohydrate, 824mg sodium*

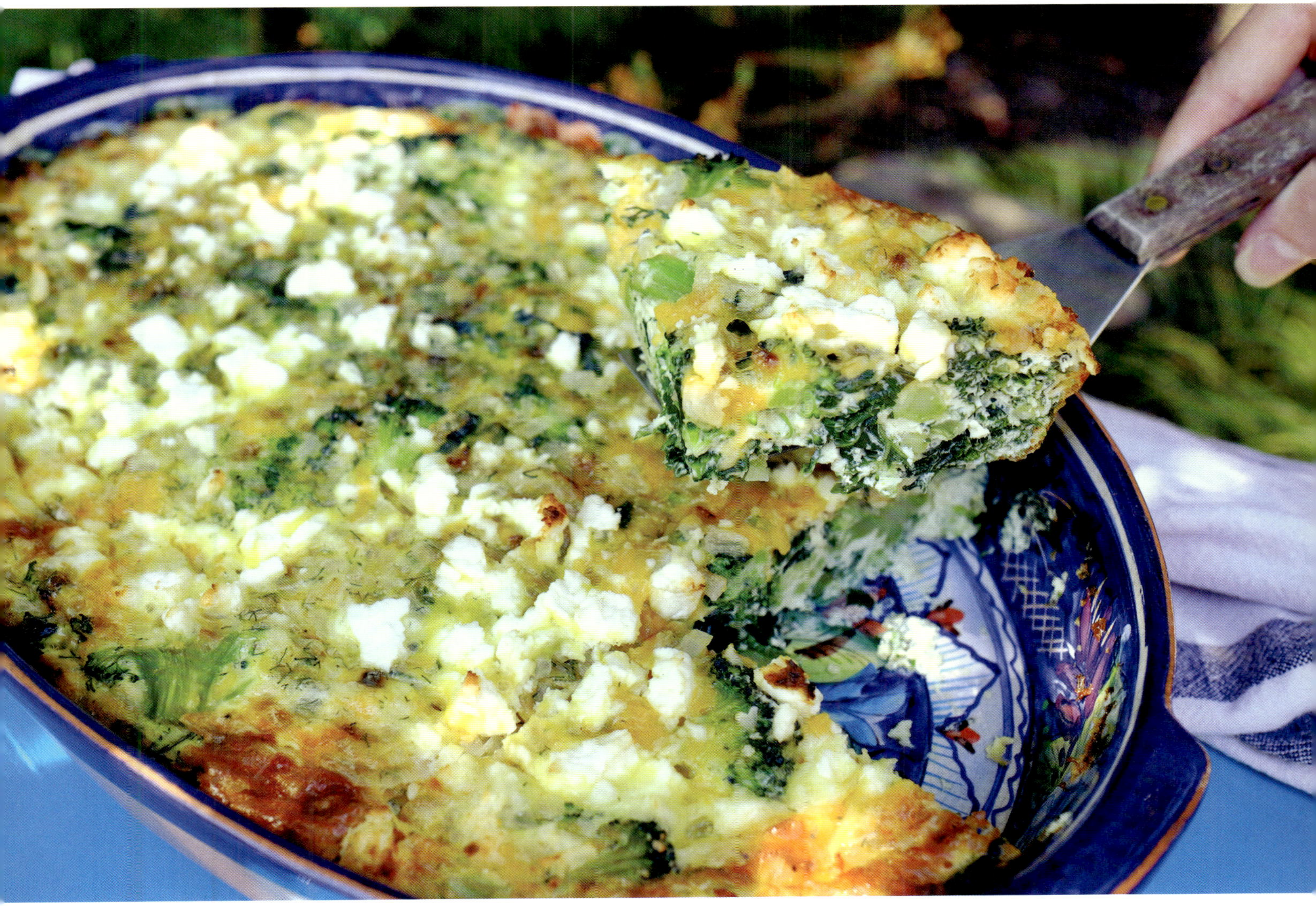

Cauliflower Mushroom Casserole

This is comfort food of the highest order. Roasting the vegetables before baking in the casserole results in a deeply satisfying vegetarian dish.

— Chef John Littlewood, Ceres Community Project

Serves: 6
Prep time: 20 minutes
Cooking time: 1 hour
Gluten-free

Ingredients

4 cups cauliflower florets
1 pound mushrooms, chopped
3 Tbsp olive oil, divided
1 cup finely chopped yellow onion
2 tsp minced garlic
7 eggs, lightly beaten
1 ⅛ cups grated cheddar cheese
2 Tbsp shredded parmesan cheese
1 cup kefir, or substitute yogurt thinned out with some water
¼ cup water
2 Tbsp chopped fresh parsley
¾ tsp salt
Dash ground black pepper

Instructions

Preheat oven to 350°F. Line a sheet pan with parchment paper or lightly oil. Lightly oil a 9 x 13-inch baking dish.

Toss cauliflower florets and mushrooms with 1½ tablespoons oil in a large mixing bowl until well coated. Spread out in even layer on sheet pan. Roast in oven for 20 to 30 minutes, or until the vegetables are lightly browned and caramelized, rotating the pan once halfway through cooking time.

In a large skillet, heat remaining oil over medium heat. Add onions and sauté, stirring for a few minutes until onions are translucent. Add garlic. Cook, stirring for another 3 or 4 minutes, just until garlic is lightly cooked. Remove from heat.

In a large mixing bowl combine eggs, both cheeses, kefir, water, parsley, salt and pepper. Add roasted vegetables and the sautéed onion mix. Mix well and spread in baking dish. Tap bottom of dish on table to flatten batter out and remove any bubbles. Try to ensure even thickness by spreading out flat with rubber spatula and spreading all the way into corners of pan.

Bake for 25 minutes and check for doneness by inserting a paring knife in the center. Knife will come out clean when done. If casserole is not done, turn pan around in oven so it browns more evenly, and cook another 5 to 10 minutes until cooked through. Let cool 10 minutes, then serve.

Nutrition info. *1 serving: 347 calories, 26g fat, 19g protein, 12g carbohydate, 570mg sodium*

Baked Falafel with Miso-Tahini Sauce

This is a classic Ceres vegetarian dish, and a client favorite. Adding miso to the traditional tahini sauce makes it more nutritious and adds depth of flavor. This versatile dipping sauce lasts well in the fridge and adding a dash of vinegar transforms it into a yummy salad dressing.

— **Chef John Littlewood, Ceres Community Project**

Serves 5
Prep time: 15 minutes, plus overnight for soaking beans
Cooking time: 1 to 1 ½ hours
Gluten-free
Dairy-free

Ingredients

Falafel

1 ⅛ cups dried chickpeas
½ cup chopped parsley
1 ½ Tbsp minced garlic
2 tsp ground cumin
½ tsp ground coriander
½ tsp salt
½ tsp baking soda
½ cup finely chopped yellow onion
2 Tbsp brown rice flour
2 eggs, beaten
1 ½ Tbsp olive oil

Miso-Tahini Sauce

1 Tbsp minced shallots
1 clove garlic, minced
2 Tbsp lemon juice
2 Tbsp chickpea miso
¼ cup tahini
2 Tbsp olive oil
½ cup water

Instructions

Soak chickpeas overnight in 4 times as much water as beans. Drain and rinse chickpeas. Cook chickpeas in 3 times as much water as beans until they are VERY soft. The time will vary depending on the freshness of your beans. Check after 45 minutes and then every 10 to 15 minutes. Drain and cool to room temperature.

Preheat oven to 350°F. Line sheet pan with parchment paper or lightly oil.

Place chickpeas, parsley, garlic, cumin, coriander, salt, and baking soda in a food processor fitted with the metal blade. Process until the mixture is coarsely puréed.

Squeeze out as much moisture as possible from the onions. Combine chickpeas and onion in a bowl; stir in the flour and eggs. Shape mixture into ¼ cup round patties and place on sheet pans. Brush each patty with olive oil. Bake for 8 minutes. Turn patty over and brush the other side with olive oil. Bake for 7 minutes more, or until golden brown.

For sauce, combine shallot, garlic, lemon juice, miso, tahini, olive oil and water in blender. Blend until smooth.

Serve warm falafels with sauce on the side.

NOTE: Canned chickpeas can also be used. Use 3 ½ cups drained and rinsed chickpeas and skip the soaking and cooking steps.

Nutrition info. *2 falafels and 2 ounces sauce: 407 calories, 21g fat, 15g protein, 41g carbohydrate,*

Roasted Veggie Enchilada Casserole

Roasting peppers turns them smoky-sweet and makes peeling a snap. To do it, place whole peppers in a single layer in your broiler or on a gas grill on high heat. Cook until the skins are blistered and have begun to blacken, turning frequently to char all sides. Then let them steam in a covered bowl or closed bag until cool. Slip off the skins and they're ready to use in this enchilada sauce, salads, scrambled eggs and dozens of other ways.

— The Healing Meals Community Project

Serves 8
Prep time: 60 minutes
Cooking time: 90 minutes
Gluten-free

Ingredients

Roasted veggies

2 sweet potatoes, peeled and diced
2 red bell peppers, diced
2 onions, diced
2 Tbsp olive oil
2 tsp ground cumin
¼ tsp each salt and ground black pepper

Enchilada Sauce

1 Tbsp olive oil
1 onion, diced
2 red peppers, roasted, peeled and chopped
2 tsp minced garlic
2 (28-ounce) cans tomato sauce
¼ cup chopped cilantro
2 Tbsp ground cumin
2 tsp ground coriander
2 tsp smoked paprika
2 Tbsp chili powder
salt and ground pepper to taste

15 corn tortillas, halved
2 cups cooked wild rice
2 (15-ounce) cans black beans, rinsed and drained
2 cups packed baby spinach leaves
2 cups corn, fresh or frozen
½ cup chopped cilantro
3 cups shredded Monterey Jack cheese

Instructions

Preheat the oven to 400°F. Line 2 sheet pans with parchment paper or lightly oil.

For the roasted veggies, place sweet potato, bell peppers and onion on sheet pans, drizzle with olive oil, cumin, salt and pepper, and toss to combine. Bake until the vegetables are tender and caramelized on the edges, about 30 minutes.

Meanwhile, prepare the enchilada sauce. In a large pan, heat oil over medium heat. Add the onion and sauté for 4 minutes until soft and translucent. Add garlic and roasted pepper and cook for another minute or two. Add the remaining ingredients, bring to a simmer and cook for 20 to 30 minutes, stirring every few minutes. Sauce can be made a day ahead.

Reduce oven to 350°F. Lightly oil a 9 x 13-inch baking dish.

To assemble casserole, spread 1 cup sauce evenly over the bottom of the baking dish. Add a single layer of halved tortilla pieces, arranged so they completely cover the sauce. Top with ⅓ each of rice, beans, roasted vegetables, spinach, corn, cilantro and cheese. Repeat to create three layers, ending with a sprinkling of cheese.

Bake 25 to 30 minutes, until bubbling and golden brown. Cool for 10 minutes before cutting.

Nutrition info. *1 serving: 574 calories, 21g fat, 26g protein, 76g carbohydrate, 582mg sodium*

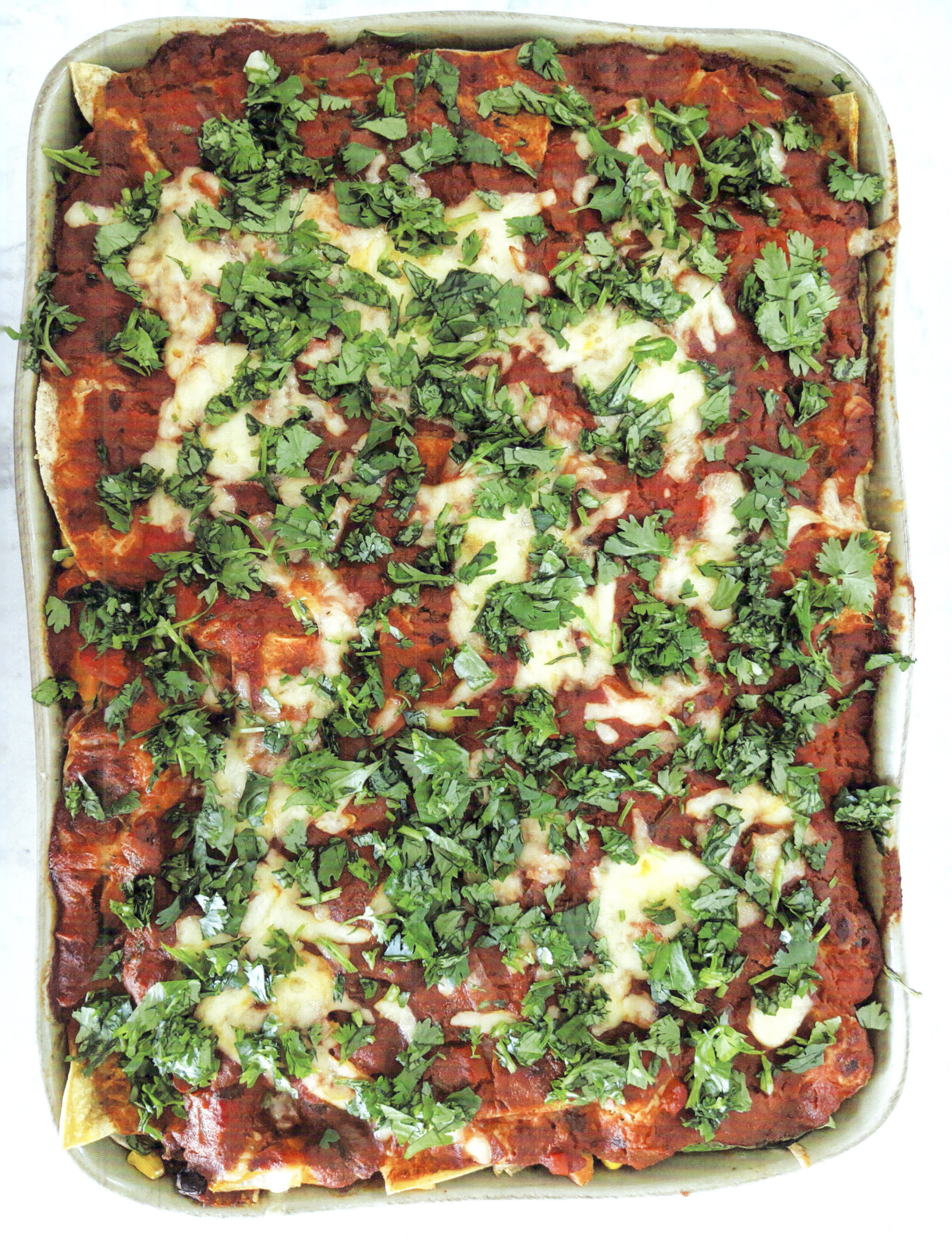

Crowd-Pleasing Tex-Mex Casserole

This is the perfect crowd-pleasing vegetarian dish—even for your most meat-loving friends and family! It combines the familiar flavors of many Tex-Mex dishes while including a plethora of vegetables, whole grains, and legumes.

— Chef Molly Evans, Fox Valley Food for Health

Serves 6
Prep time: 1 hour
Cooking time: 20 to 25 minutes
Gluten-free

Ingredients

1 Tbsp chili powder
1 tsp ground cumin
1½ tsp ground coriander
1 tsp smoked sweet paprika
½ tsp cayenne or ground hot pepper
1 tsp salt
1 Tbsp olive oil
1 red onion, diced
2 cloves garlic, minced
1 orange bell pepper, diced
1 red bell pepper, diced
1 jalapeno, seeded and minced
2 cups chopped baby spinach
½ cup frozen corn, thawed
1 (14-ounce) can diced tomatoes, not drained
1 cup tomato purée
1 (15-ounce) can or 1 cup cooked black beans, drained
3 cups cooked brown rice
1 cup shredded Mexican cheese blend or Monterey Jack cheese, divided into two portions
Salt and ground black pepper to taste

Garnish (Any or all):

Corn chips
Cilantro
Lime juice
Fresh avocado or guacamole, salsa

Instructions

Preheat oven to 375°F. Oil a 9 x 13-inch baking dish.

In a small bowl, combine chili powder, cumin, coriander, paprika, cayenne and salt. Set aside.

In a large skillet, heat oil over medium heat, add onions and cook for 5 minutes.

Add garlic, bell peppers, and jalapeno; continue cooking for 5 minutes.

Add spinach and cook for 2 minutes.

Add reserved spice blend, corn, diced tomatoes, tomato purée, beans and rice. Heat for 3 minutes.

Stir in half of the shredded cheese.

Pour mixture into prepared baking dish and smooth top. Sprinkle the remaining half of the cheese over the casserole. Cover with foil, tenting if needed to keep cheese from sticking.

Bake for 15 minutes. Uncover and bake for 5 to 10 minutes more, or until bubbly and slightly golden around the edges.

Serve with garnishes of your choice.

Nutrition info. *1 serving: 314 calories, 16g fat, 15g protein, 32g carbohydate, 612mg sodium*

Walnut Mushroom Enchilada Casserole

Always a favorite of our clients, this meatless entrée takes the crunchiness of walnuts and marries it with meaty mushrooms for a fabulous meat substitute. The spiciness can be adjusted to your liking!

— The Caring Kitchen Project Team

Serves 8
Prep time: 15 to 20 minutes
Cooking time: 30 to 35 minutes
Gluten-free

Ingredients

2 ½ cups walnut halves and pieces
1 lb cremini mushrooms
½ cup olive oil
1 ½ cups diced onions
1 Tbsp minced garlic
1 pound broccoli stems and florets, chopped
1 small bunch kale, de-stemmed and chopped
1 tsp ground cumin
1 ½ tsp salt, divided
¼ tsp ground black pepper, divided
1 ½ cups cooked black beans
3 cups mild red enchilada sauce or 2 cans
1 ½ cups shredded cheddar cheese
1 ½ cups shredded jack cheese
12 6-inch corn tortillas, cut in half

Instructions

Preheat oven to 350°F. Oil a 9 x 13-inch baking dish.

In a food processor fitted with the metal blade, pulse the walnuts and mushrooms until chopped well, about the consistency of cooked ground meat. Set aside.

In a large skillet, heat the olive oil. Add the onions and cook until translucent and lightly browned, about 2 to 3 minutes. Add the garlic and cook another minute.

Add the mushroom and walnut mixture to the skillet. Cook for 10 to 20 minutes, or until the liquid from the mushrooms is cooked off, scraping the bottom of the pan frequently. You may need to add a small amount of water if the mixture sticks.

Add the broccoli and kale and cook another 2 minutes. Add the cumin, salt, pepper, and black beans. Stir well to combine and cook another minute, then turn off the heat. Set aside.

Combine cheeses in a medium bowl and mix well.

To assemble casserole, spread one-third of the enchilada sauce in the baking dish, cover with a layer of one-third of the tortillas, then one-half of the mushroom and broccoli mixture, then sprinkle on one-third of the cheese. Repeat this step for the second layer. For the final layer, spread the remaining tortillas, the remaining enchilada sauce, and the remaining cheese.

Cover dish with foil and bake for 20 minutes. Remove the foil and bake another 10 minutes, until cheese is golden brown and bubbling.

Nutrition info. *1 serving: 656 calories, 47g fat, 25g protein, 41g carbohydrate, 1g sodium*

Sweet Potato Black Bean Tacos with Roasted Corn Salsa & Avocado Crema

The peels on citrus carry health benefits that are often overlooked. We try not to waste anything here, so the zest is a win-win — adding both flavor and nutritional benefits.

— The Positive Community Kitchen Team

Serves 4
Prep & cooking time: 45 minutes
Vegan (using vegan cheese)
Gluten-free

Ingredients

Roasted Vegetables

2 small to medium sweet potatoes or yams, peeled and cut into ¾" cubes, about 2 cups
1 Tbsp olive oil
¾ tsp smoked paprika
¼ tsp cayenne pepper, optional
¼ tsp fine salt

2 medium ears of corn, or 1 ½ cups frozen corn kernels
½ Tbsp olive oil
¼ tsp salt
¼ tsp ground black pepper

Filling

½ Tbsp olive oil
½ cup finely chopped onion
1 garlic clove, minced
1 tsp ground cumin
¼ tsp chili powder
1 (14-ounce) can black beans, rinsed and drained (or 1½ cups cooked black beans)
¼ tsp salt
¼ tsp ground black pepper, to taste

Salsa

1 large tomato, seeded and diced
¼ cup minced red onion
1 garlic clove, minced
¼ cup chopped cilantro
1 lime, zested and then juiced
1 ½ tsp olive oil
1 Tbsp red wine vinegar
1 ½ tsp chili powder
1 ½ tsp paprika
½ tsp ground cumin
¼ tsp salt
Roasted corn (see above)

Avocado Crema Sauce

¼ cup cashews, soaked in ½ cup water for at least 2 hours then drained and chopped coarsely
½ small avocado, diced
1 garlic clove, minced
Juice of ½ lime
2 to 4 Tbsp water
¼ tsp salt
¼ tsp ground black pepper, to taste

8 taco-sized corn tortillas
2 cups shredded purple cabbage
½ cup crumbled vegan or regular cotija cheese (optional)
Cilantro leaves for garnish

Instructions

Roasted Vegetables

Preheat oven to 425°F.

Toss sweet potatoes with olive oil, paprika, cayenne and ¼ tsp salt. Spread on baking sheet lined with parchment paper or lightly oiled.

Shuck and clean your corn if using fresh ears. Place ears on a second oiled baking sheet, drizzle with ½ to 1 tablespoon olive oil and season with salt and pepper. If you are using frozen corn, toss with ½ tablespoon of olive oil, salt and pepper and spread evenly on the second baking sheet.

Place sweet potato and corn in the oven and roast for about 20 minutes, tossing half-way through the baking to help everything cook evenly.

Filling

In a 2-quart saucepan, heat the olive oil over medium heat. Add onion and garlic and cook, stirring often, for about five minutes or until onion is translucent and tender. Add cumin and chili powder and cook, stirring, for 30 seconds. Add black beans and heat until warmed through. Cover and turn off the heat. When the roasted sweet potatoes are tender, add them to the pan and toss to combine. If needed, warm gently before serving.

Salsa

In a small bowl, combine all ingredients except corn and toss to mix. When your corn is tender, let it cool slightly. If using fresh ears, cut the kernels from the cob, then add the corn to the salsa ingredients and mix gently to combine.

Avocado Crema Sauce

Combine in a blender: chopped cashews, diced avocado, garlic, lime juice and 2 table-spoons water. Blend until smooth and creamy, adding more water as needed to get a thick but creamy consistency. Season to taste with salt and pepper.

Assembly

When ready to serve, warm tortillas on a grill. Fill each tortilla with about ½ cup of the filling mixture. Top with salsa, avocado crema, shredded purple cabbage and crumbled cheese. Garnish with cilantro leaves. Enjoy!

NOTES: This is a great recipe to make in the summer when fresh corn and tomatoes are at their peak, but you can make it any time of year with roma tomatoes and frozen corn, or even omit the tomatoes from the salsa and replace them with 1 cup chopped red or green bell pepper roasted along with the corn.

While it looks like a lot of steps, they are all simple and the recipe comes together in about 40 to 45 minutes (including washing the dishes). You can make this over a day or two as all the components keep well in the refrigerator. To serve, simply warm the filling mixture while you are preparing the tortillas.

If you are making this for one or two people, serve half the filling and salsa as tacos the first night. The next night, combine the remaining filling and salsa with 1 to 1 ½ cups cooked quinoa. Warm in a 350°F oven for 20 minutes, and top with the remaining avocado crema. Serve with a green salad.

Nutrition info. *2 tacos: 417 calories, 17g fat, 10g protein, 63g carbohydrate, 680mg sodium*

Eggplant Ragù with Quinoa Pasta

"This hearty recipe is loaded with good ingredients and heightened flavor with beloved herbs basil and oregano. The pasta and white beans create an especially nourishing, complete vegetable protein."

— Meals 4 Health and Healing Client

Serves 4
Prep time: 15 minutes
Cooking time: 45 minutes
Vegan
Gluten-free

Ingredients

3 Tbsp olive oil or coconut oil
1 small red onion, diced
1 celery rib, diced
1 carrot, shredded
½ tsp sea salt
¼ tsp ground black pepper
3 large garlic cloves, minced
3 cups diced fresh tomatoes, or diced canned tomatoes in juice (28-ounce can)
1 medium eggplant cut into ½ inch pieces (about 1 pound)
¼ - ½ cup chopped fresh basil
3 Tbsp chopped fresh oregano
3 Tbsp liquid aminos or low-sodium tamari
1 cup cooked white beans, or canned white beans, rinsed and drained

3 cups cooked quinoa pasta (any shape)

Instructions

Heat oil in a medium saucepan over medium-high heat. Add onion, celery and carrot and sauté with a pinch of salt and pepper until tender, about 5 minutes.

Add garlic and sauté for another minute, until aromatic.

Add tomatoes, eggplant, herbs and liquid aminos. Cook until eggplant is tender and sauce is thickened, about 30 minutes.

Transfer half of the eggplant mixture to a food processor fitted with the metal blade and purée until smooth.

Add this mixture back to the eggplant mixture in the pot. Add the cooked beans.

Heat until ragù is warmed and serve over cooked quinoa pasta.

Nutrition info. *1 serving: 321 calories, 12g fat, 7g protein, 51g carbohydrate, 485mg sodium*

Meals 4 Health and Healing volunteers packing meals.

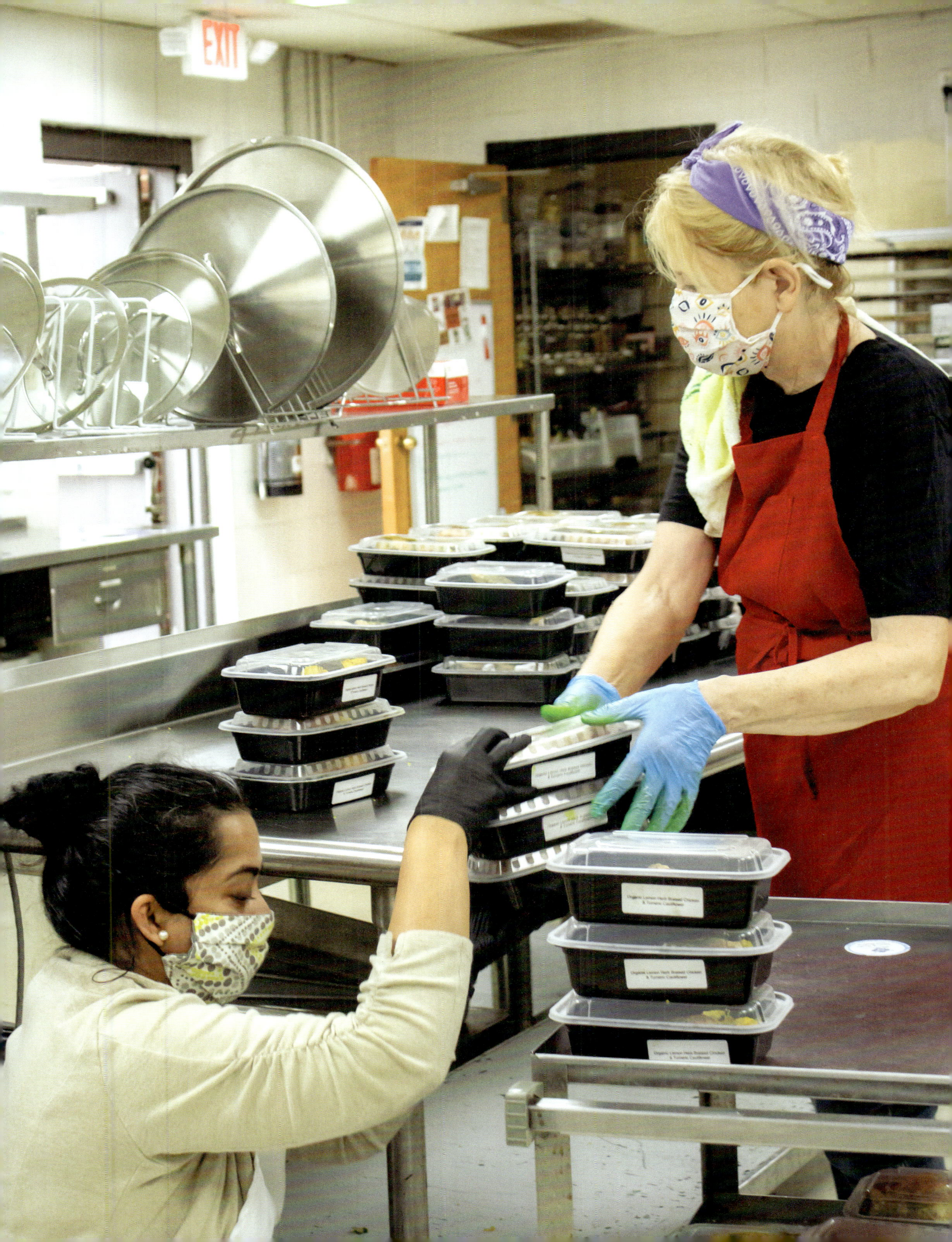
EXIT

Quinoa Pasta Mac and "Cheese"

We remember how Teen Mentor Chef Ryan loved sampling this dish. He loved it even more when he made it completely by himself one Tuesday cooking day!

— The Meals 4 Health and Healing Team

Serves 6
Prep time: 10 minutes
Cooking time: 25 minutes
Vegan
Gluten-free

Ingredients

"Cheese" Sauce

½ cup raw cashews
½ cup minced garlic cloves
½ cup carrots, chopped into large chunks
2 to 3 cups vegetable broth, as needed
1 ¼ cups almond milk
2 tsp chickpea miso
1 Tbsp nutritional yeast (more to taste if needed)
¼ tsp paprika
¼ tsp each salt and ground black pepper

1 pound quinoa elbow pasta
4 cups finely chopped broccoli
2 Tbsp chopped fresh chives

Instructions

Place cashews, garlic and carrots in a medium saucepan and cover with 2 cups vegetable broth. Bring to a boil, then reduce to a simmer and cook, partially covered, for 10 to 15 minutes, until carrots are fully softened.

Remove from heat, drain, rinse, then add to a blender or food processor. Slowly incorporate almond milk and blend until smooth. Add the miso, nutritional yeast and paprika and purée to combine. Add vegetable broth if needed to thin sauce. Season to taste with salt and pepper.

While the cheese sauce is cooking, bring a large pot of salted water to a boil. Drop in quinoa pasta and cook until al dente. Add the broccoli for the last 1 to 2 minutes. When pasta and broccoli are tender, drain.

In a large bowl, toss cooked pasta and broccoli with vegan cheese sauce.

Serve garnished with chopped chives.

Nutrition info. *1 serving: 400 calories, 6g fat, 12g protein, 77g carbohydrate, 314mg sodium*

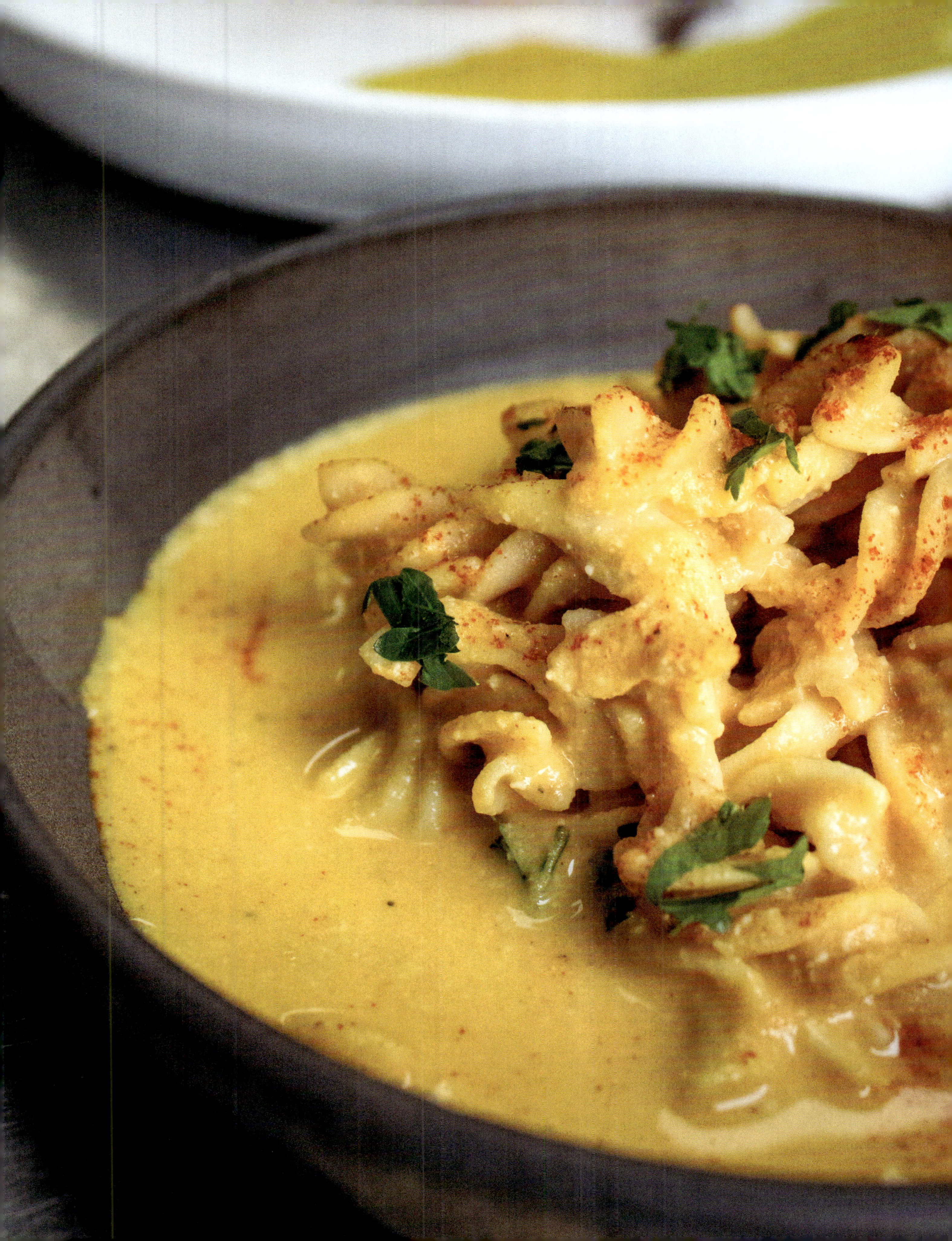

Lentil Meatballs with Seasonal Pesto

This recipe always reminds us of client Angie, who confessed that she loved this dish so much that she ate not only her portion as soon as her meal bag was delivered, but also ate her husband's portion before he got home!

— The Meals 4 Health and Healing Team

Serves 6
Prep time: 15 minutes
Cooking time: 25 minutes
Gluten-free

Ingredients

Pesto

1 garlic clove
2 cups packed raw seasonal greens (kale, spinach, etc.)
¼ cup toasted pine nuts
2 Tbsp lemon juice
1 cup grated Parmesan cheese
¼ cup extra virgin olive oil

Meatballs

2 Tbsp olive oil, plus more for baking meatballs
1 onion, chopped
¼ tsp salt
¼ tsp ground black pepper
3 garlic cloves, minced
8 oz cremini mushrooms, pulsed in the food processor until finely chopped
3 cups cooked brown or green lentils, drained
½ cup nutritional yeast
½ cup chopped fresh parsley
1 tsp dried oregano
1 Tbsp coconut aminos or low-sodium tamari
2 eggs

Instructions

Preheat the oven to 350°F and line a baking sheet with parchment paper or lightly oil.

Turn on food processor and drop in garlic clove to mince. Add in greens, pine nuts, lemon juice and cheese; pulse until minced. Drizzle in olive oil until a pesto-like consistency is reached. Taste, adjust seasoning and set aside.

Warm a skillet over medium-high heat. Add 1 tablespoon of oil and sauté onions with a pinch of salt and pepper until tender, about 5 minutes. Add garlic and sauté until aromatic, about 30 to 60 seconds longer.

Stir in mushrooms and remaining tablespoon of oil; sauté until tender. Remove cooked vegetables from pan and let cool.

Mix cooked vegetables with remaining ingredients and form into 12 equal-sized balls. Arrange evenly on baking sheet, drizzle with olive oil, and bake until firm to the touch, about 20 minutes.

Serve hot with the pesto.

Nutrition info. *2 meatballs: 565 calories, 33g fat, 25g protein, 45g carbohydrate, 533g sodium*

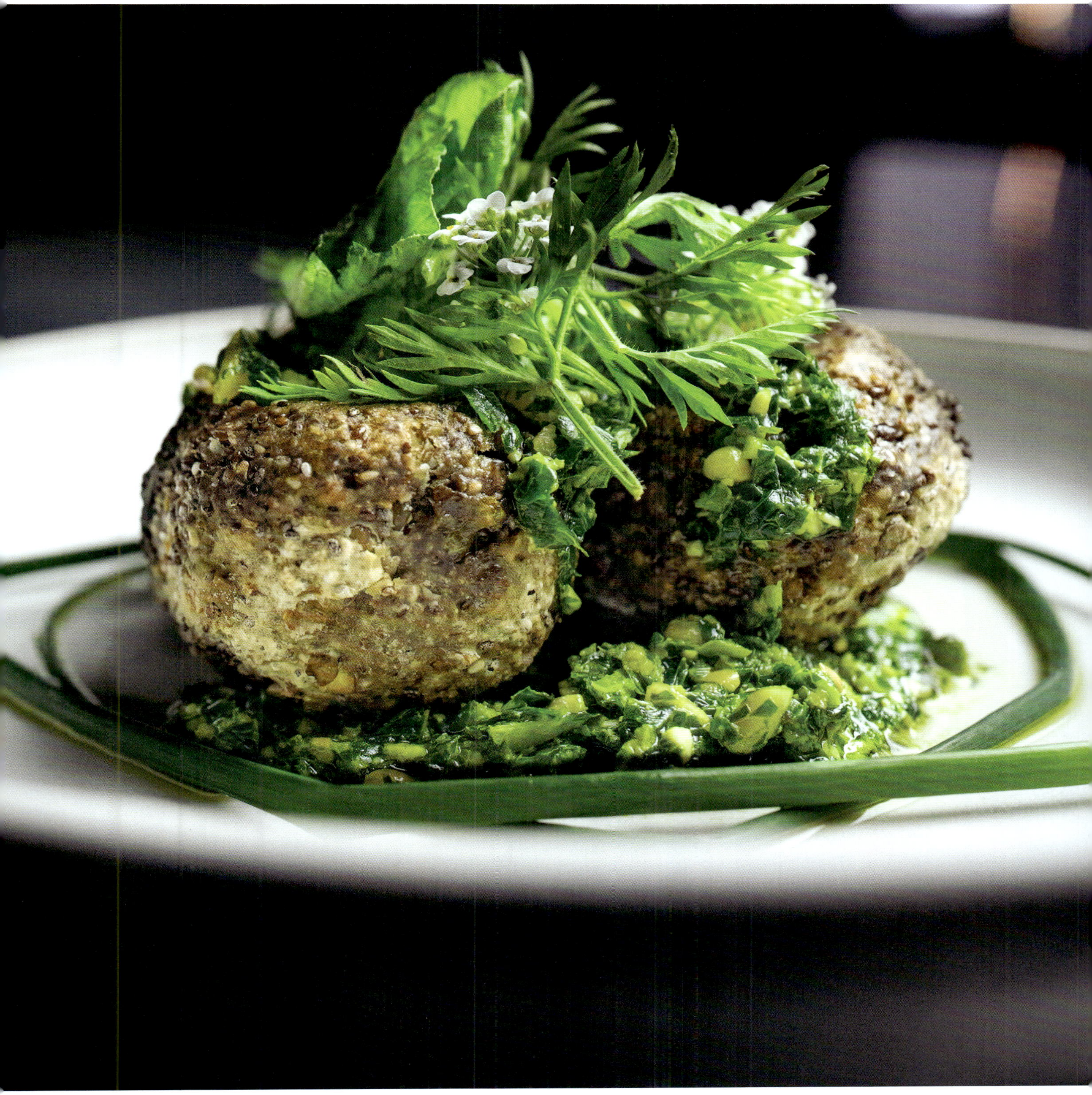

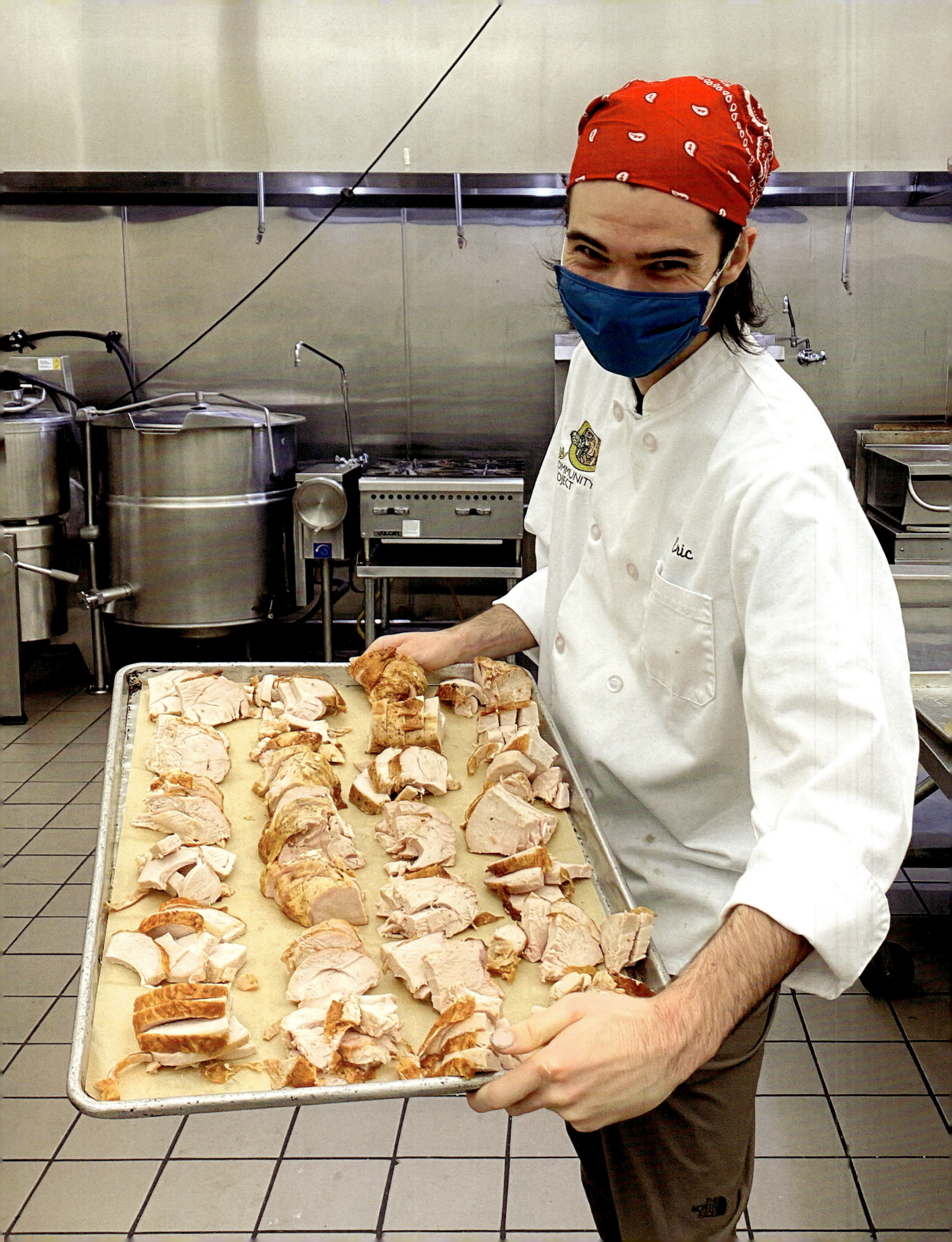

POULTRY & BEEF

Roast Chicken with Herbs and Mustard Gravy

This rich chicken recipe is just the thing for a cool autumn evening. While the oven is already hot, roast some vegetables to complete the meal—brussels sprouts or carrots would be delicious.

— The Revive & Thrive Project team

Serves 6
Prep time: 10 minutes
Cooking time: 45 minutes
Gluten-free

Ingredients

1 Tbsp unsalted butter
3 Tbsp olive oil
8 cloves garlic, peeled
8 chicken thighs, seasoned with salt and pepper
8 baby red or Yukon gold potatoes, peeled
2 Tbsp chopped fresh herbs (any of these: parsley, tarragon, thyme, rosemary, dill, or a blend)

Mustard Gravy

½ lemon, juiced
1 Tbsp Dijon mustard
1 tsp corn starch, dissolved in 1 Tbsp of water
¼ cup chicken stock, plus more as needed
1 tsp salt
½ tsp ground black pepper to taste

Nutrition info. *1 serving: 581 calories, 25g fat, 53g protein, 40g carbohydrate, 713mg sodium*

Instructions

Preheat the oven to 375°F.

Melt the butter with the olive oil over medium heat in a large oven-safe skillet. Add the garlic cloves and cook, stirring occasionally, until lightly golden. Remove garlic and set aside.

Increase heat, then add chicken to skillet and cook for 5 minutes on each side, until the skin is crisp and golden brown. Add the garlic and potatoes and sprinkle with fresh herbs. Place the skillet in the oven and roast for about 25 to 35 minutes, until chicken reaches an internal temperature of 165°F.

Remove the chicken and garlic cloves, leaving any liquid in the skillet. If the potatoes are cooked through, remove them from the skillet using a slotted spoon. If not, return to oven and let them finish cooking in the liquid, adding a bit of broth if needed.

To make the gravy, place skillet with pan drippings on stove over medium heat. Add the stock, lemon juice, and mustard. Stir to combine, then stir in the liquid corn starch and heat for a couple of minutes until it starts to come to a boil and thickens.

Serve the roasted chicken, garlic, and potatoes with the mustard gravy.

A roast chicken dish from Meals 4 Health and Healing with an edible flower garnish.

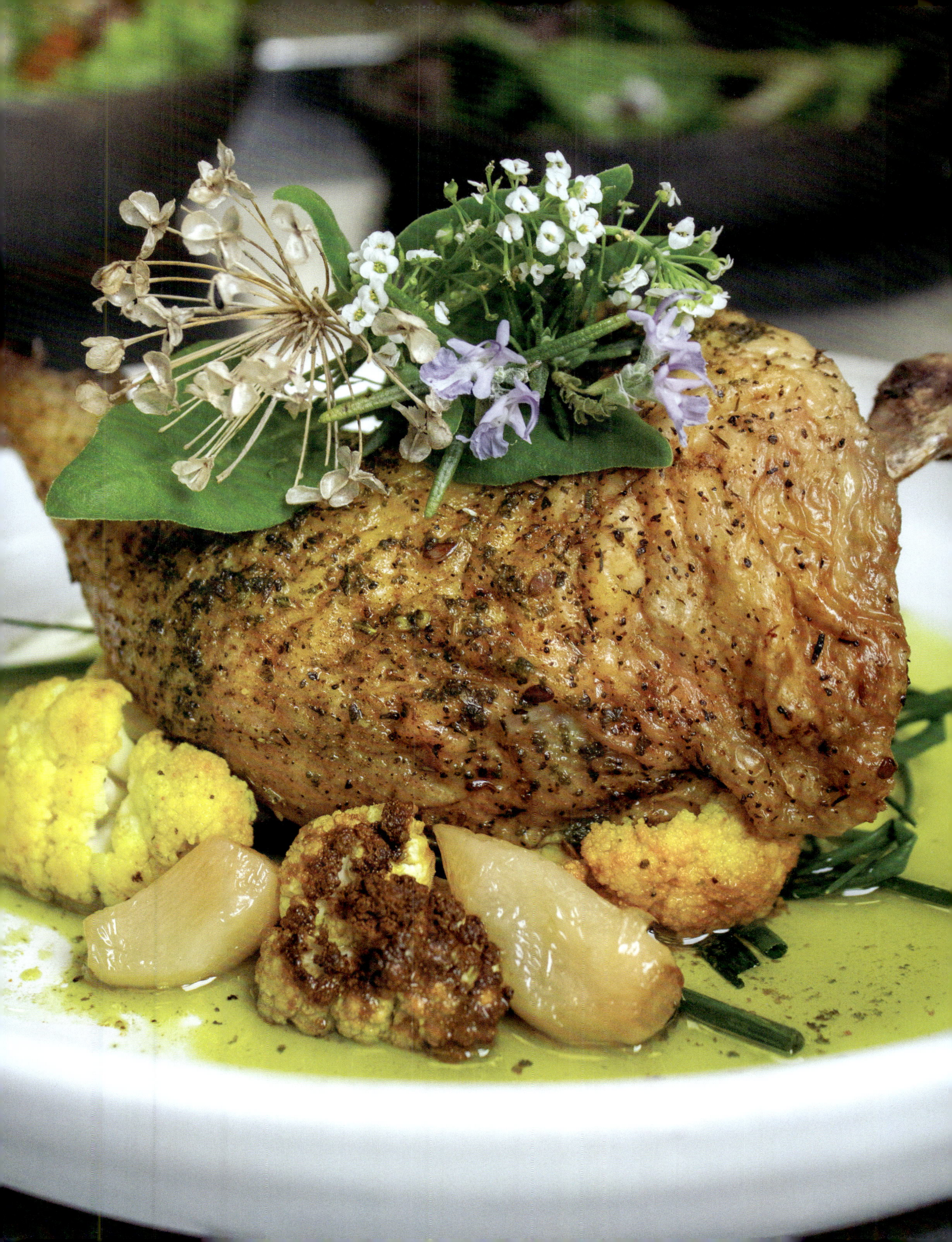

Oven "Fried" Buttermilk Chicken

This healthy version of "fried" chicken has been a client favorite since our founding. Marinating the chicken in kefir and seasonings makes it wonderfully tender and flavorful.

— Chef John Littlewood, Ceres Community Project

Serves 6
Prep time: 3 hours or overnight
Cooking time: 45 minutes
Gluten-free, if using gluten-free breadcrumbs

Ingredients

Marinade

⅔ cup kefir, buttermilk or yogurt, thinned with a bit of water if necessary to a pourable consistency
2 tsp olive oil
2 tsp Dijon mustard
Splash Tabasco sauce
1 tsp granulated garlic
½ tsp salt
½ tsp ground black pepper
2 tsp granulated onion
2 pounds boneless skinless chicken breast

1 ¼ cup breadcrumbs
¼ cup grated Parmesan cheese
2 Tbsp rice flour
1 tsp thyme
½ tsp paprika
1 Tbsp olive oil

Instructions

In a large bowl or baking dish, mix together the kefir, olive oil, mustard, Tabasco, garlic, salt, pepper, and onion. Add the chicken pieces and turn to coat evenly. Cover and chill for at least 3 hours or, preferably, overnight.

Preheat the oven to 425°F. Line a sheet pan with parchment paper or lightly oil.

Combine the breadcrumbs, Parmesan, flour, thyme and paprika in a wide, shallow bowl.

Remove the chicken from the marinade, allowing any excess to run off. Coat the chicken in the breadcrumb mixture and place it on the prepared sheet pan.

Drizzle each piece with some of the olive oil.

Bake the chicken until it is crisp and golden and reaches an internal temperature of 165°F, about 25 to 35 minutes.

Nutrition info. *1 serving: 324 calories, 13g fat, 29g protein, 25g carbohydrate, 496mg sodium*

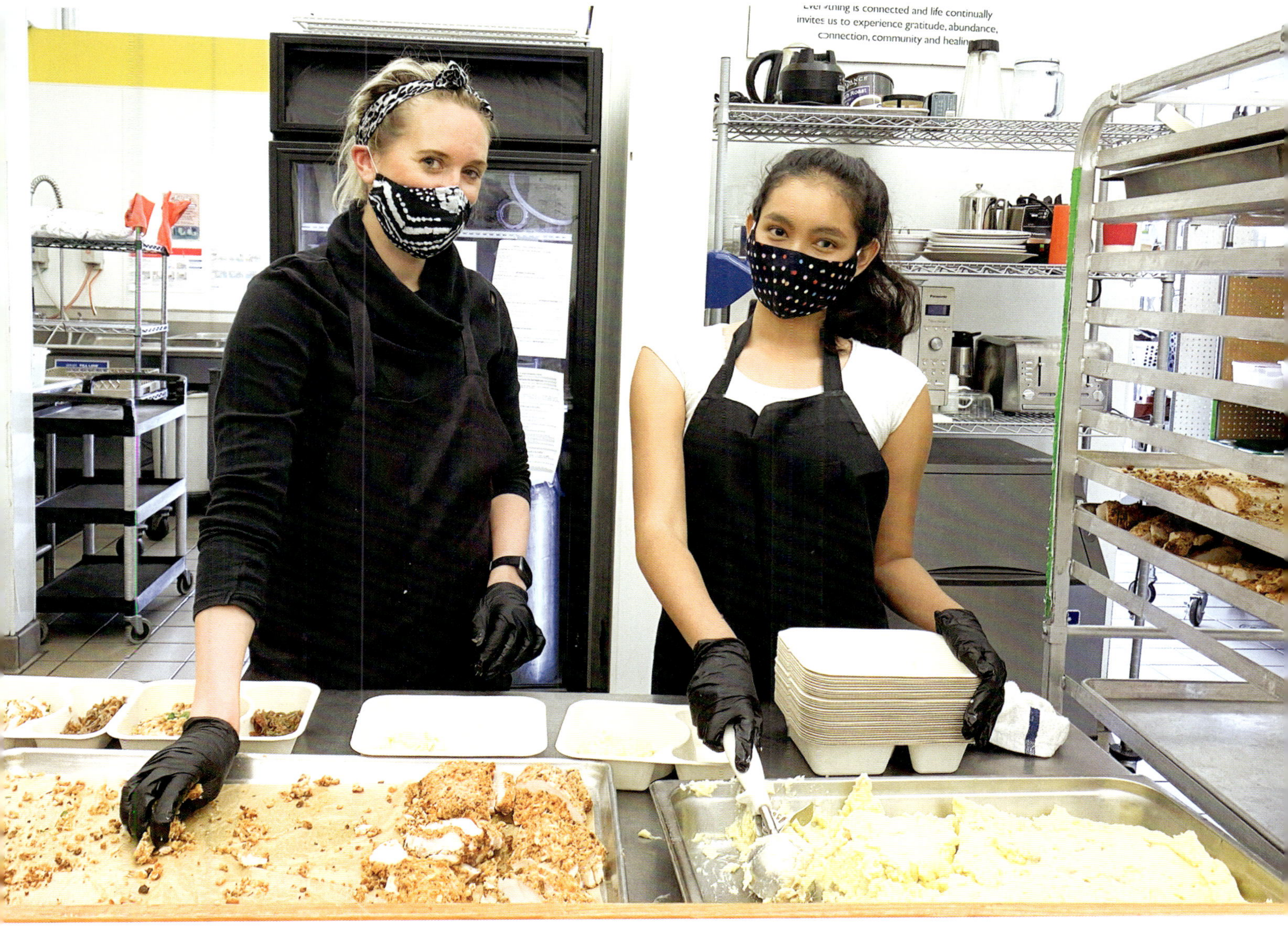

Cooking Oven "Fried" Buttermilk Chicken at Ceres kitchen.

Boller I Karry
Chicken Meatballs in Curry Veggie Sauce with Oriental Rice Salad

Meatballs in curry sauce is considered one of Denmark's national dishes. Many families eat it several times a month. This recipe is a lightened-up version of the original with more veggies, healthier fats, and chicken instead of pork. The rice salad goes nicely with mango chutney and toasted coconut.

— Det Kærlige Måltid Team

Serves 8
Prep time: 30 minutes
Cooking time: 1 hour
Gluten-free

Ingredients

Rice salad
1 ½ cups brown rice
1 ½ cups shelled edamame beans
⅔ cup diced red bell pepper
⅔ cup cubed fresh pineapple
¼ tsp salt

Curry sauce
2 Tbsp coconut oil
2 potatoes, peeled and roughly chopped (about 2 ½ to 3 cups)
1 ¾ cups roughly diced onion
4 ½ cups grated carrots
1 apple, roughly chopped
3 garlic cloves, minced
2 Tbsp curry powder
1 cup vegetable broth
2 ¾ cups coconut milk
¼ tsp salt
¼ tsp ground black pepper
Apple cider vinegar to taste

Meatballs
2 cups grated onion
½ cup low-fat milk
1 ½ tsp salt
3 eggs whites
⅔ cup flour
2 tsp ground black pepper
1 ½ pounds ground chicken
4 cups water
4 cups chicken broth

Instructions

To prepare the rice salad, cook rice according to package. Let cool. In a salad bowl, combine rice, edamame, bell pepper, pineapple and salt; toss together.

To prepare the curry sauce, heat coconut oil in a large saucepan over medium heat. Add the potatoes. Cook for a few minutes, then add the onions. Cook onions until just translucent, stirring to prevent potatoes from sticking. Add carrots, apple, and curry powder, and sauté until golden. Add the vegetable broth, coconut milk, and salt. Bring to a simmer and cook, uncovered, until the vegetables are tender.

Nutrition info. *1 serving: 642 calories, 29g fat, 30g protein, 70g carbohydrate, 624mg sodium*

Blend the sauce with an immersion blender until the texture is to your liking. Taste, and add salt, pepper and apple cider vinegar as needed. Keep the sauce warm over low heat until ready to serve.

While the sauce is simmering, prepare the meatballs. Mix grated onion with the milk and set aside. In a large bowl, whisk salt and egg whites to combine. Add flour and pepper, and mix until evenly distributed. Add the onion and milk mixture, slowly whisking to combine.

Finally, add the ground chicken and mix to combine everything evenly.

In a large pot, bring water and broth to a boil, then lower the heat to a gentle simmer. Form chicken mixture into balls, about 3 Tbsp each. Simmer meatballs carefully, about 13 to 15 minutes, until the internal temperature reaches 165°F.

Put the meatballs in the warm sauce and heat over a low flame. Serve with rice salad on the side.

A client family happily receives a meal from Det Kærlige Måltid in Denmark.

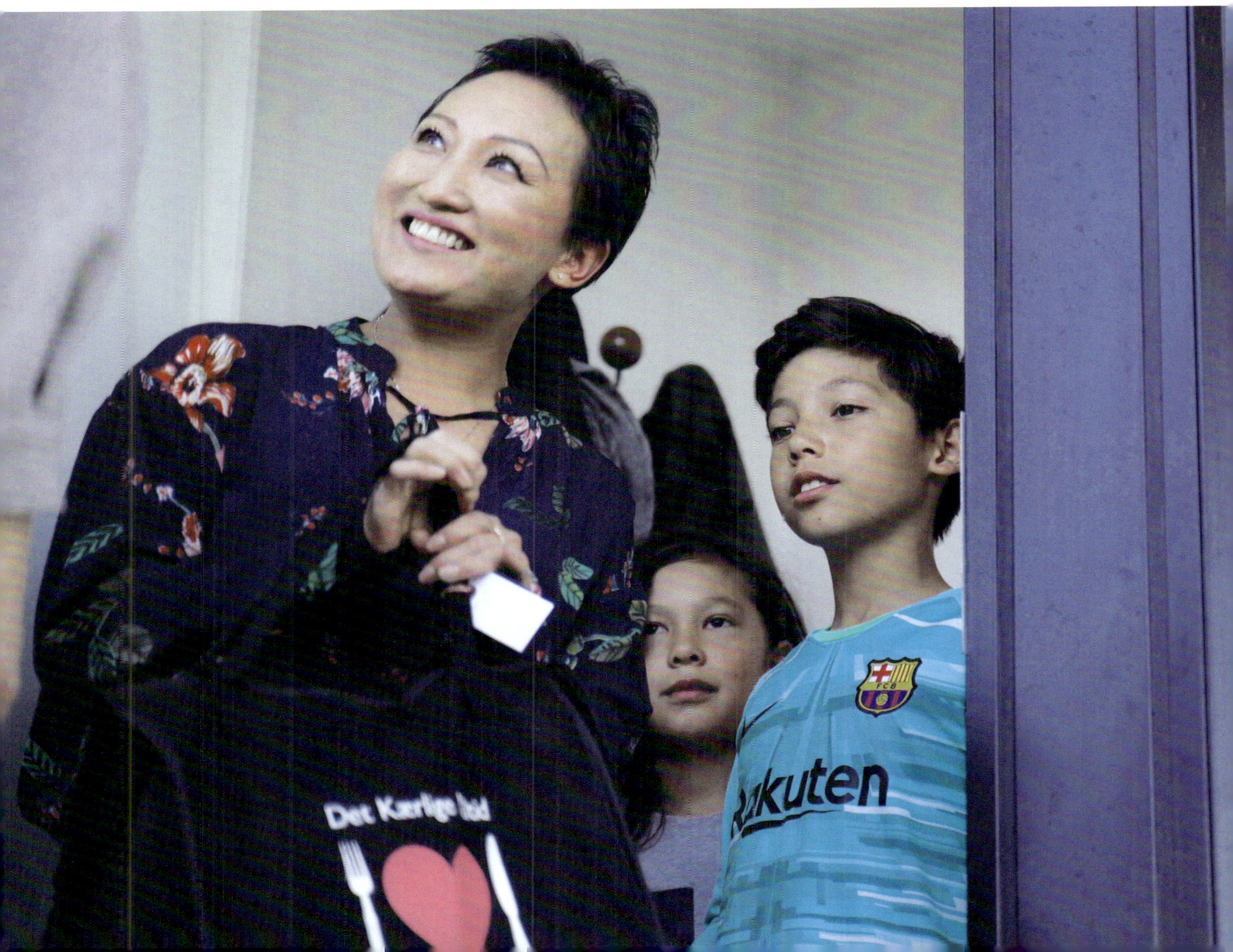

Asian Chicken with Rice Noodles and Cilantro Pesto

Like international travel, this dish requires some work but will surely take you to new places. Cilantro, basil, garlic and ginger blend together to create a flavor that is more than the sum of its parts.

— Chef John Littlewood, Ceres Community Project

Serves 8
Prep time: 1 hour, or overnight
Cooking time: 45 minutes
Dairy-free

Ingredients

4 Tbsp sesame oil, divided
2 Tbsp chickpea miso
1 ½ Tbsp rice wine vinegar
1 Tbsp rice wine (mirin)
5 tsp peeled and minced ginger, divided
2 ½ pounds boneless skinless chicken breast
1 ½ cups chopped cilantro
¾ cup chopped basil
½ cup unsalted cashew butter
¼ cup lime juice
½ cup olive oil
1 Tbsp minced garlic clove
½ tsp salt
1 pound rice noodles, not cooked

Instructions

Whisk together 2 tablespoons sesame oil, miso, rice vinegar, mirin and 2 teaspoons ginger. Marinate chicken in this mixture, refrigerated, for at least an hour, or preferably overnight.

Preheat oven to 375°F. Line sheet pan with parchment paper or lightly oil.

Remove chicken from marinade, place on sheet pan and bake until just cooked through, about 20 to 25 minutes until an instant-read thermometer placed in the thickest part of the breast reads 165°F, being careful not to overcook. Cool, then slice.

In a food processor fitted with the metal blade, add the cilantro, basil, cashew butter, lime juice, remaining sesame oil, olive oil, garlic, remaining ginger and salt. Process until the pesto is creamy.

Bring a large pot of salted water to a boil. Cook the noodles according to the package directions until they are just tender. Rinse under cold water to stop the cooking. Drain well.

Toss the noodles with the pesto and serve, topped with sliced chicken.

NOTE: You can also substitute part of the chicken for an assortment of steamed or sautéed fresh vegetables.

Nutrition info. *1 serving: 620 calories, 31g fat, 30g protein, 53g carbohydrate, 431mg sodium*

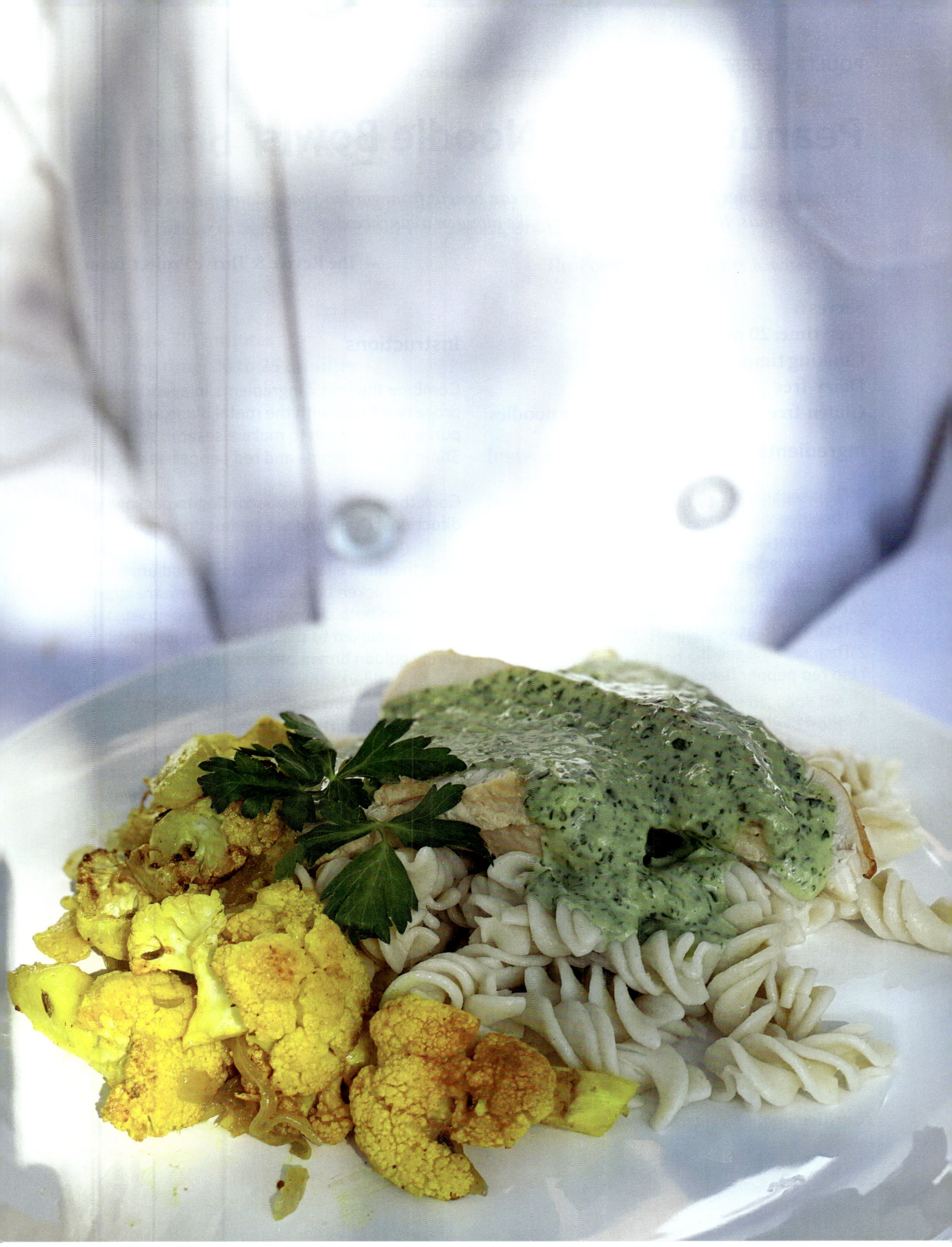

Turkey Stuffed Peppers

We love making these just as bell peppers come into season. They feel like a celebration of summer!

— The Revive & Thrive Project Team

Serves 6
Prep time: 20 minutes
Cooking time: 30 minutes
Gluten-free

Ingredients

6 large bell peppers, any color
1 Tbsp olive oil
2 cloves garlic, minced
1 small yellow onion, diced
1 pound ground turkey
1 tsp salt
½ tsp ground black pepper
1 (14-ounce) can crushed tomato
2 cups cooked brown rice
½ tsp Italian seasoning
1 ½ cups shredded mozzarella cheese, divided
1 tsp chopped fresh parsley
1 tsp chopped fresh basil

Instructions

Preheat oven to 350°F. Lightly oil a baking dish that is large enough to hold all 6 peppers. Cut off the tops of the peppers and remove the seeds. Trim the bottoms of the peppers to help them stand up in the baking dish.

Heat a pot of water to boiling. Blanch the peppers for 5 minutes, remove from water and turn upside down onto a paper towel to dry.

Heat olive oil in a large skillet over medium heat. Sauté the garlic and onion until tender, about 5 minutes. Add the turkey, salt and pepper, and brown until thoroughly cooked.

Add the crushed tomatoes, cooked rice, Italian seasoning, and ½ cup of the shredded cheese and stir until blended.

Divide the turkey mixture between the peppers. Place in the baking dish. Bake, uncovered, for 25 to 30 minutes. Top with the remaining cheese and bake for an additional 5 to 8 minutes, or until the cheese is melted.

Nutrition info. *1 serving, 1 bell pepper: 406 calories, 18g fat, 23g protein,29g carbohydrate, 661mg sodium*

Mushroom Turkey Meatloaf

"We are thankful from the bottom and top of our hearts, and we will forever be grateful. The food is always amazing."

— Healing Meals Community Project Client

Serves 6
Prep time: 35 minutes
Cooking time: 30 minutes
Gluten-free
Dairy-free

Ingredients

1 Tbsp olive oil
1 medium onion, finely chopped
8 ounces mushrooms, finely chopped
2 cloves garlic, minced
1 Tbsp coconut aminos or soy sauce
5 Tbsp ketchup, divided
1 cup gluten-free breadcrumbs
2 eggs, beaten
1 tsp salt
½ tsp ground black pepper
1 pound ground turkey

Instructions

Heat oven to 375°F. Lightly oil a sheet pan or line with parchment paper.

Heat oil in a large skillet over medium heat. Add the onion, mushrooms, and garlic. Cook about 10 minutes until soft. (Alternatively, toss these ingredients together, spread them on a sheet pan and roast 10 to 15 minutes until golden). Transfer the onions and mushrooms to a large bowl, and stir in the coconut aminos and 3 tablespoons of the ketchup. Set aside to cool for 5 minutes.

Stir the breadcrumbs and eggs into the mushroom mixture. Using a fork or your hands, gently mix in the turkey, salt, and pepper. The mixture will be very wet. Divide the mixture into 6 portions. Form each into a mini-meatloaf shape and place evenly spaced on your prepared sheet pan. Divide the remaining 2 tablespoons ketchup among each loaf and spread to coat the tops.

Bake the meatloaf until an instant-read thermometer inserted into the thickest part of the meatloaf registers 170°F, about 20 minutes.

Nutrition info. *1 Serving: 526 calories, 18g fat, 28g protein, 66g carbohydrate, 1g sodium*

Turkey Applesauce Meatloaf

The applesauce makes this meatloaf moist and flavorful. Pair it with a simple green salad and you have a great weekday dinner.

— The Revive & Thrive Project Team

Serves 4
Prep time: 10 minutes
Cooking time: 1½ hours
Dairy-free
Gluten-free, if using gluten-free breadcrumbs

Ingredients

1 pound ground turkey
½ cup finely chopped onion
1 clove garlic, minced
1 egg, beaten
½ cup applesauce
½ cup plain breadcrumbs
2 Tbsp ketchup (optional)
1 tsp salt
¼ tsp ground black pepper

Instructions

Preheat oven to 350°F. Lightly grease a 9x5x3-inch loaf pan. In a large bowl, combine all ingredients and mix well. Pat the meatloaf mixture into the prepared pan. Bake for 1 ½ hours. Let cool 10 minutes; remove to a platter and slice.

Nutrition info. *1 serving: 489 calories, 19g fat, 29g protein, 51g carbohydrate, 1g sodium*

Adult volunteer Kim and teen volunteer Alex in the Positive Community Project kitchen.

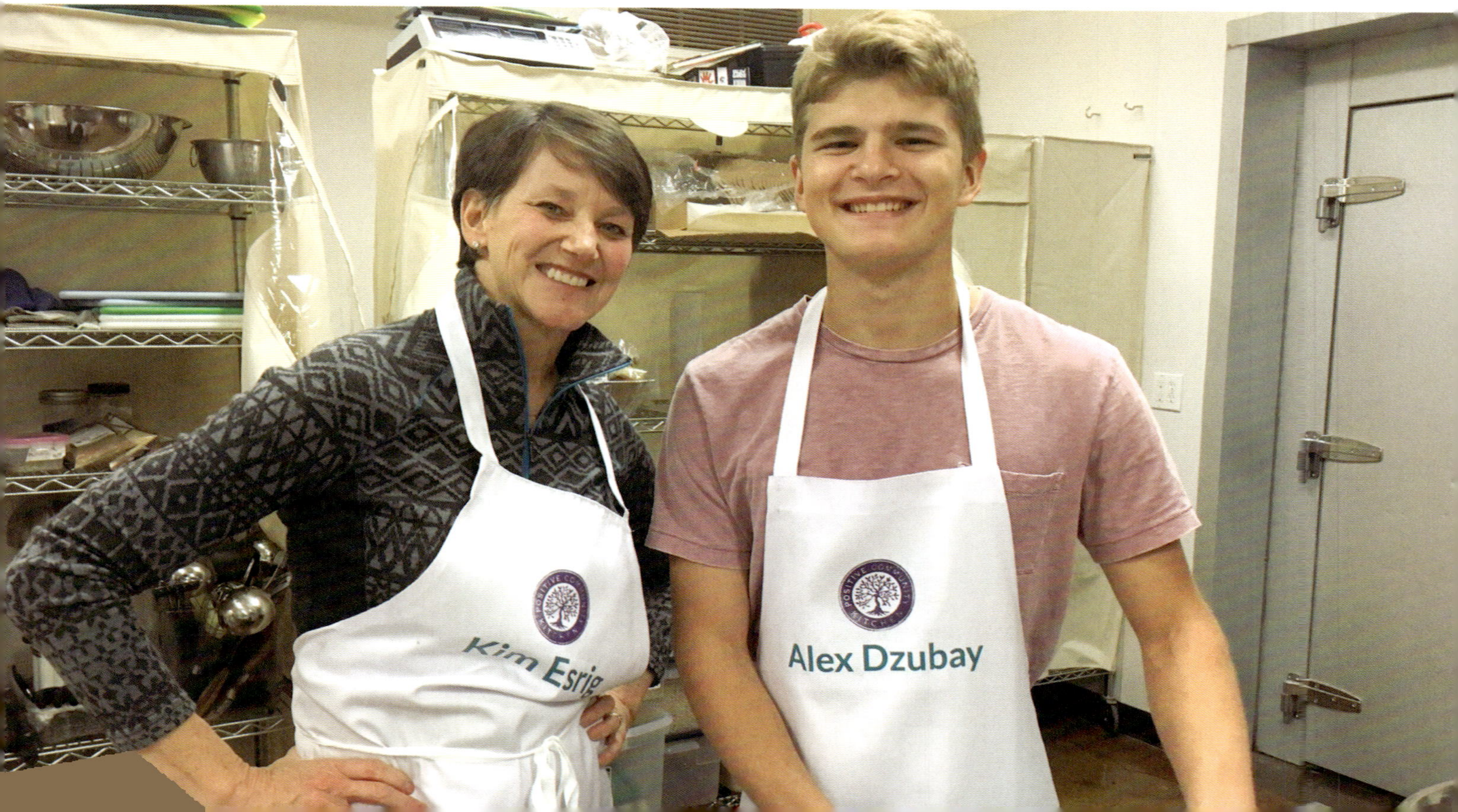

Beef Stew

"Today our chefs have been able to introduce grass-fed beef to our menu which I studied in my Econ class and brought to a Circle presentation for my team. Turns out, for our economy and our planet, there's a lot of benefit in grass-fed beef, but it's not yet widely practiced."

— Teen Chef, Positive Community Kitchen

Serves 4
Prep time: 20 minutes
Cooking time: 4 hours
Gluten-free
Dairy-free

Ingredients

2 Tbsp avocado oil
1 ½ pounds beef stew meat
½ cup small diced yellow onion
½ cup peeled and small diced celery root
½ cup carrot, sliced into half moons
1 ½ cups thinly sliced mushrooms
2 tsp minced garlic clove
3 Tbsp red wine
1 ½ Tbsp tomato paste
2 ½ cups beef broth
1 bay leaf
1 tsp dried thyme (or 2 tsp fresh thyme)
1 ½ tsp salt
¼ tsp pepper

Instructions

In a braising pan or dutch oven, heat the avocado oil over medium heat. Sprinkle the meat with 1 tsp salt and sear it until golden on all sides. This may to be done in batches, depending on the size of your pan. Remove the meat with a slotted spatula and set aside.

In the same pan, add the onion, celery root, carrot, mushroom, and garlic. Toss to combine and let the veggies cook for a few minutes, until slightly softened.

Add the red wine and cook until reduced by half. Add the tomato paste, beef broth, bay leaf, thyme, remaining salt and pepper. Return the meat and any accumulated juices to the pan. Bring to a boil and then reduce to low simmer.

Cover and let cook for 3 to 4 hours until meat is tender. If you like your stew to be very thick, you may need to uncover the pan and let the juices reduce until you've reached your desired consistency.

Nutrition info. *1 serving: 298 calories, 13g fat, 39g protein, 8g carbohydrate, 872mg sodium*

Meatloaf with Tomato and Dijon Glaze

"Positive Community Kitchen is about more than a meal. It's not like when you order a pizza. It's someone showing up at your door, someone who cares, and letting you know, everything is going to be alright."

— **Positive Community Kitchen Client**

Serves 8
Prep time: 15 minutes
Cooking time: 45 minutes
Gluten-free
Dairy-free

Ingredients

Meatloaf

2 Tbsp avocado or sunflower oil
1 small onion, minced
1 carrot, minced
1 stalk celery, minced
2 tsp minced garlic
2 pounds ground beef
1 egg
2 slices gluten-free bread, torn into bite-sized pieces
½ cup tomato sauce
1 tsp salt
½ tsp ground black pepper
2 tsp dried oregano

Glaze

½ cup tomato sauce
1 Tbsp Dijon mustard
2 Tbsp apple cider vinegar
2 Tbsp coconut palm sugar

Instructions

Preheat oven to 350°F. Line a sheet pan with parchment paper or lightly oil.

Heat oil in a skillet over medium heat. Add onion, carrot, celery and garlic and sauté until soft.

In a large bowl, combine the ground beef, egg, bread, tomato sauce, cooked veggies and seasonings. Mix gently to combine. Form into a loaf and bake on sheet pan for 10 minutes.

While meatloaf is cooking, combine the glaze ingredients.

After the meatloaf has baked for 10 minutes, baste with the glaze and return to the oven for 30 minutes.

Check the temperature and baste again. Bake until the meatloaf reaches an internal temperature of 165°F. Let rest for 10 minutes before slicing.

Nutrition info. *1 serving: 352 calories, 19g fat, 32g protein, 16g carbohydrate, 501mg sodium*

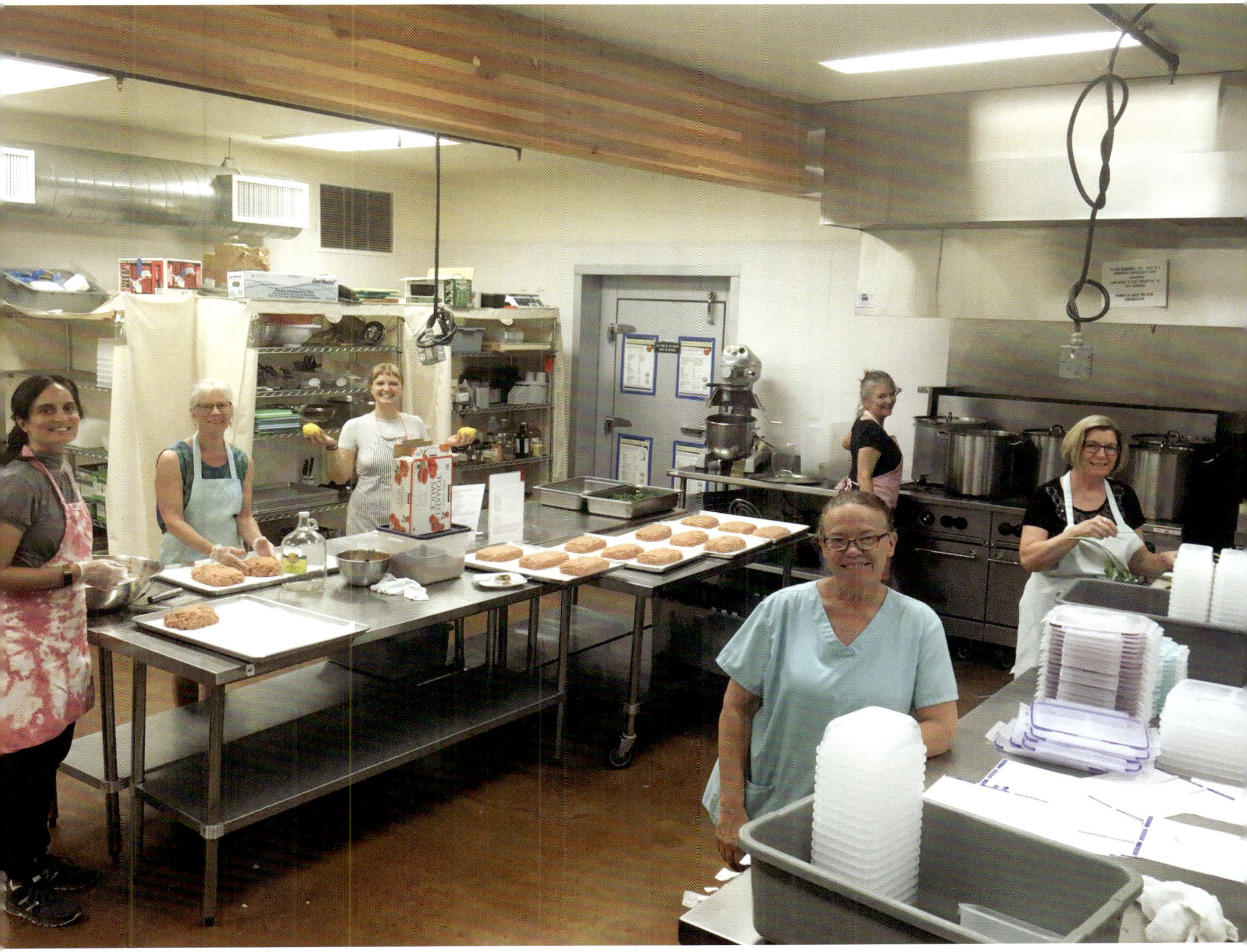

The team at Positive Community Kitchen preparing meatloaf.

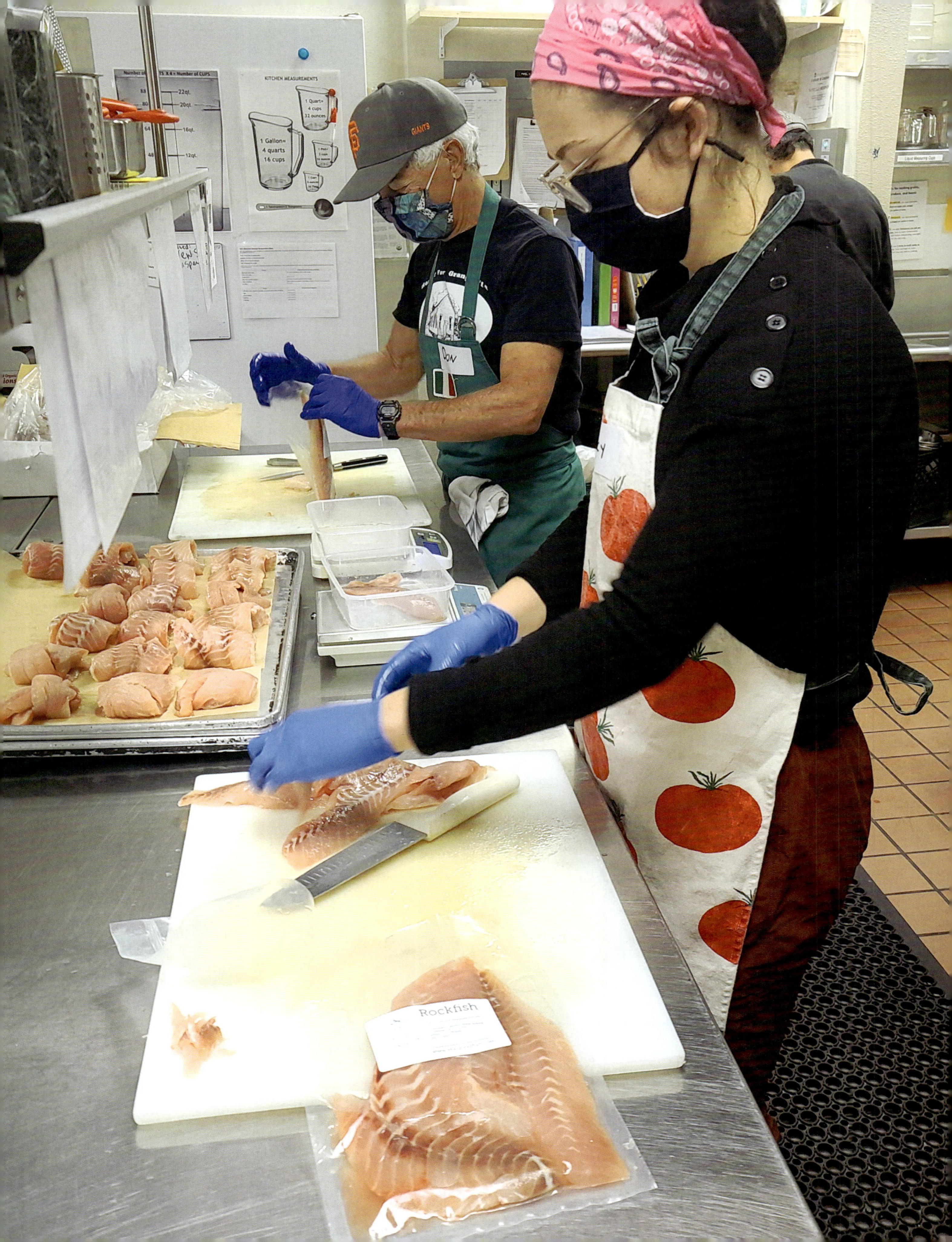
KITCHEN MEASUREMENTS
1 Quart=
4 cups
32 ounces
1 Gallon=
4 quarts
16 cups
GIANTS
Rockfish

SEAFOOD ENTREES

Fiske Frikadeller

Traditional Danish Fish Cakes with Pickled Vegetable Remoulade and Citrus Cabbage Salad

In Denmark, we eat remoulade with French fries, hot dogs, on sandwiches, and with fish. Danish remoulade has a mild, sweet-and-sour taste and a light-yellow color. It is made using a base of marinated veggies and mayonnaise. Serve with crusty bread or boiled potatoes.

— Det Kærlige Måltid Team

Serves 4
Prep time: 1 hour
Cooking time: 20 minutes
Gluten-free, if made with gluten-free flour

Ingredients

Remoulade

1 cup very small cauliflower florets
⅓ cup small diced carrots
2 Tbsp olive oil
2 Tbsp balsamic vinegar
2 tsp Dijon mustard
2 tsp turmeric
2 pinches tarragon
¼ tsp salt
¼ tsp ground black pepper
2 large dill pickles, chopped
6 Tbsp mayonnaise
6 Tbsp plain Greek-style yogurt or sour cream

Fish cakes

½ cup finely chopped onion
½ cup chopped fresh parsley
½ cup chopped fresh dill
1 clove garlic, minced
1 tsp salt
½ tsp ground black pepper
3 to 4 Tbsp flour (regular or gluten-free)
½ cup half and half
2 large eggs, whisked
1 ¼ pounds white fish, roughly chopped
Butter and olive oil, to coat pan

Citrus cabbage salad

2 cups shredded carrots
2 cups shredded green cabbage
⅓ cup raisins
1 grapefruit
Juice of one orange
1 Tbsp honey

Instructions

Remoulade

Blanch the cauliflower florets and diced carrots in lightly salted boiling water until just tender, about three to four minutes. Drain and rinse under cold water to stop the cooking. Drain well.

While the vegetables are blanching, make a marinade by whisking together the olive oil, balsamic vinegar, Dijon, turmeric, tarragon, salt, and pepper. Toss the drained vegetables with the marinade and refrigerate for at least 30 minutes and up to several hours.

Drain off any excess marinade. Mix in the pickle, yogurt and mayonnaise, and stir to combine evenly. Refrigerate until ready to serve. Remoulade can be made a day ahead.

Fish Cakes

In a food processor fitted with the metal blade, pulse the onion, parsley, dill, and garlic until minced and combined. Add the salt, pepper, 3 tablespoons of flour, half and half, and eggs. Pulse to combine everything evenly.

Add in chopped fish and pulse until just combined. Be careful not to overmix. Let the mixture rest for an hour in the refrigerator. Adjust the consistency with a little more flour if needed to be able to form a patty that holds together.

Preheat oven to 325°F. Line a sheet pan with parchment paper or lightly oil.

Form the fish mixture into 8 equal patties. In a large skillet, heat just enough butter and olive oil to coat the bottom evenly. Working over medium high heat, fry the fish cakes until golden brown, about two minutes on each side. Place on sheet pan and finish in the oven until cooked through, about 15 to 20 minutes.

Cabbage Salad

While the fish cakes are in the oven, prepare the salad. Combine the shredded carrots and cabbage in a large bowl with the raisins.

Peel the grapefruit, being careful to remove all the white pith. Section the grapefruit, remove any seeds, and cut each section into three or four pieces. Add to the salad and toss to combine.

Whisk together the orange juice and honey, pour over the salad and toss to combine. It will seem at first like there isn't enough dressing, but as the cabbage begins to wilt it will become wetter.

NOTES: The remoulade can be made up to several days ahead. The fish cake mixture can be made up to 4 hours ahead. Make the salad within an hour of the meal as the cabbage will wilt considerably over time. The fish cakes can be frozen.

If you make the fish cakes slightly larger, they are delicious on a whole-grain bun with thick slices of tomato, arugula and the remoulade.

Nutrition info. *Serving size, 2 fish cakes, cabbage salad and remoulade: 555 calories, 30g fat, 32g protein, 47g carbohydrate, 1.5g sodium*

Rock Cod Veracruz

The combination of tomatoes, green olives, and capers reflects Mexico's Spanish heritage. They also marry together beautifully in this simple, flavor-packed dish.

— Chef John Littlewood, Ceres Community Project

Serves 6
Prep time: 10 minutes
Cooking time: 30 minutes
Dairy-free
Gluten-free

Ingredients

¼ cup olive oil, divided, plus extra for greasing pan
⅝ salt, divided
⅛ tsp ground black pepper
6 (5-ounce) portions cod
½ cup small diced yellow onions
2 tsp minced garlic
1 ½ cups canned diced tomato, including liquid
1 tsp thyme
1 ½ tsp lemon zest
⅓ cup green olives
¾ tsp oregano
1 ½ Tbsp capers, drained
½ cup Healing Vegetable Broth (page 106)

Instructions

Preheat the oven to 350°F. Line sheet pan with parchment paper and brush lightly with oil.

In a small bowl, mix 2 tablespoons of the olive oil, ⅛ teaspoon salt, and pepper and set aside.

Debone and portion the cod and arrange on sheet pan, leaving ½-inch space between pieces. Brush each piece of fish with the oil, salt, and pepper mixture so each piece is lightly coated. Keep cold until ready to bake.

Heat a large skillet over medium-high heat. Add the remaining oil and immediately add the yellow onion and cook, stirring often, until it softens (about 5 minutes). Add the garlic and cook for another minute or two, stirring.

Add the tomatoes, thyme, lemon zest, olives, oregano, capers and ½ teaspoon salt. Add broth, reduce the heat as low as possible, cover, and simmer for about 10 to 15 minutes. If sauce seems very thick, add a little more broth. If sauce seems thin, uncover and simmer until it thickens to desired consistency.

While the sauce is simmering, bake the fish for 10 to 12 minutes or until it reaches an internal temperature of 135°F. The length of time will depend on the thickness of the fish.

Serve fish with sauce on top.

Nutrition info. *1 serving: 198 calories, 12g fat, 18g protein, 5g carbohydrate, 874mg sodium*

Ceres teen chef Genevieve prepares Rock Cod Veracruz.

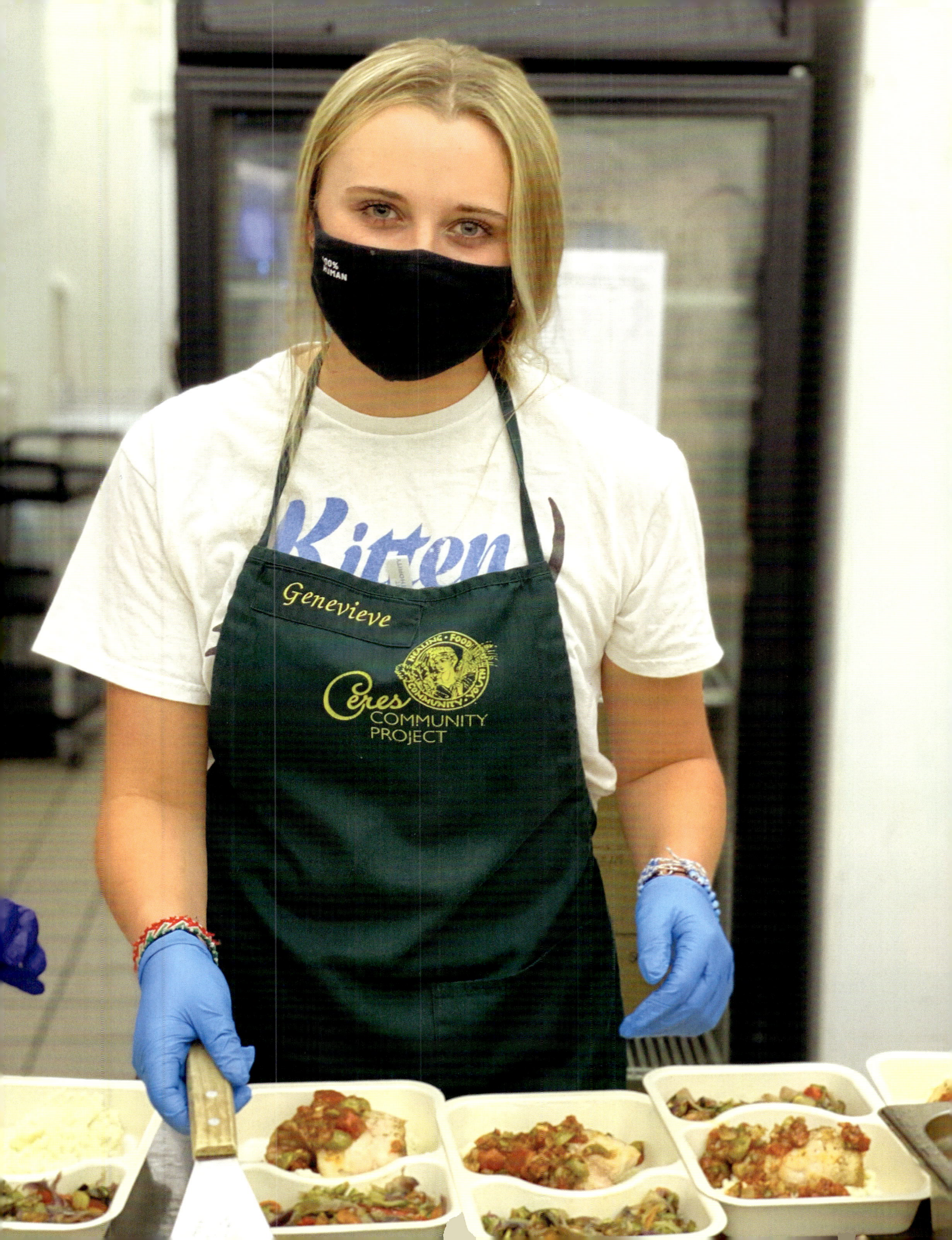
Kitten
Genevieve
Ceres
COMMUNITY
PROJECT

Ginger Orange Glazed Salmon over Braised Greens

Our Meals 4 Health and Healing volunteers love making this nutritious dish for our clients. Flavorfully prepared, it is also a beautiful creation of color and texture.

— The Meals 4 Health and Healing Team

Serves 4
Prep time: 20 minutes
Cooking time: 10 to 12 minutes
Gluten-free
Dairy-free

Ingredients

Salmon

4 (4-ounce) wild-caught salmon fillets
1 large orange
1 Tbsp avocado or olive oil
1 Tbsp peeled and minced fresh ginger
3 Tbsp low-sodium tamari
Ground black pepper, to taste

Braised Greens

2 Tbsp olive oil
1 small red onion, halved then sliced thinly
¼ tsp salt
¼ tsp ground black pepper
4 cloves garlic, minced
2 bunches of hearty greens (kale, Swiss chard, beet tops, turnip greens, etc.), stemmed and chopped
2 tsp apple cider vinegar
1 tsp honey
Splash of vegetable broth
Chopped parsley or cilantro, for garnish

Instructions

For the fish, preheat the oven to 375°F and line a baking sheet with parchment paper or lightly oil. Evenly arrange salmon fillets on it and set aside.

Zest and then juice orange. Combine the zest and ¼ cup of juice with oil, ginger, tamari and ground black pepper in a small bowl. Brush about half over salmon fillets. Put remaining glaze in a small pan on a low burner. Simmer until reduced and slightly thickened.

Bake salmon for 5 minutes, then brush with reduced glaze and bake for another 5 to 8 minutes, until fish is just cooked through.

While salmon is cooking, prepare the greens. Heat a large skillet or wok over medium-high heat and coat the bottom with the oil. Add onion and a pinch of salt and pepper and sauté until onion is tender, about 3 to 5 minutes. Stir in garlic and cook another 30 seconds until aromatic.

Add chopped greens in batches and cook until wilted, adding more as space becomes available in the pan.

Stir in apple cider vinegar, honey, and vegetable stock and cook until greens are tender and flavors combine. Taste and adjust seasoning by adding more vinegar and/or honey, then keep on very low heat until the fish is cooked through.

Serve salmon on a bed of greens, garnished with chopped parsley or cilantro.

Nutrition info. *1 serving: 295 calories, 17g fat, 26g protein, 8g carbohydrate, 609mg sodium*

Romesco Salmon with Parsley Rice

Salmon contains omega-3s, selenium, vitamins D and B-12, which are important nutrients involved in genetic stability and DNA repair. Plus, it's an anti-inflammatory protein. It is stunning paired with Romesco sauce made from roasted tomatoes, garlic, toasted almonds, peppers, and olive oil, on a bed of parsley brown rice.

— The Meals 4 Health and Healing Team

Serves 4
Prep time: 20 minutes
Cooking time: 50 minutes
Gluten-free
Dairy-free

Ingredients

Rice

2 tsp olive oil
½ small yellow onion, diced
Salt and ground black pepper
2 cloves garlic, minced
1½ cups brown rice, rinsed and drained well
3 cups low-sodium vegetable broth
2 Tbsp chopped fresh parsley

Sauce

¼ cup raw almonds, lightly toasted and cooled
1 small clove garlic, smashed
½ roasted red bell pepper, seeds removed and roughly chopped
¼ cup diced fresh tomato
1 ½ tsp sherry vinegar
1 Tbsp chopped fresh parsley
2 Tbsp olive oil
Vegetable broth or water (if needed)
Salt and ground black pepper

Salmon

4 (4-ounce) wild-caught salmon fillets
1 ½ tsp melted coconut oil
Salt and ground black pepper to taste
Chopped fresh parsley as garnish

Instructions

For the rice, coat the bottom of a small saucepan with olive oil and heat over medium-high heat until hot. Sauté onions with a pinch of salt and pepper until tender. Stir in garlic and sauté until aromatic.

Stir in brown rice and then add vegetable stock. Bring to a boil, then turn down to low and cook, covered, until rice is tender (about 45 minutes). Stir in minced parsley and keep warm until needed.

While rice is cooking, make the Romesco sauce. Using a food processor fitted with the metal blade, finely chop toasted almonds and garlic.

Add roasted red pepper, tomato, vinegar and parsley and process to combine. Drizzle in olive oil and process until you reach a pesto consistency, using vegetable broth or water if needed to thin sauce. Season to taste with salt and pepper.

Preheat the oven to 350°F and line a baking sheet with parchment paper or lightly oil.

Season salmon with salt and pepper. Arrange on prepared baking sheet. Top with an even layer of Romesco (about 1 ½ teaspoons per fillet). Drizzle with a little melted coconut oil and bake until Romesco is browned nicely and salmon is bright pink and cooked through, about 12 to 15 minutes.

Serve salmon over rice and top with parsley garnish. Serve with remaining Romesco sauce.

Nutrition info: *1 serving: 560 calories, 24g fat, 32g protein, 60g carbohydrate, 309mg sodium*

Salmon with Arugula Pesto and Sweet Potato Gnocchi

The bitterness of the arugula balances out the sweet nuttiness of the sweet potato in this rich, delicious, and filling meal from Revive & Thrive Project. Though it's involved, the effort of making gnocchi from scratch always pays off. Both the pesto and the gnocchi can be prepared early in the day or even the day before.

— The Revive & Thrive Project Team

Serves 6
Prep time: 30 minutes
Cooking time: 1 hour

Ingredients

Pesto

½ cup walnuts
1 clove garlic, minced
2 cups arugula, packed
½ cup fresh basil, packed
½ cup freshly grated Parmesan cheese
1 cup extra-virgin olive oil
¼ tsp salt

Gnocchi

1 pound sweet potatoes
1½ cups unbleached all-purpose flour, plus more for dusting
1 large egg, room temperature, beaten
1½ tsp salt
1 Tbsp olive oil

Salmon

1½ pound salmon fillets
¼ tsp salt
¼ tsp pepper

Instructions

Pesto

Preheat oven to 375°F. Lightly toast the walnuts in the oven for about 5 minutes. Combine walnuts, garlic, arugula, basil, cheese, salt, and olive oil in a food processor fitted with a metal blade. Process until mostly smooth. Add salt to taste. Set aside.

Gnocchi

Cover sweet potatoes with at least an inch of cold water in a large pot. Bring to a boil and cook until fork tender, about 20 to 25 minutes. Drain and let cool. Peel the potatoes and let cool completely.

Run the potatoes through a food mill, or puree in food processor. Place them in a bowl. Add flour, egg, and salt to bowl and gently stir until a ragged dough forms, being careful not to overwork. Overworking will produce tough gnocchi.

On a floured work surface, gently knead dough to even out the color and flour. If dough is sticky (sweet potato gnocchi are notorious for requiring extra flour), sprinkle with flour and fold it in gently, until dough is just workable.

Nutrition info. *1 serving: 780 calories, 53g fat, 34 protein, 42g carbohydrate, 1045mg sodium*

Divide dough into 4 to 6 pieces; roll each one out into a ¾ inch diameter rope. Cut crosswise into ½-inch thick gnocchi. With floured fingers, press a dimple into each gnocchi or roll over the tines of a fork. Transfer to a baking sheet lined with parchment paper and floured.

Cook the gnocchi in boiling salted water in batches. For each batch, drop the gnocchi in, let it cook until it rises to the surface, and cook about 30 seconds more. Remove with a slotted spoon, transfer to ice water and chill until fully cooled. Drain.

Salmon

When you are ready to make dinner, preheat oven to 375°F. Line a sheet pan with parchment paper or lightly oil.

Place the salmon on your prepared pan. Season lightly with salt and pepper, lightly brush with a little of the pesto, then roast for 12 to 15 minutes, until just cooked through.

While the salmon is cooking, heat a tablespoon of oil in a non-stick pan until hot. Add the gnocchi to the pan in a single layer. Season with salt and pepper. Cook on one side until lightly browned, then toss and cook the other side. Total cooking time will depend on the size of the pan and how many gnocchi you put into it, about 5 to 7 minutes.

When the salmon is finished, plate it, top with a generous dollop of the arugula pesto, and serve with the gnocchi. Serve more pesto on the side.

A client family of Revive & Thrive enjoying their meals.

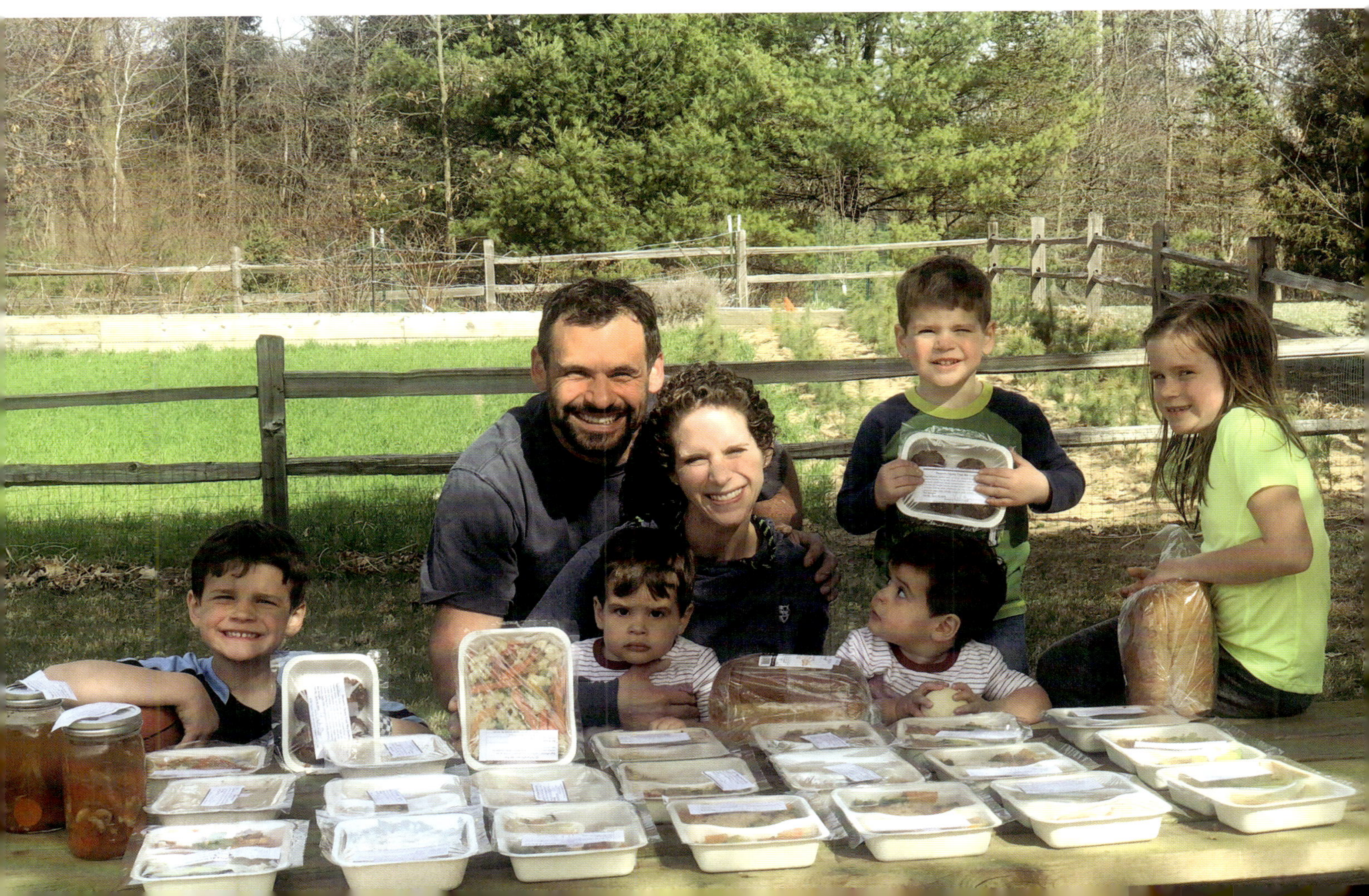

Roasted Salmon with Tomato-Mango Salsa

This is always one of the first dishes we have on our menu when tomatoes are in season in late summer. The tomatoes and mangoes plus fresh herbs are the perfect finishing touch to a roasted or grilled salmon. This dish is also delicious made with peaches in place of mango.

— Chef Molly Evans, Fox Valley Food for Health

Serves 4
Prep time: 35 minutes
Cooking time: 12 minutes
Dairy-free
Gluten-free

Ingredients

1 cup peeled and chopped ripe mango
¾ cup quartered or halved cherry tomatoes
¼ cup thinly vertically sliced red onion
3 Tbsp coarsely chopped fresh mint
3 Tbsp coarsely chopped fresh basil
2 Tbsp lemon juice
1 Tbsp olive oil, plus more for drizzling on fish
1 Tbsp honey
1 jalapeño pepper, seeded and thinly sliced
1 tsp kosher salt, divided
1 ½ pounds wild-caught salmon fillets with skin on
¼ tsp ground black pepper

Instructions

In a large bowl, combine mango, tomatoes, onion, mint, basil, lemon juice, olive oil, honey, jalapeño and ½ tsp salt; toss gently.

Preheat oven to 400°F. Line a baking sheet with parchment paper or lightly oil. Place salmon fillets on prepared sheet and sprinkle with remaining ½ tsp salt and ¼ tsp black pepper. then drizzle with olive oil.

Roast, uncovered, in preheated oven for 12 to 15 minutes or until salmon is just cooked through (internal temperature of 145°F). To serve, portion the salmon and spoon salsa over each serving.

Nutrition info. *1 serving size, 6 oz: 327calories, 14g fat, 38g protein, 12g carbohydrate, 677mg sodium*

Teen chef at Fox Valley prepares salmon for roasting.

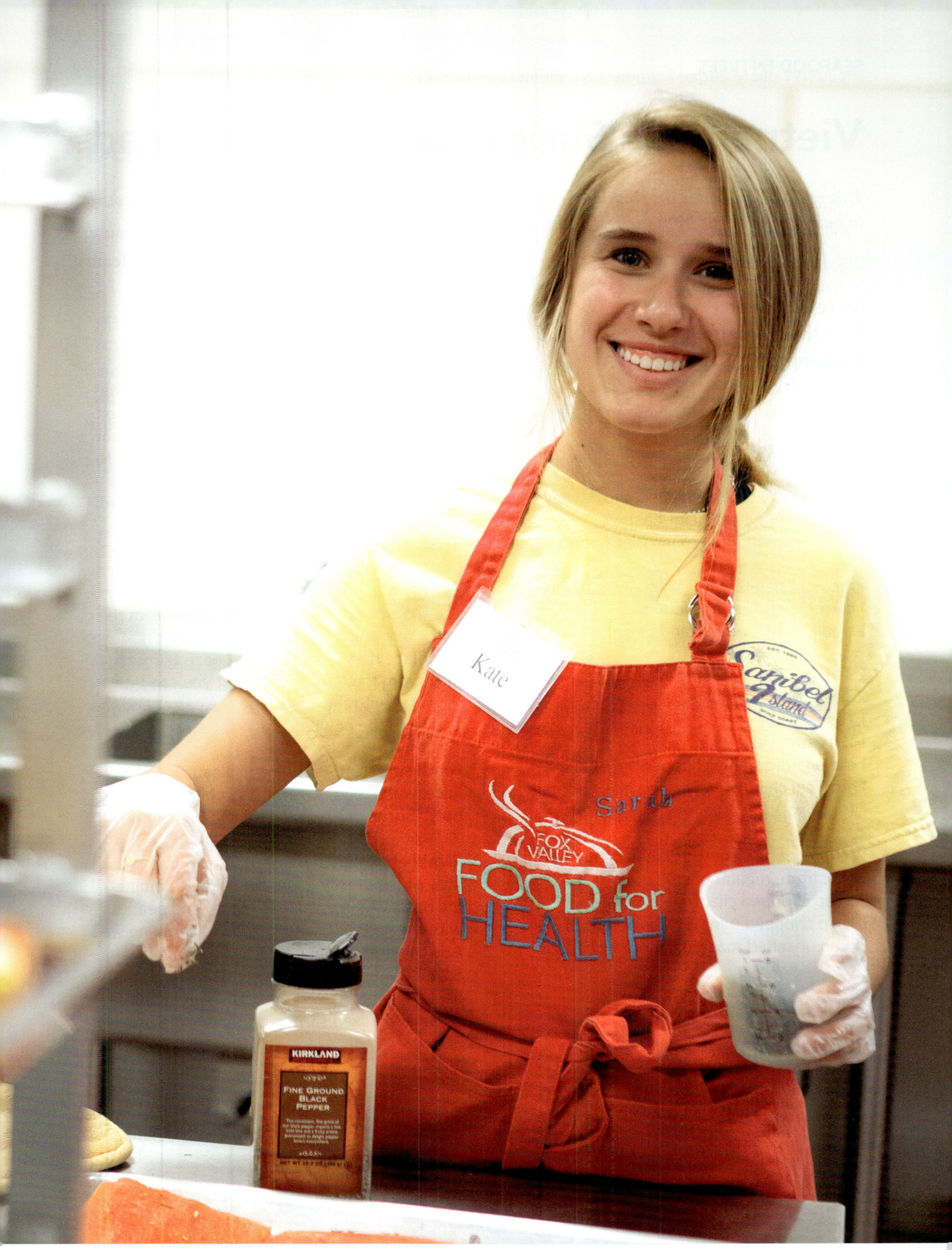
Kate
Sarah
FOX VALLEY
FOOD for
HEALTH
Sanibel Island
KIRKLAND
FINE GROUND
BLACK
PEPPER

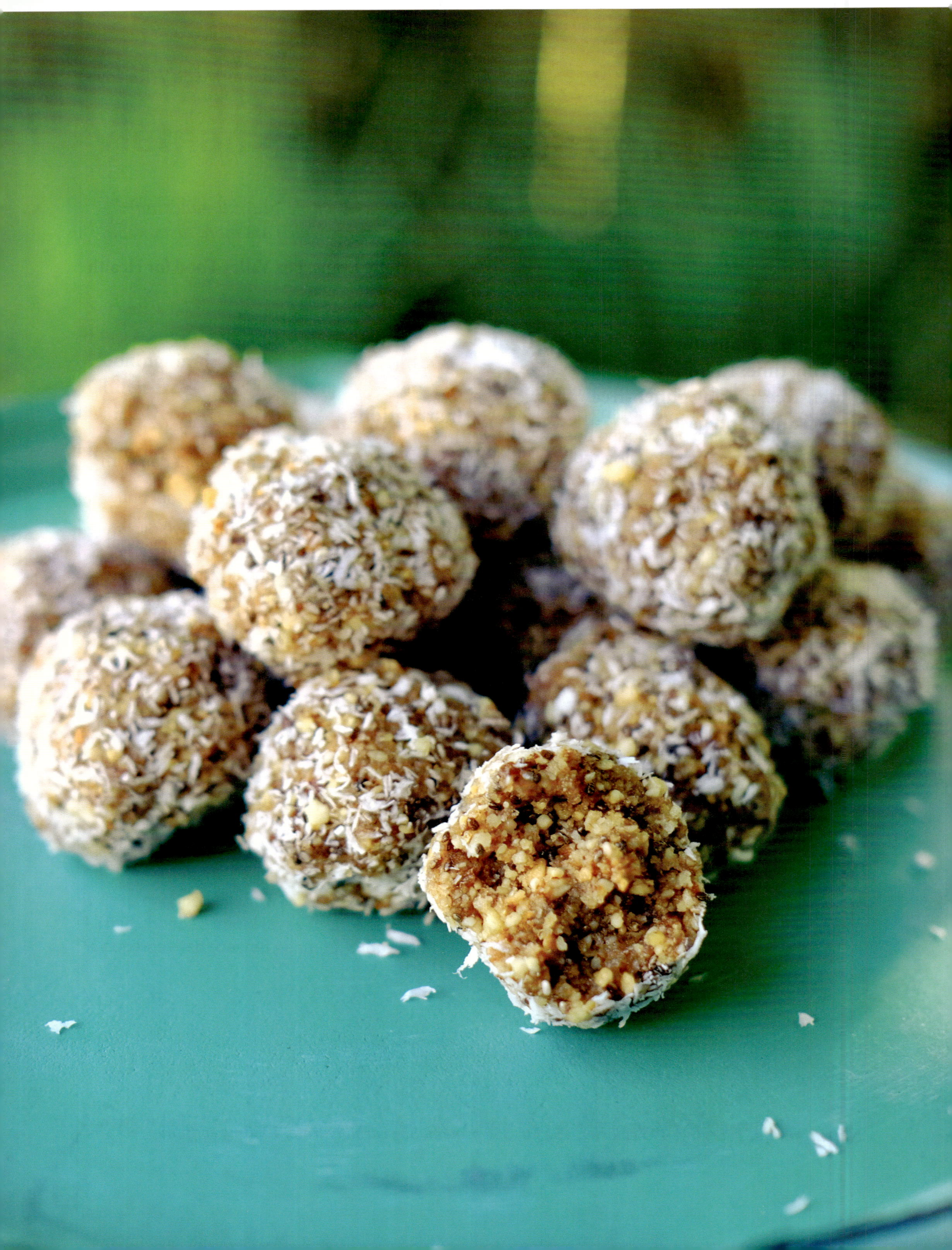

DESSERTS

Grilled Peaches with Mascarpone and Honey

This dessert is the perfect way to end your summertime dinner with peaches found at the farmers' market. Be sure to choose firm peaches for best results; very ripe peaches will become too mushy when grilled. Grilled rosemary makes a beautiful garnish.

— The Revive & Thrive Project Team

Serves 6
Cook time: 15 to 20 minutes
Gluten-free

Ingredients

3 peaches, freestone variety
1 tsp avocado or sunflower oil
8 ounces mascarpone cheese
2 Tbsp honey
2 ounces slivered almonds, toasted

Instructions

Split the peaches, remove the pits and brush the cut edges with oil. Place the peaches on the grill, cut side down and grill for 2 to 3 minutes over medium heat, until colored. Flip them onto the rounded side and cook them for 3 to 4 minutes, until cooked through, but still firm enough to be handled.

Plate the peaches, cut side up. Fill each with a dollop of mascarpone, dividing the cheese evenly between peaches. Drizzle with honey, about 1 teaspoon per serving. Sprinkle with the almonds. Serve warm.

Nutrition info. *Serving size, ½ peach: 272 calories, 22g fat, 4g protein, 16g carbohydrate, 20mg sodium*

Cashew Cardamom Balls

A holiday and teen favorite, you'll find this recipe at almost every Ceres event. This comes together quickly and easily with a food processor and provides a delicious and nourishing treat.

— The Ceres Community Project Team

Serves 6
Prep time: 5 minutes
Cooking time: 4 to 8 minutes
Vegan
Gluten-free

Ingredients

1 cup unsweetened shredded coconut
1 cup cashews, lightly roasted, chopped roughly
1 cup chopped dates
¼ tsp ground cardamom
1 Tbsp orange zest
¼ cup unsalted cashew butter

Instructions

Preheat oven to 325°F. Line a baking sheet with parchment paper.

Spread coconut evenly on baking sheet and toast 4 to 8 minutes, until just turning golden. Cool.

Place a steel blade in the work bowl of a food processor. Add the cashews and about ⅔ of the coconut and process until the cashews are ground to about the texture of very coarse sand. Transfer to a mixing bowl.

Add the dates to the work bowl and process until they come together in a ball and are finely chopped. Add to cashew mix.

Stir in the cardamom, orange zest, and cashew butter. Knead the mixture with your fingers until uniform, then roll into twelve 1 ½-inch balls. Place the remaining coconut on a plate and roll the balls in the coconut to coat.

NOTE: If mixture is too dry and fails to stick together in ball form, add a bit of melted coconut oil or cashew butter. Cashew butter can be used in place of some of the cashews. Use no more than half cashew butter, or balls will be too soft.

Previous page: Cashew Cardamom Balls

Nutrition info. *Serving size, 2 balls: 331 calories, 23g fat, 7g protein, 31g carbohydrate, 9mg sodium*

Caramel Coconut Fudge Delights

"The food is delicious, and it makes our life a little easier. Most importantly, we're feeling the love which we need and appreciate."

— Client, Healing Meals Community Project

Serves 10
Prep time: 15 minutes
Cooking time: 15 minutes
Vegan
Gluten-free

Ingredients

1 cup unsweetened shredded coconut
1 cup pitted Medjool dates
⅓ cup dark chocolate (chips or a chopped bar)
½ tsp coconut oil

Instructions

Pre-heat oven to 375°F. Spread the shredded coconut onto a baking sheet. Place in oven to toast for 5 minutes, until coconut is a light golden-brown color.

Place dates and toasted coconut into the bowl of a food processor fitted with metal blade. Pulse until mixture is combined and starts to form a ball.

Remove from food processor, roll tablespoon-size pieces of dough into a ball and then shape into a round cookie. Using a straw or chopstick, punch a small hole in the middle of each cookie.

Place cookies on a baking sheet lined with parchment paper. Reshape as necessary and transfer to the freezer to firm up.

While cookies are in the freezer, add chocolate and coconut oil to a shallow microwave-safe bowl and microwave in 30-second increments until the chocolate is melted enough to drizzle. If you do not have a microwave, warm the chocolate in a glass bowl set over a saucepan of hot water (do not let the bowl touch the hot water), stirring frequently until melted and smooth.

Take cookies from the freezer and dip each one in the chocolate to coat the bottom. Place cookies on the parchment and use remaining chocolate to drizzle decorative lines over top the cookies. Transfer cookies back into the freezer for 15 minutes.

Nutrition info. *Serving size, 1 cookie: 123 calories, 7g fat, 1g protein, 16g carbohydrate, 4mg sodium*

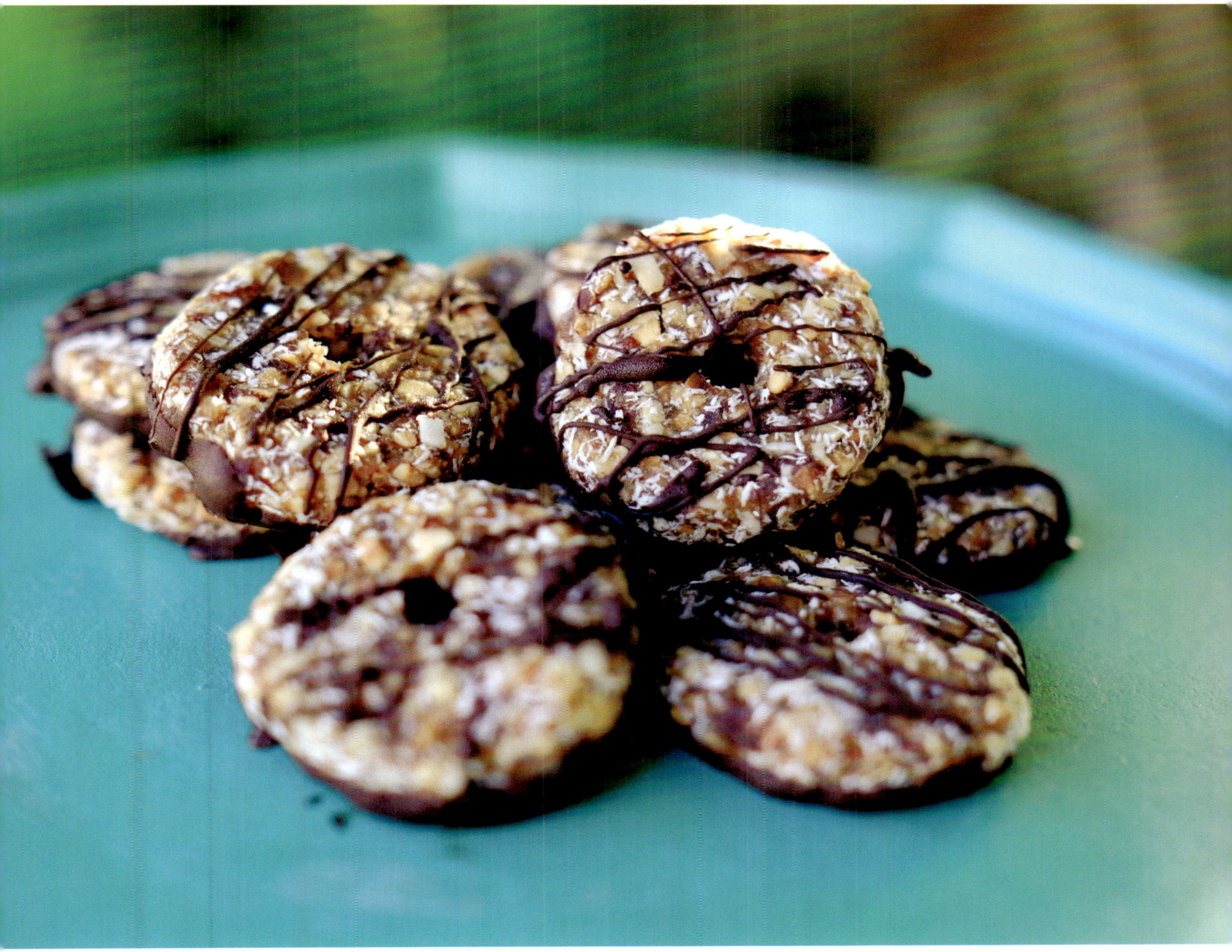

Pillowy Pumpkin Snacking Cookies

These cookies have become a fall favorite in our kitchen. They are easy to make, contain antioxidant rich pumpkin purée, warm fall spices, and have a soft texture that everyone loves.

— **Chef Molly Evans, Fox Valley Food for Health**

Serves 6
Prep time: 30 minutes
Baking time: 12 to 14 minutes
Dairy-free

Ingredients

3 Tbsp coconut oil, softened
½ cup honey
⅓ cup unsweetened pumpkin purée
½ tsp vanilla extract
2 tsp ground cinnamon
2 tsp ground flaxseed
¾ tsp ground ginger
½ tsp baking soda
½ tsp freshly grated nutmeg
⅛ tsp ground cloves
⅛ tsp ground cardamom
¼ tsp salt
1 ¼ cup spelt flour

Instructions

Preheat oven to 350° F. Line a large baking sheet with parchment paper or lightly oil.

Using an electric mixer, beat together coconut oil, honey, pumpkin, and vanilla until smooth. Add cinnamon, ground flaxseed, ginger, baking soda, nutmeg, cloves, cardamom and salt. Beat until combined. Add flour and beat again until combined. The dough should be moist slightly sticky and easy to roll into balls.

Shape the dough into large balls, about 2 packed tablespoons each (you should have 12 total). Place the balls 2 to 3 inches apart on prepared baking sheet. Do not flatten the balls (or cookies will not be as fluffy).

Bake for 12 to 14 minutes or until cookies have puffed up, rotating trays once. Some might be lightly cracked on the surface. Let cool on pan for 5 minutes before transferring to cooling rack to cool completely.

Nutrition info. *Serving size, 2 cookies: 264 calories, 11g fat, 4g protein, 39g carbohydrate, 328mg sodium*

Fudgy Black Bean Brownies

These delicious brownies come together so quickly, and they're easy to take along in your lunch-box for a little treat.

— The Revive & Thrive Project Team

Serves 8
Prep time: 15 minutes
Baking time: 20 minutes
Gluten-free

Ingredients

- 1 ½ cups cooked black beans (or one 15-ounce can, rinsed and drained)
- ½ cup gluten-free quick oats
- ½ cup dark chocolate chips
- 2 Tbsp cocoa powder
- ⅓ cup honey
- ¼ cup coconut oil
- 1 egg
- 1 tsp vanilla extract
- ½ tsp baking soda
- ¼ tsp sea salt
- ¼ cup finely chopped walnuts

Instructions

Preheat the oven to 350°F. Oil a 9x9-inch baking pan.

Grind the oats in a food processor until they resemble flour.

Place all the ingredients in a blender or food processor and blend until smooth.

Spread into prepared pan.

Bake for 17 minutes, or until a tester inserted in middle of pan comes out clean.

Allow to cool for 30 minutes before cutting into squares.

Nutrition info. *Serving size, 1 square: 247 calories, 9g fat, 7g protein, 37g carbohydrate, 76mg sodium*

Chocolaty No-Bake Brownies

Studies have increasingly documented the potential health benefits associated with chocolate. The flavonoid antioxidants may lower the risk of cancer, diabetes, stroke, and heart disease, along with boosting cognitive function. Keep in mind that the darker the chocolate, the more antioxidants—and usually less sugar—it contains.

— Assistant Chef Marcie Carlson, Fox Valley Food for Health

Makes 16 squares
Prep time: 30 minutes
Chill time: 2 hours
Gluten-free
Dairy-free if using coconut oil

Ingredients

Brownies

2 ½ cups loosely packed, pitted dates
1 ½ cups walnuts
6 Tbsp cocoa powder
1 ½ tsp vanilla extract
2 tsp water
Scant ½ tsp salt

Frosting

¼ cup cocoa powder
¼ cup pure maple syrup
2 Tbsp unsalted butter (or coconut oil), melted
½ tsp vanilla extract

Instructions

Brownies

Lightly grease or line a 9-inch square baking pan with parchment paper.

Place a steel blade in the work bowl of a food processor. Add dates, walnuts, cocoa powder, vanilla, water, and salt; process until completely smooth.

Transfer brownie mixture to prepared pan and press very firmly to evenly distribute.

Frosting

Combine cocoa powder, maple syrup, melted butter or coconut oil, and vanilla in a medium bowl.

Stir or whisk mixture vigorously until thoroughly combined and smooth. Spread frosting evenly over brownies in pan. Refrigerate at least 2 hours before cutting into squares.

Store in an airtight container in refrigerator for up to 2 weeks or 1 to 2 months in the freezer.

Nutrition info. *Serving size, 1 square: 176 calories, 9g fat, 7g protein, 37g carbohydrate, 76mg sodium*

Fox Valley volunteer melting chocolate.

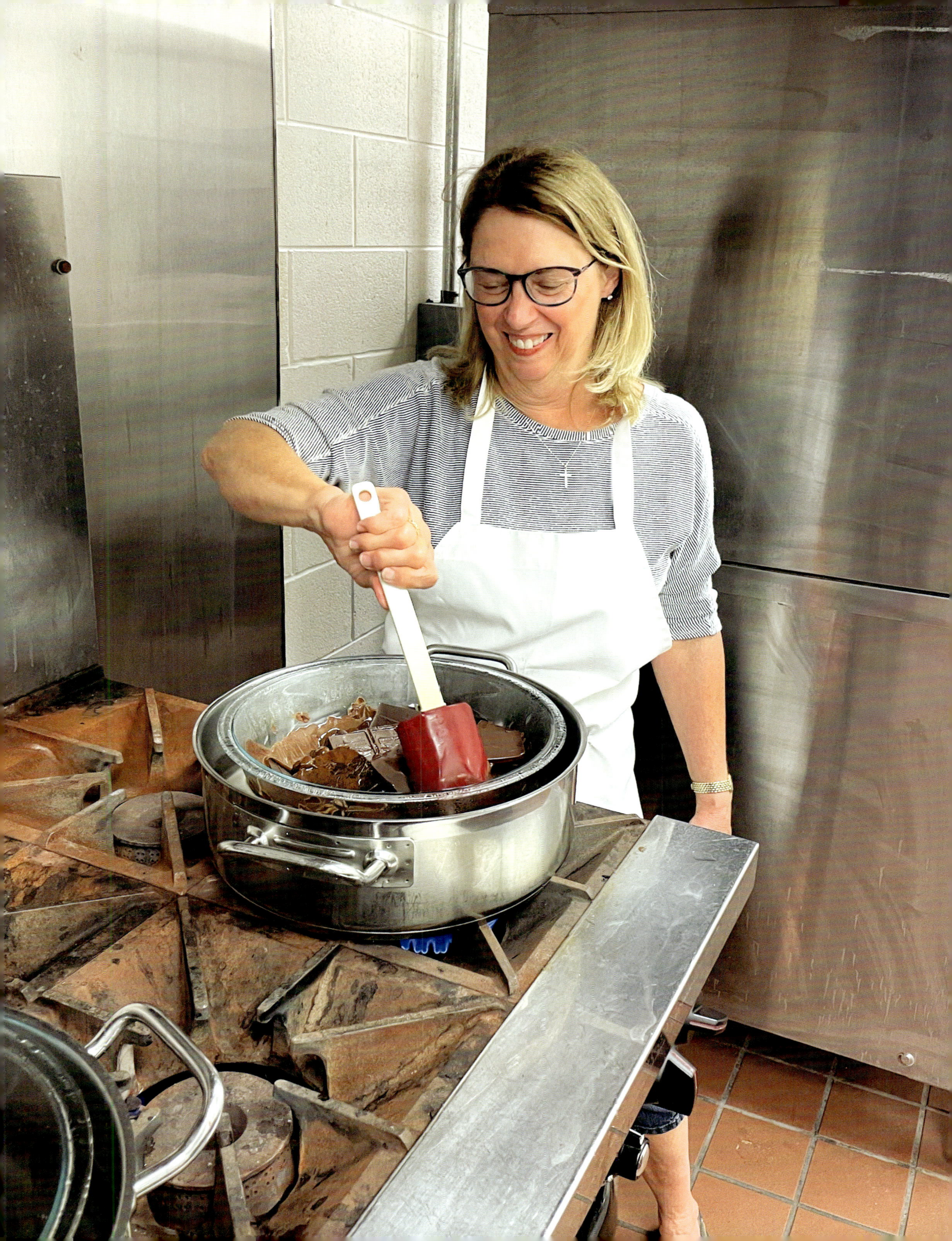

Date Bars

"Being a part of such an amazing organization has made me realize the importance of the work that I am doing. While I cook or package each meal, I think of the individuals and families struggling to cope with an illness."

— Rachel, Healing Meals Community Project Youth Volunteer

Serves 16
Prep time: 15 minutes
Bake time: 18 minutes
Gluten-free, if made with gluten-free oats
Dairy-free

Ingredients

Filling

1 ½ cups rolled oats (divided)
½ cup unsweetened coconut
5 to 6 pitted Medjool dates (4 ounces)
¼ tsp salt
½ tsp baking soda
½ cup almonds, chopped
1 egg
2 Tbsp ground flax seed
¼ cup melted coconut oil

Topping

18 pitted Medjool dates (12 ounces), broken into quarters
1 tsp lemon juice
¼ tsp salt

Instructions

Preheat oven to 325°F. Line an 8×8-inch pan with parchment paper or lightly oil.

For the filling, add 1 cup oats to a food processor bowl fitted with a metal blade, and process to a flour-like consistency. Add coconut, pitted dates, salt, and baking soda; process until the dates are fully broken up. Dates can be added through processor feed tube for easier blending.

Add the remaining ½ cup oats and the almonds. Pulse 8 to 10 times, until the nuts are chopped, but still a bit chunky. Add the egg, ground flax seed and coconut oil to the food processor bowl and pulse until combined.

Reserve ½ cup of this oat mixture to use as a topping. Add the rest to the prepared pan and press down into an even layer.

For the topping, rinse out the food processor, then add the 18 dates, lemon juice and salt. Pulse 10 to 15 times, until the dates are broken up. Then process for another 3 to 4 minutes, until the dates take on a light, whipped caramel color. If dates are firm and difficult to process, add 1 to 2 tablespoons of hot water to get a smoother mix.

Carefully spread the topping mixture over the filling layer, using wet hands to press mixture down and smooth it without pulling up the cookie layer. Crumble the reserved ½ cup of oat mixture over the top.

Bake for 18 minutes. Cool completely before slicing. Date bars may be stored in the freezer and served frozen.

Nutrition info. *Serving size, 1 bar: 184 calories, 8g fat, 3g protein, 28g carbohydrate, 103mg sodium*

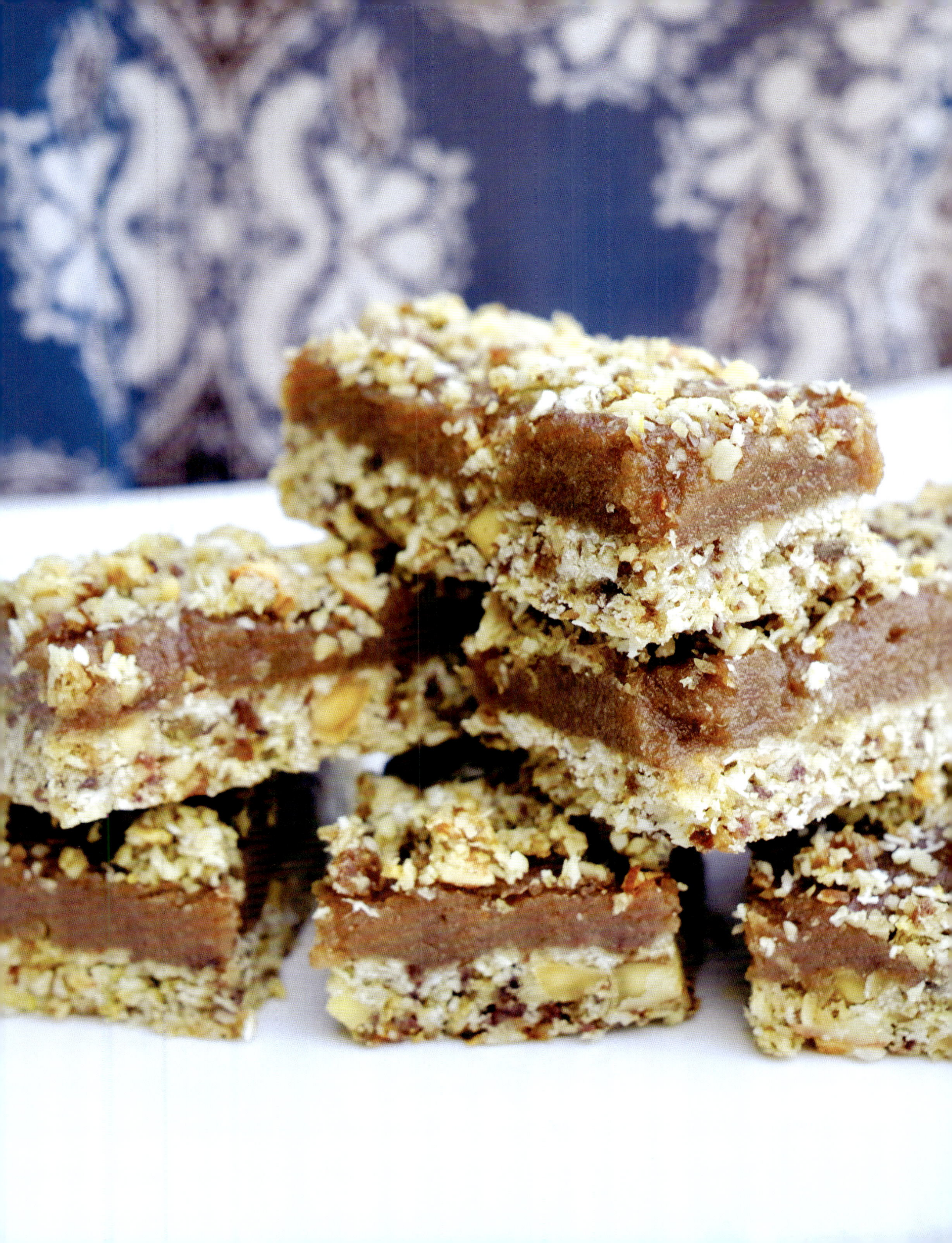

Lily's Coconut Pumpkin Pudding

Lily Mazzarella, a clinical herbalist who's been supporting Ceres since our founding, shared her coconut pudding recipe with our founder Cathryn back in 2007. We consider this a Ceres classic. The pumpkin variation was developed for Thanksgiving one year. A "crust" can easily be added by crumbling graham crackers or toasted pecans on top before serving. Give thanks!

— Ceres Founder Cathryn Couch and Chef John Littlewood

Serves 6
Prep time: 5 minutes
Cooking time: 20 minutes
Dairy-free
Gluten-free

Ingredients

¼ cup cornstarch
2 eggs
1 cup canned pumpkin or fresh pumpkin purée
3 ½ cups coconut milk (two 14-ounce cans)
½ cup + 2 Tbsp maple syrup
½ tsp cinnamon
½ tsp nutmeg
⅛ tsp salt
2 tsp vanilla extract
4 Tbsp gluten-free graham cracker crumbs or toasted chopped pecans, optional

Instructions

Whisk cornstarch with eggs and pumpkin in mixing bowl. Set aside.

Combine coconut milk, maple syrup, spices, and salt in a stainless pan with a heavy bottom, then bring to a simmer over medium heat.

Whisk about ¾ of the hot coconut milk mix into the egg and pumpkin mixture, a little at a time, to bring the temperature of the egg mix up slowly. Add the egg mixture into the milk mix in the pan and whisk to combine. Heat on medium, whisking frequently, until pudding thickens. It should thicken visibly. You may see a bubble here and there, but do not to let it come to a boil.

Remove from heat and mix in vanilla, then immediately scrape pudding into shallow bowl. Cover surface of pudding with parchment paper. Chill for at least 2 hours before serving.

If topping, sprinkle about 2 teaspoons of garnish of choice on each serving.

Nutrition info. *1 serving: 384 calories, 30g fat, 5g protein, 28g carbohydrate, 182mg sodium*

Deep Dark Chocolate Budino

This is by far the favorite dessert of all our volunteers and clients. We often serve it at events and with just a few simple ingredients, you can have a dessert that is a showstopper. We love using dark chocolate chips in this recipe.

— Chef Molly Evans, Fox Valley Food for Health

Serves 6
Prep time: 30 minutes
Vegan
Gluten-free

Ingredients

10 ounces (about 2 cups) chocolate chips, preferably at least 63% dark chocolate
2 Tbsp coconut palm sugar
¾ tsp vanilla extract
2 cups coconut milk (not lite coconut milk)
¼ cup toasted slivered almonds (optional)
¼ cup cacao nibs (optional)

Instructions

In a large bowl, combine chocolate chips, sugar, and vanilla.

In a heavy saucepan, bring coconut milk to a simmer over medium-high heat. Do not boil. Pour over chocolate mixture. Using a whisk and starting at the center of the bowl, stir the mixture in small concentric circles. Continue stirring in ever-widening concentric circles until the last circle reaches the edges of the bowl and mixture is a smooth, velvety liquid.

Pour into an 8 x 8-inch glass dish or 6 individual serving dishes; cover and chill.

To serve, sprinkle with toasted slivered almonds and cacao nibs.

Nutrition info. *1 Serving, ½ cup: 465 calories, 36g fat, 5g protein, 32g carbohydrate, 15mg sodium*

Heart Beet Cake

On rotation year-round in our kitchen and a recipe we always have handy to share!

— The Positive Community Kitchen Team

Serves 9
Prep time: 10 minutes
Cooking time: 90 minutes
Gluten-free

Ingredients

For the cake:
3 beets (about 2″ diameter)
2 to 3 Tbsp water
1 ½ Tbsp coconut oil
⅓ cup cocoa powder, plus extra for lining pans
1 cup + 2 Tbsp almond flour
½ tsp baking soda
½ tsp cinnamon
¼ cup dark chocolate chips
¾ tsp apple cider vinegar
¾ tsp vanilla extract
3 eggs, at room temperature
1 cup coconut palm sugar
¾ tsp salt

For the glaze:
½ cup dark chocolate chips
1 ½ Tbsp coconut oil
½ tsp vanilla extract
Pinch salt

Instructions

Cook beets in a large pot of boiling unsalted water until tender, 30 to 40 minutes, depending on size. Drain and rinse under cold water until cool enough to handle. Cut off stem end, then peel and cut beets into large pieces. Transfer to a blender and add 2 tablespoons water. Blend, adding water 1 tablespoon at a time as needed, until a smooth purée forms. It should be the consistency of applesauce. Measure out ¾ cup purée.

Preheat oven to 350° F. Line bottom of 8x8-inch cake pan with parchment. Grease with coconut oil, then dust with cocoa powder, tapping out excess.

Whisk almond flour, baking soda, cinnamon, and ⅓ cup cocoa powder in a medium bowl; set aside.

Nutrition info. *1 slice: 310 calories, 17g fat, 6g protein, 37g carbohydrate, 319mg sodium*

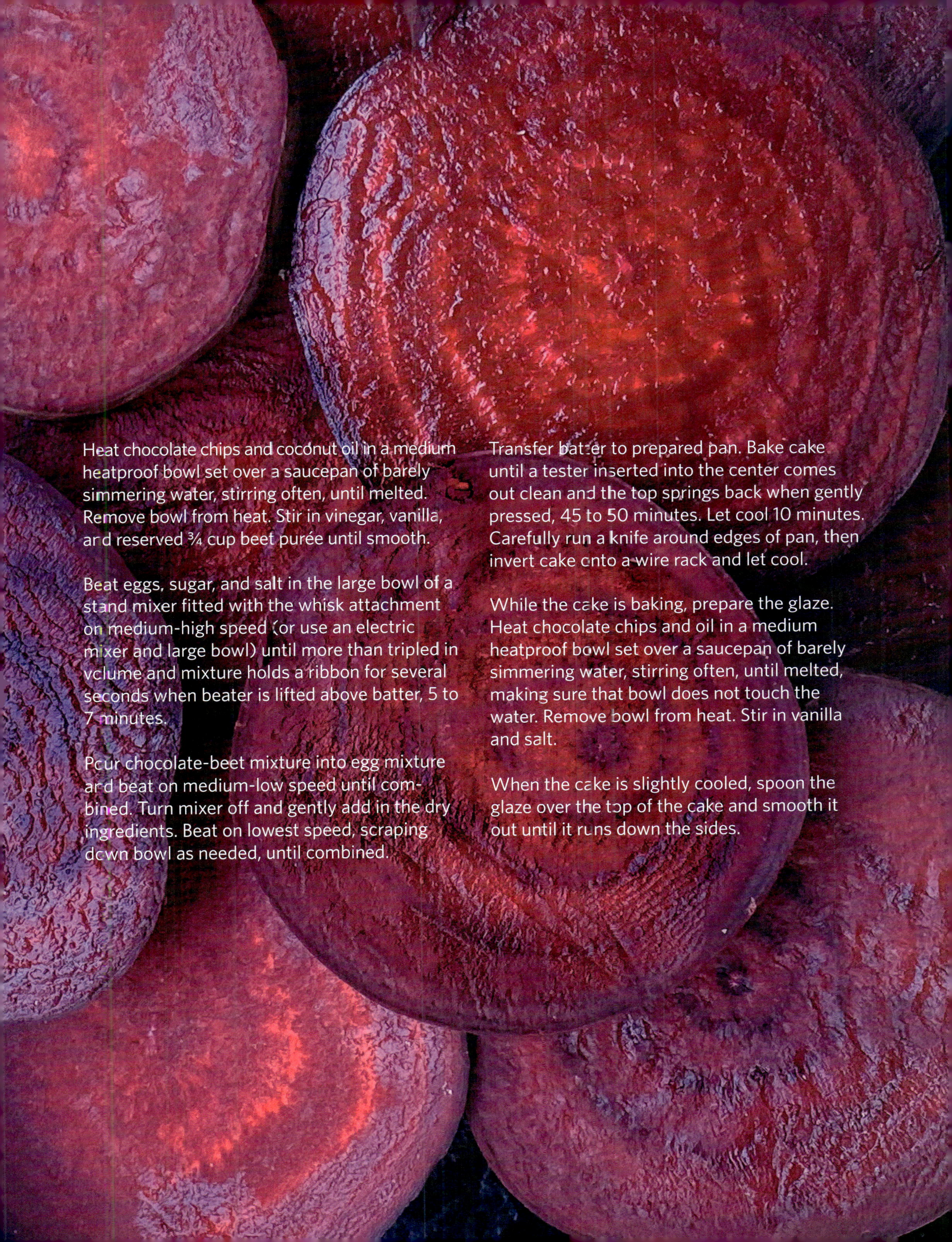

Heat chocolate chips and coconut oil in a medium heatproof bowl set over a saucepan of barely simmering water, stirring often, until melted. Remove bowl from heat. Stir in vinegar, vanilla, and reserved ¾ cup beet purée until smooth.

Beat eggs, sugar, and salt in the large bowl of a stand mixer fitted with the whisk attachment on medium-high speed (or use an electric mixer and large bowl) until more than tripled in volume and mixture holds a ribbon for several seconds when beater is lifted above batter, 5 to 7 minutes.

Pour chocolate-beet mixture into egg mixture and beat on medium-low speed until combined. Turn mixer off and gently add in the dry ingredients. Beat on lowest speed, scraping down bowl as needed, until combined.

Transfer batter to prepared pan. Bake cake until a tester inserted into the center comes out clean and the top springs back when gently pressed, 45 to 50 minutes. Let cool 10 minutes. Carefully run a knife around edges of pan, then invert cake onto a wire rack and let cool.

While the cake is baking, prepare the glaze. Heat chocolate chips and oil in a medium heatproof bowl set over a saucepan of barely simmering water, stirring often, until melted, making sure that bowl does not touch the water. Remove bowl from heat. Stir in vanilla and salt.

When the cake is slightly cooled, spoon the glaze over the top of the cake and smooth it out until it runs down the sides.

Apple Walnut Cake

This is a wonderfully moist cake with a touch of cinnamon and chunks of apple inside. And the gluten-free version is equally tempting.

— Chef John Littlewood, Ceres Community Project

Serves 12
Prep time: 10 minutes
Cooking Time: 35 minutes
Gluten-free, if using gluten-free flour
Dairy-free

Ingredients

2 cups whole wheat flour or 1 ¾ cups of your favorite gluten-free flour blend
½ tsp baking soda
¼ tsp salt
1 ½ tsp cinnamon
3 eggs
1 ¼ cups unrefined cane sugar, such as rapadura
¾ cup melted coconut oil
1 tsp vanilla extract
¼ cup water
1 cup walnuts, toasted
4 cups tart apples, peeled, cored, and diced into ½-inch cubes

Instructions

Preheat oven to 325°F. Lightly grease a 9x13-inch baking dish.

Mix flour, baking soda, salt, and cinnamon in a mixing bowl and set aside.

In a large bowl, whisk eggs, sugar, coconut oil, vanilla, and water until smooth. Using a rubber spatula or wooden spoon, stir flour mixture, nuts and apples into wet ingredients until just combined.

Pour batter into baking dish. Bake for 25 minutes, then check for doneness. Cake is done when a toothpick or small knife inserted into the center of the cake comes out clean. If cake is still moist, bake another 5 to 10 minutes. Remove from oven and cool completely before cutting.

Nutrition info. *1 serving: 400 calories, 21g fat, 5g protein, 49g carbohydrate, 215mg sodium*

The joy of cooking! A volunteer at Positive Community Kitchen.

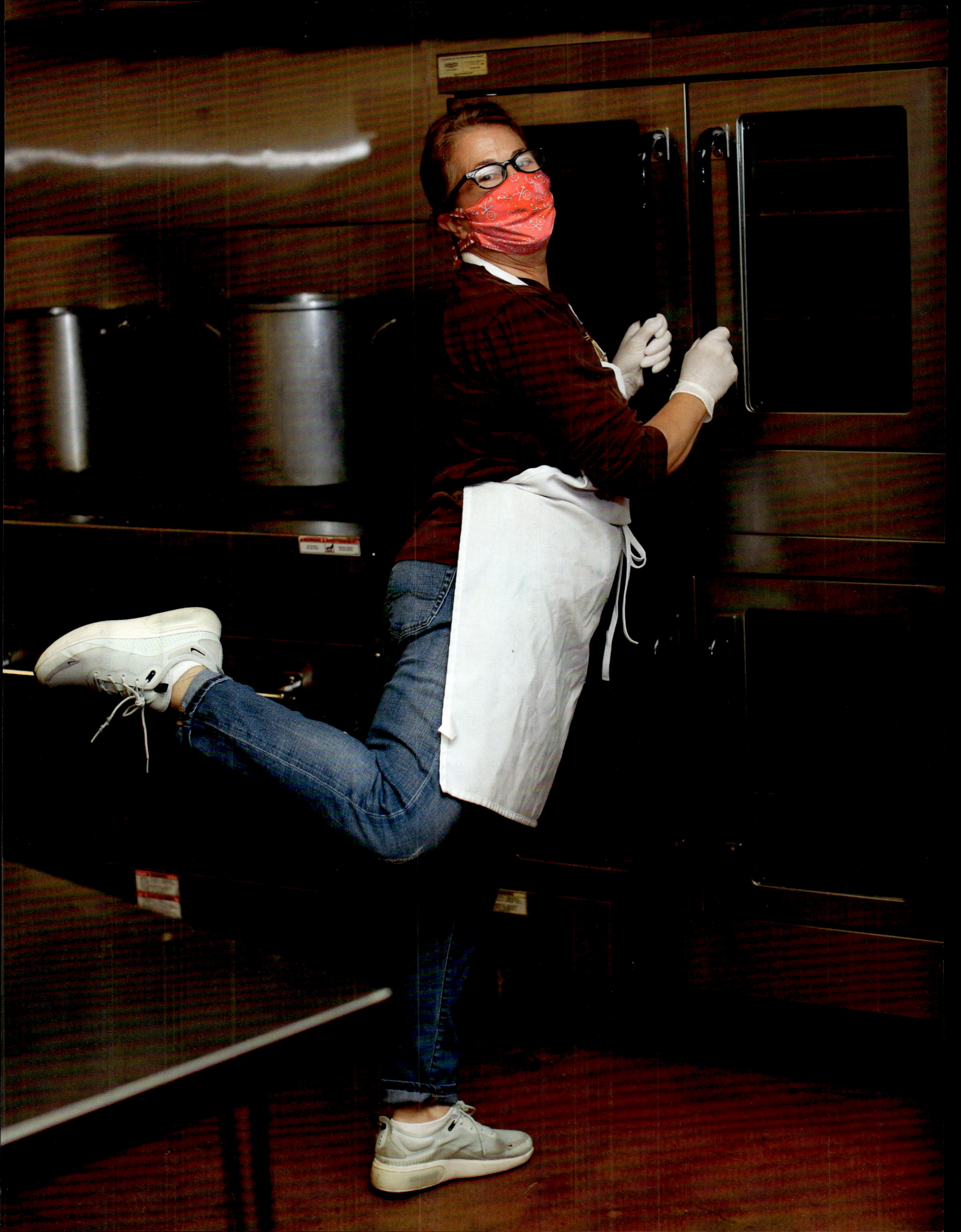

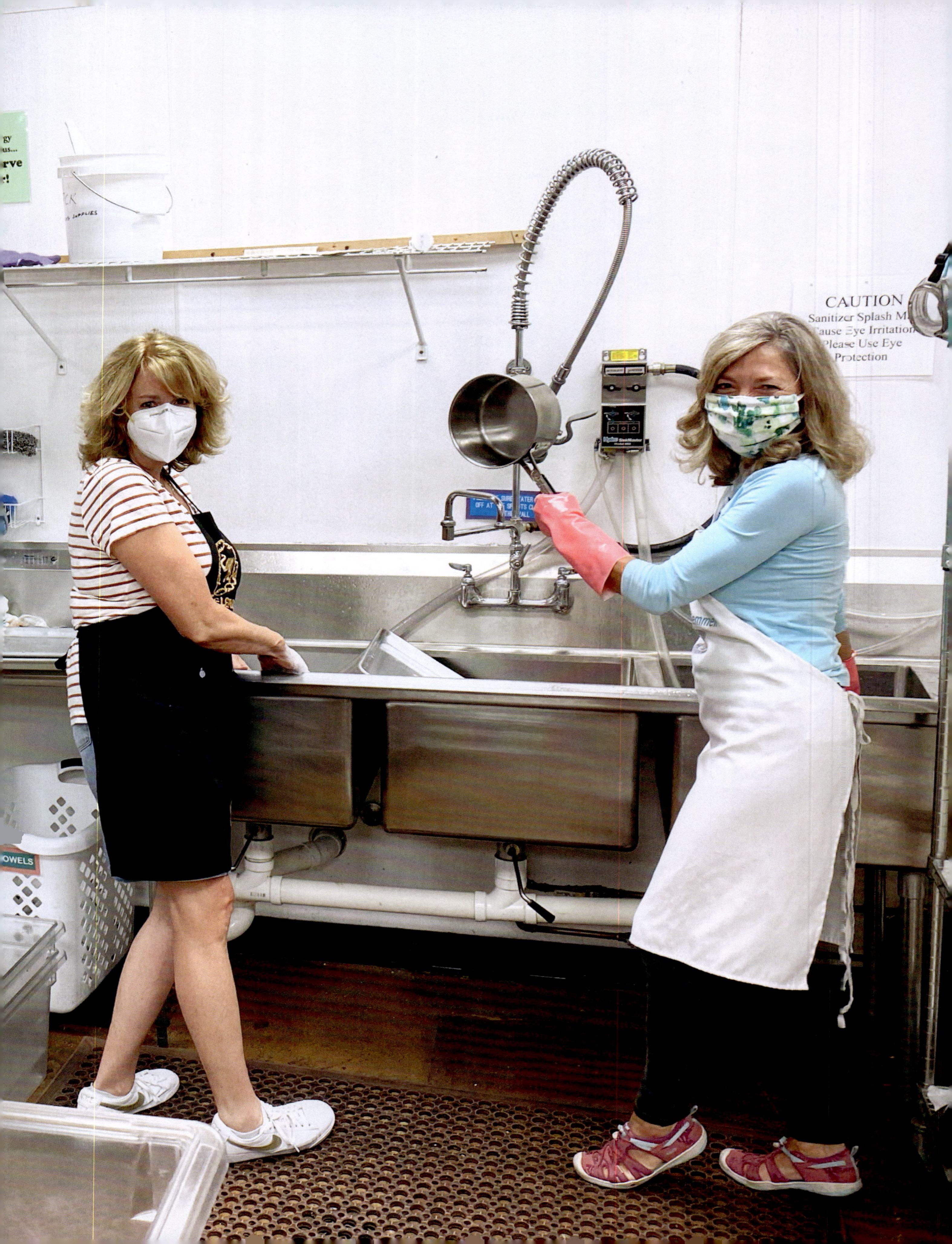
CAUTION
Please Use Eye
Protection

AFFILIATE RESOURCES

About Us

Our programs share a unique, integrated model that:

- Supports individuals who are living with a serious health challenge with free or low-cost, nutrient-rich and mostly organic prepared meals, nutrition education, and a community of caring.
- Involves young people as volunteer gardeners and chefs, giving them direct, hands-on experience of the difference that fresh, healthy foods and community make, and of their own capacity to contribute.
- Educates the broader community about the connection between fresh healthy food, strong social networks, healing and wellness.
- Connects people of all ages and from all walks of life to one another, and to their value as an integral part of the community.
- Supports a just and sustainable food system through prioritizing organic and locally raised foods.

Where to find us

Ceres Community Project
Serving Marin and Sonoma counties, California
www.ceresproject.org
info@ceresproject.org tel: 707.829.5833

Det Kærlige Måltid

Det Kærlige Måltid (The Loving Meal)
Aarhus, Denmark
detkaerligemaaltid.dk
charlotte@detkaerligemaaltid.dk tel: +45 40 35 68 39

Fox Valley Food for Health
Geneva, Illinois
www.fvffh.org
info@fvffh.org tel: (630) 377-078

Healing Meals Community Project
Bloomfield, Connecticut
www.healingmealsproject.org
info@healingmealsproject.org tel: (860) 549-2099

Meals 4 Health and Healing
Nashville, Tennessee
www.hfmeals.org
info@hfmeals.org tel: (615) 730-5632

North Coast Opportunities Caring Kitchen Project
Ukiah, California
www.ncoinc.org/programs/caring-kitchen-project
acunningham@ncoinc.org tel: (707) 467-3212

Positive Community Kitchen
Eugene, Oregon
www.positivecommunitykitchen.org
info@positivecommunitykitchen.org tel: (541) 249-4942

Revive & Thrive Project
Grand Rapids, Michigan
www.reviveandthriveproject.org
info@reviveandthriveproject.org tel: (616) 229-0205

Join Us!

Learn about joining the Ceres Affiliate Partner program, including training and ongoing support, by visiting CeresProject.org/affiliate-partner-network

Recipes by Affiliate

Ceres Community Project

Det Kærlige Måltid (The Loving Meal)

Fox Valley Food for Health

Healing Meals Community Project

Meals 4 Health and Healing

North Coast Opportunities Caring Kitchen Project

Positive Community Kitchen

Revive & Thrive Project

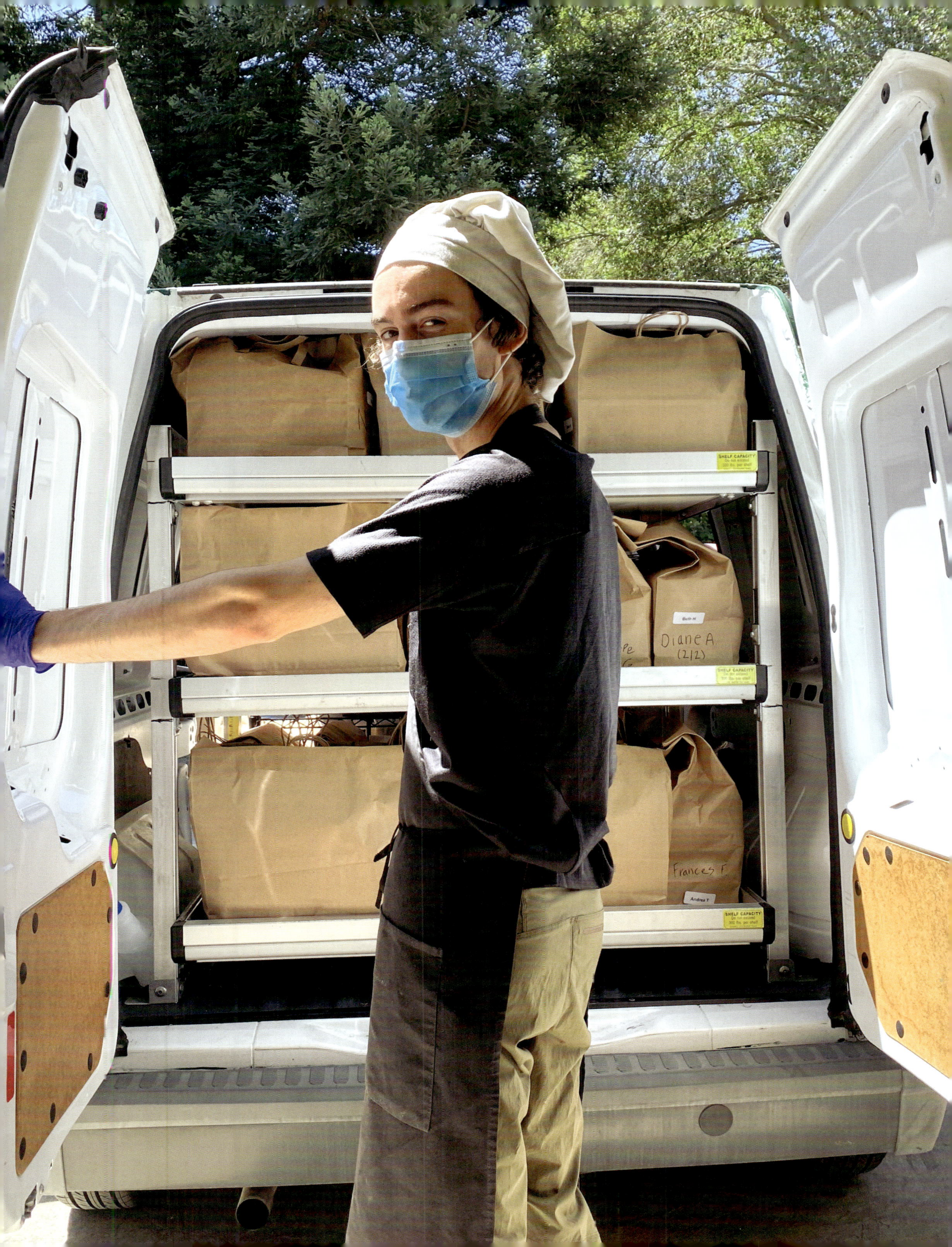

Diane A
(2/12)
Frances F

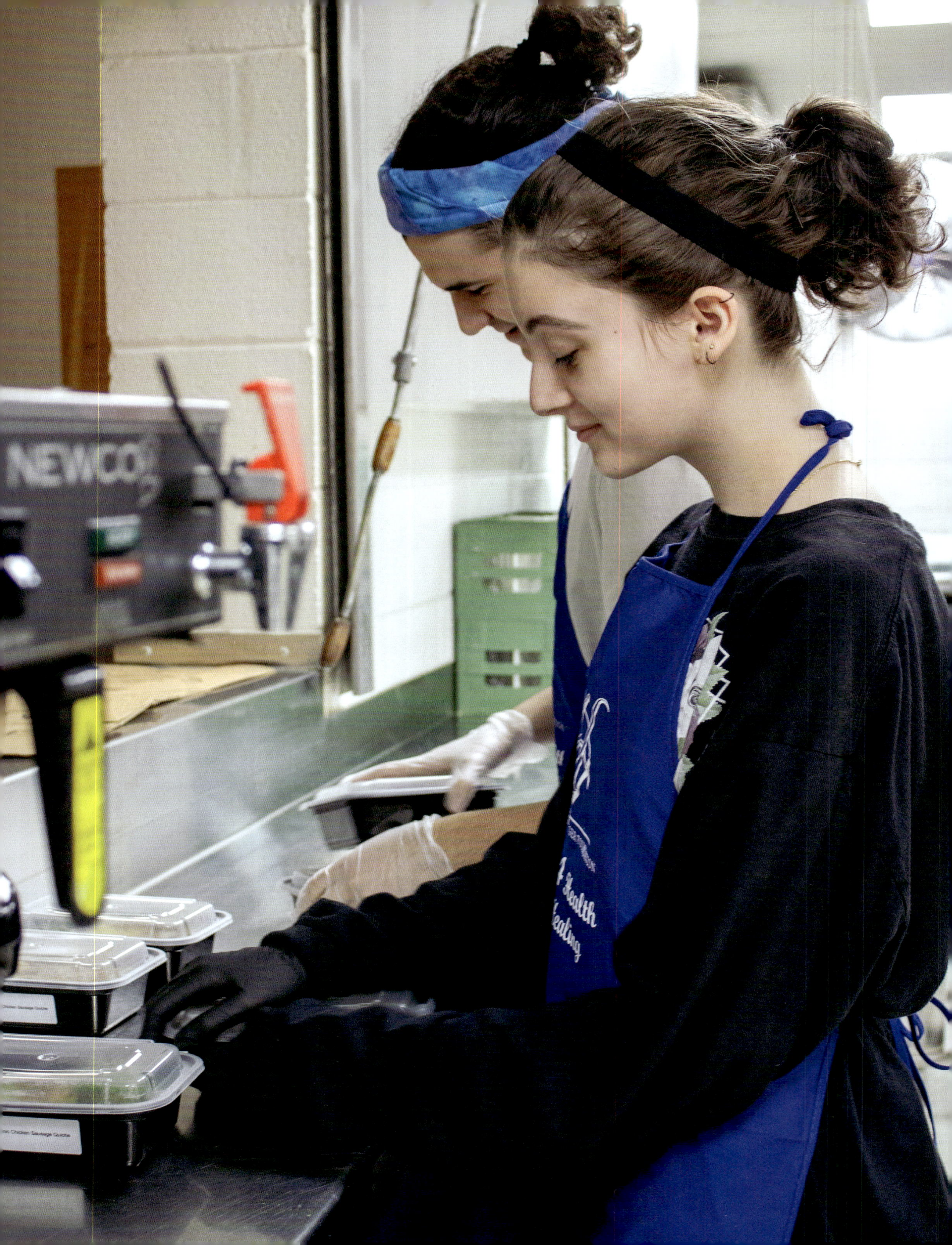
NEWCO

Acknowledgements

To all the marvelous people who helped to make this book happen, including:

Recipe Testers: Anna Ransome, Beverly Shirley, Cathryn Couch, Dawn Bryan, Deborah Green-Jacobi, Deirdre Lordan, Evie Facendini, Jenny Belforte, Kassidy Ford, Laura Lee, Linda Hahn, Lorraine Fuentez, Maile Shubin, Martin Reed, Mary Gonnella, Matt Cadigan, Michaela Worona, Monnet Zubieta, Nathan Myers, Nicole Sadaah, Paula, Rayne Dessayer, Reilly Briggs, Sara McCamant, Shannon Wesley, Sharon Meckman, Stephanie LaPlante, Susan Bryer Shelton, Susan Hirsch, Tamara Evans, Tiann Lordan

Editing and Proofreading: Beth Lamb, Jane Frances, Janice Sunday, Mary Miller

Photography
Ai Kojima, Connecticut Headshots, Elijah Rawlings, Felicity Crush, Kelly Lyon of Kelly Lyon Photography, Neil Parkin, Rob Brodman (cover), Tommy Quinn

Food Styling
Skylar Bush, Sylvie Parkin

and of course, to all our amazing staff, volunteers and donors, past and present.

INDEX

A

B

C

D

E

F

G

H

I

J

K

L

M

N

O

P

Q

T

V

W

Z

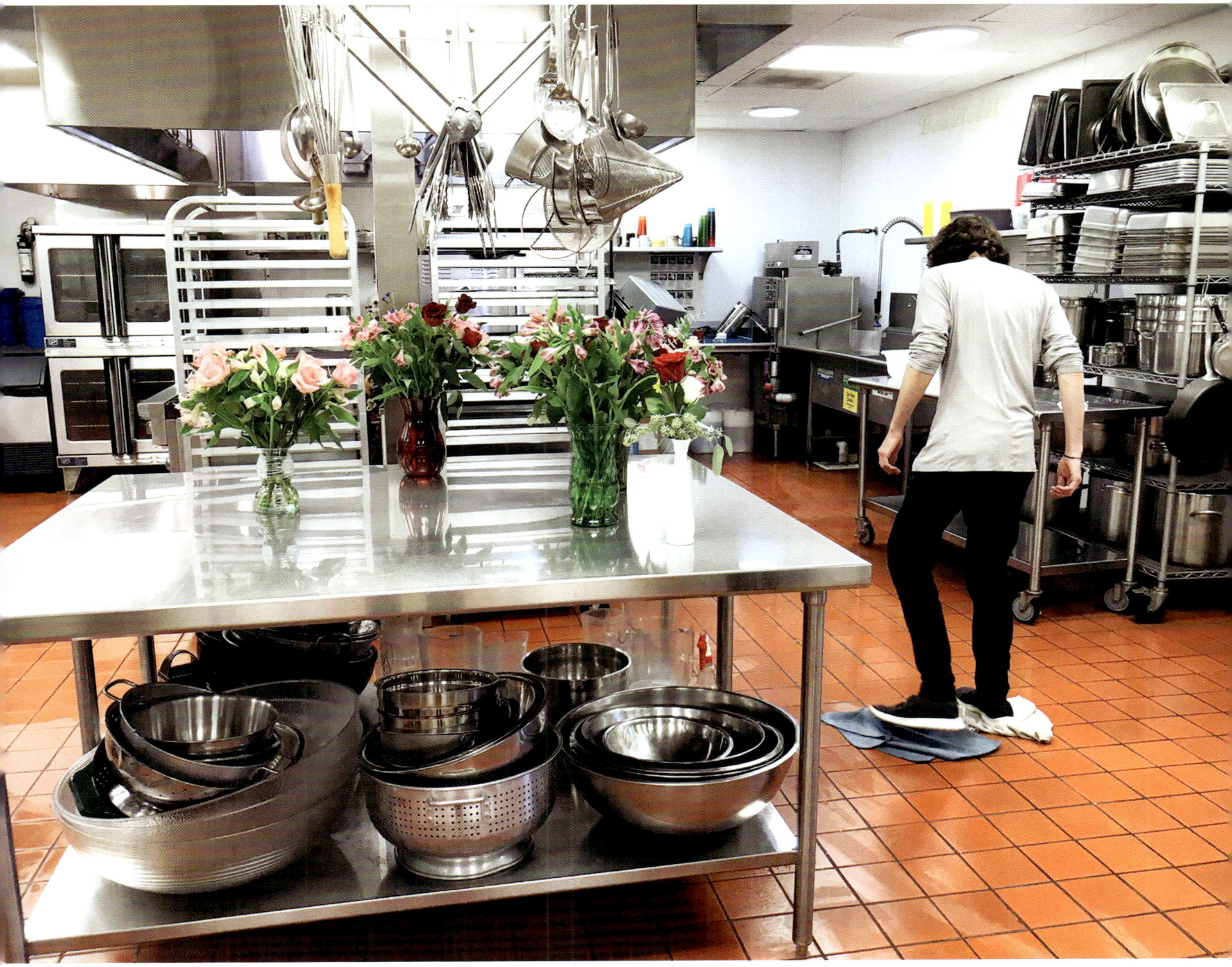

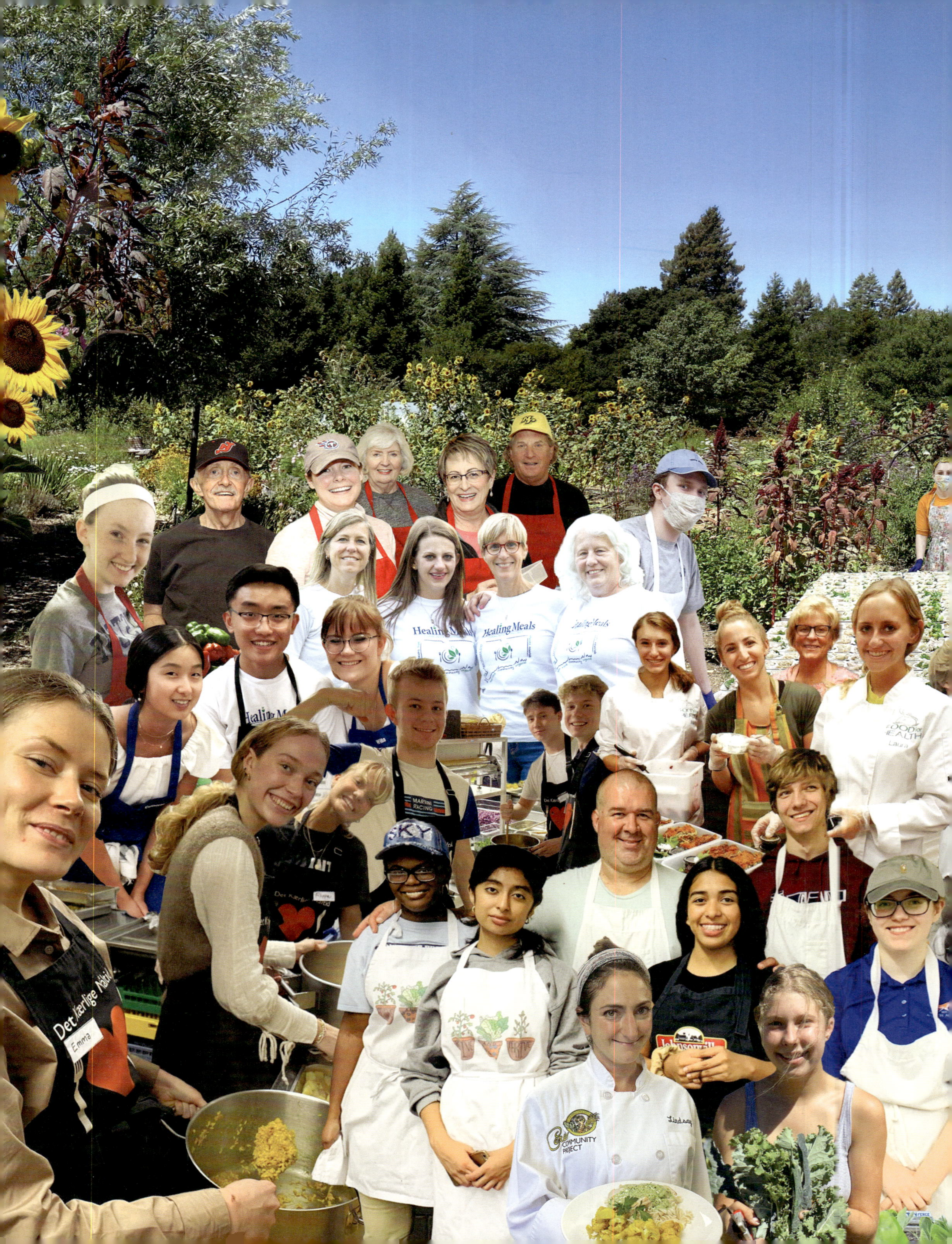
Healing Meals
Healing Meals
FOOD for HEALTH
Emma
MARTINI RACING
SKY
COMMUNITY PROJECT